W9-CFK-603

Pediatric Nursing
CLINICAL GUIDE

Terri Kyle, MSN, CPNP
Associate Director of Nursing
Herzing University - Orlando
Winter Park, Florida

Susan Carman, MSN, MBA
Professor of Nursing
Most recently, Edison Community College
Fort Myers, Florida

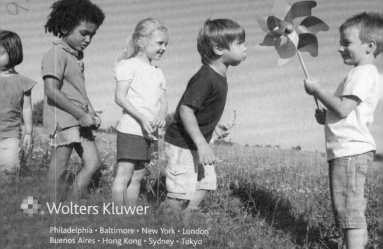

Wolters Kluwer

Philadelphia · Baltimore · New York · London
Buenos Aires · Hong Kong · Sydney · Tokyo

Gift $39.99
9/14/2017

Acquisitions Editor: Natasha McIntyre
Product Development Editor: Annette Ferran
Production Project Manager: Marian Bellus
Editorial Assistant: Dan Reilly
Design Coordinator: Joan Wendt
Illustration Coordinator: Jennifer Clements
Manufacturing Coordinator: Karin Duffield
Prepress Vendor: Aptara, Inc.

9 8 7 6 5 4 3 2 1

Printed in China

Library of Congress Cataloging-in-Publication Data
Names: Kyle, Terri, author. | Carman, Susan, author. | Kyle, Terri.
   Essentials of pediatric nursing. Adaptation of (expression):
Title: Pediatric nursing clinical guide / Terri Kyle, Susan Carman.
Description: 2nd edition. | Philadelphia : Wolters Kluwer, [2017] |
   Adaptation of: Essentials of pediatric nursing / Terri Kyle, Susan Carman.
   Third edition. [2017]. | Includes bibliographical references and index.
Identifiers: LCCN 2015041729 | ISBN 9781451192414
Subjects: | MESH: Pediatric Nursing–Outlines.
Classification: LCC RJ245 | NLM WY 18.2 | DDC 618.92—dc23
LC record available at http://lccn.loc.gov/2015041729

CCS1215

Reviewers

Elizabeth Aycock, MSN, RN
Professor of Nursing
Middle Georgia State University
Cochran, Georgia

Patricia Braun, DNSC, MSN, MA, BSN
Assistant Professor
Northern Illinois University
DeKalb, Illinois

Claire Creamer, PhD, RN, CPNP-PC
Assistant Professor
Rhode Island College School of Nursing
Providence, Rhode Island

Sandra B. Englert, MSN, RN, CNE
Assistant Professor
D'Youville College School of Nursing
Buffalo, New York

Niki Fogg, MS, RN, CPN
Assistant Clinical Professor
Texas Woman's University
The Houston J. and Florence A. Doswell College of Nursing
Dallas, Texas

Nancy Gasper, MSN, RN, CPNP
Assistant Professor of Nursing
Cuyahoga Community College
Cleveland, Ohio

Leslie E. (Swaim) Guthrie, MS, RN
Assistant Professor
Tulsa Community College/Nursing Division
Tulsa, Oklahoma

Laura Kubin, PhD, RN, CPN, CHES
Associate Professor
Texas Woman's University
The Houston J. and Florence A. Doswell College of Nursing
Dallas, Texas

Preface

The pediatric clinical setting is an environment that changes constantly due to rapid turnover in patient census. There is a clear need to have a readily accessible, reliable tool that will help nurses and nursing students provide thorough and safe patient care. The goal of *Pediatric Nursing Clinical Guide* is to answer this need.

Adapted from *Essentials of Pediatric Nursing*, 3rd edition, this pocket-sized book is the perfect clinical reference guide for students and practicing nurses to have on hand while providing nursing care to children and their families, or as a resource for studying need-to-know content. Essential, clinically relevant information is presented in a concise outline format for quick access in a way that makes sense and is easy to follow. An alphabetical listing is used to show nursing management for commonly encountered childhood illnesses and disorders. Common diagnostic tests and nursing procedures are also included.

Organization
The handbook consists of three sections and is primarily organized in an outline format for ease of locating and applying content.

Part I. Principles of Nursing Care in Children
Part I presents foundational material to help promote understanding of how nursing care of the child differs from that of the adult. The following content areas are covered:

- General concepts related to **growth and development** include nutritional needs and information about motor, language, and psychosocial development across age groups. While caring for children in the clinical setting, students will have a handy reference to assist them with promoting developmentally appropriate care.
- **Health supervision** includes key elements related to health supervision visits, developmental surveillance, various screening tests used to identify certain conditions in the pediatric client, and immunizations.
- **Health assessment** covers health history and physical examination to help with learning differences in nursing assessment when caring for children versus caring for adults. This section also discusses a variety of pain assessment tools and pain management techniques.
- The section on **medication administration** and intravenous therapy provides information about pediatric dosage calculation and developmental approaches to administering medications to children.

- Content related to **managing pediatric emergencies** is also included. Students are often concerned about emergency care for children, as it differs from emergency care of the adult. This section breaks down emergency care that providers need to know in a way that makes concepts easy to grasp.

Part II. Nursing Care for Common Health Disorders

Part II provides information related to health disorders more commonly encountered in the pediatric clinical setting. Disorders are alphabetized and provided in a structured, bulleted format for quick access and to help commit key points to memory. Readers can expect the following content for each disorder:

- Brief description, pathophysiology, and a to-the-point explanation of typical therapeutic management.
- Nursing assessment guidelines including assessment of health history, physical examination, and common laboratory and diagnostic findings.
- Possible nursing interventions.
- Child and family teaching guidelines to help promote communication and understanding.

Part III. Common Diagnostic Tests and Nursing Procedures

Part III includes common diagnostic tests along with information on results and important nursing considerations, as well as common nursing procedures with an explanation of purpose. In addition, Part III also discusses consent for care in children and provides guidance for provision of nursing care related to diagnostic testing and nursing procedures. This section is important because it delivers content with a focus on developmentally appropriate and atraumatic care, which are critical factors in every pediatric care setting.

Recurring Features

To provide readers with exciting and user-friendly text, a number of recurring features have been developed.

Atraumatic Care

These highlights provide tips for delivering atraumatic care to children in particular situations related to the topic being discussed. Their inclusion in the handbook permits quick access to helpful tips while caring for children. For example, the child with cancer often undergoes a large number of painful procedures related to laboratory specimens and treatment protocols. This handbook offers suggestions, such as providing distraction in the form of reading a favorite book or playing a favorite movie or musical selection, to assist the child to cope with these procedures.

Take Note

This feature shows new or critically relevant information related to information being discussed. For example, under the section caring for a child with a cast, the take note states that persistent complaints of pain may indicate compromised skin integrity under the cast.

Teaching Guidelines

Teaching guidelines serve as valuable health education tools. The guidelines raise the student's awareness, provide timely and accurate information, and are designed to ensure the student's preparation for educating children and their families about various issues.

Comparison Charts

These charts compare two or more disorders or other easily confused concepts. They serve to provide an explanation that clarifies the concepts for the student.

Tables, Boxes, Illustrations, and Photographs

Tables and boxes are included throughout the sections to summarize key content areas. Beautiful illustrations and photographs help the student to visualize the content. These features allow the student to quickly and easily access information.

References

References that were used in the development of the text are provided at the end of each section. The listings allow the student to further pursue topics of interest.

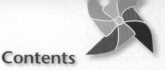

Contents

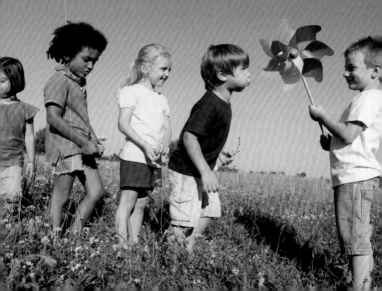

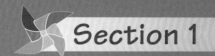
Principles of Nursing Care in Children

GROWTH AND DEVELOPMENT

Growth and development are interrelated, ongoing processes in infancy and childhood. Growth refers to an increase in physical size. Development is the sequential process by which infants and children gain various skills and functions. Maturation refers to an increase in functionality of various body systems or developmental skills. Noting adequacy of growth and development at various ages is an important part of the nursing assessment of infants and children.

Infant Growth and Development

Infants exhibit phenomenal increases in their gross and fine motor skills over the first 12 months of life. Gross motor skills develop in a cephalocaudal fashion (from the head to the tail). In other words, the baby learns to lift the head before learning to roll over and sit. Fine motor skills develop in a proximodistal fashion (from the center to the periphery). The infant fist grabs in a whole-hand fashion and eventually progresses to a fine pincer grasp.

Psychosocial Development

The infant is in Erikson's (1963) period of trust versus mistrust. The infant is completely dependent upon a parent or caregiver. Caregivers respond to the infant's basic needs by feeding, changing diapers, and cleaning, touching, holding, and talking to the infant. This creates a sense of trust in the infant. If the infant is neglected or his or her needs are not met, then mistrust may develop. As the nervous system matures, infants realize they are separate beings from their caregivers. Over time, the infant learns to tolerate small amounts of frustration and trusts that although gratification may be delayed, it will eventually be provided.

Motor and Language Skill Development

Gross motor, fine motor, and language skill acquisition develop sequentially over time. Refer to Tables 1.1 and 1.2 for details.

Nutritional Guidelines

Adequate nutrition is essential for growth and development. Breast-feeding and bottlefeeding of iron-fortified infant formula are both acceptable means of nutrition in the newborn and infant. Breast milk or formula supplies all of the infant's daily nutritional requirements until 4 to 6 months of age (AAP, 2012; Stettler, Bhatia, Parish, & Stallings, 2011).

Newborns may only take 0.5 to 1 ounces per feeding initially, working up to 2 to 3 ounces per feeding in the first few days. They need to feed about 6 to 10 times per day and should be fed on demand,

(text continues on page 4)

TABLE 1.1	INFANT GROSS AND FINE MOTOR SKILL MILESTONES	
Age	**Gross Motor Skills**	**Fine Motor Skills**
1 month	Lifts and turns head to side in prone position Head lag when pulled to sit Rounded back when sitting	Fists mostly clenched Involuntary hand movements
2 months	Raises head and chest, holds position Improving head control	
3 months	Raises head to 45 degrees in prone Slight head lag in pull-to-sit maneuver	Holds hand in front of face, hands open
4 months	Lifts head and looks around Rolls from prone to supine Head leads body when pulled to sit	Bats at objects
5 months	Rolls from supine to prone and back again Sits with back upright when supported	Grasps rattle
6 months	Tripod sits	Releases object in hand to take another
7 months	Sits alone with some use of hands for support	Transfers object from one hand to the other
8 months	Sits unsupported	Gross pincer grasp (rakes)
9 months	Crawls, abdomen off floor	Bangs objects together
10 months	Pulls to stand Cruises	Fine pincer grasp
12 months	Sits from standing position Walks independently	

Adapted from Feigelman, S. (2011c). The first year. In R. M. Kliegman, B. F. Stanton, J. W. St. Geme III, N. F. Schor, & R. E. Behrman (Eds.), *Nelson's textbook of pediatrics* (19th ed.). Philadelphia, PA: Elsevier, Saunders; and Goldson, E., & Reynolds, A. (2012). Child development and behavior. In W. W. Hay, Jr., M. J. Levin, R. R. Deterding, M. J. Abzug, & J. M. Sondheimer (Eds.), *Current diagnosis and treatment: Pediatrics* (21st ed.). New York, NY: McGraw-Hill.

TABLE 1.2	INFANT LANGUAGE MILESTONES
Newborn	Cries with Unmet Needs
1–3 months old	Coos, makes other vocalizations, and demonstrates differentiated crying.
4–5 months old	Makes simple vowel sounds, laughs aloud, performs "raspberries," and vocalizes in response to voices. Responds to his or her own name and begins to respond to "no."
4–7 months old	Begins to distinguish emotions based on tone of voice.
6 months old	Squeals or yells to express joy or displeasure.
7–10 months old	Babbling begins and progresses to strings (e.g., mamama, dadada) without meaning. Able to respond to simple commands.
9–12 months old	Begins to attach meaning to "mama" and "dada" and starts to imitate other speech sounds.
Average 12 month old	Uses two or three recognizable words with meaning, recognizes objects by name, starts to imitate animal sounds. Pays increasing attention to speech, tries to imitate words; may say, "uh-oh." Babbles with inflection.

Adapted from Feigelman, S. (2011c). The first year. In R. M. Kliegman, B. F. Stanton, J. W. St. Geme III, N. F. Schor, & R. E. Behrman (Eds.), *Nelson's textbook of pediatrics* (19th ed.). Philadelphia, PA: Elsevier, Saunders; and Goldson, E., & Reynolds, A. (2012). Child development and behavior. In W. W. Hay, Jr., M. J. Levin, R. R. Deterding, M. J. Abzug, & J. M. Sondheimer (Eds.), *Current diagnosis and treatment: Pediatrics* (21st ed.). New York, NY: McGraw-Hill.

whether breast- or bottlefeeding. By 3 to 4 months of age, babies feed four or five times per day and take 6 to 7 ounces per feeding.

Solid foods may be introduced at 4 to 6 months of age, when the tongue extrusion reflex begins to disappear (Dietz, & Stern, 2012). The ability to swallow solid food becomes functional at this age, as do the enzymes necessary to properly food other than breast milk or formula. Rice cereal mixed with breast milk or formula should be introduced first and fed with a spoon and then add pureed foods, introducing one new food every 4 to 7 days in case of allergy (Stettler et al., 2011). Generally, by 8 months, you may offer soft, smashed table food without large chunks and finger foods such as Cheerios, soft green bean pieces, or soft peas. Avoid hard foods that the infant may choke on. Strained, pureed, or mashed meats may be introduced at 10 to 12 months of age.

Introduce the cup at 6 to 8 months of age by offering a small amount of breast milk or formula in it. Fruit juice is unnecessary and should not be introduced until 6 months of age, at which point it should be limited to 2 to 4 ounces per day (Stettler et al., 2011).

Take Note!

Cow's milk does not provide an adequate balance of nutrients for the growing infant, especially iron. It may also overload the infant's renal system with inappropriate amounts of protein, sodium, and minerals.

Toddler Growth and Development

Toddlerhood spans the ages from 1 to 3 years. Both physical growth and acquisition of new motor skills slow somewhat during the toddler years. Refinement of motor skills, continued cognitive growth, and acquisition of appropriate language skills are of prime importance during toddlerhood.

Psychosocial Development

Erikson (1963) defines the toddler period as a time of autonomy versus shame and doubt, a time of asserting one's self to learn control and independence. Ambivalence during the move from dependence to autonomy often results in emotional lability. Activities during this period include:

- achieves autonomy and self-control
- separates from parent/caregiver
- withstands delayed gratification
- negativism abounds (often says "no" even when means "yes")
- imitates adults and playmates
- shows affection spontaneously
- increasingly enthusiastic about playmates
- cannot take turns in games until 3 years of age.

Motor Skill and Language Development

Toddlerhood continues to be a period of rapid gross motor, fine motor, and language acquisition. Refer to Tables 1.3 and 1.4 for details.

Nutritional Guidelines

During the toddler years, the ability to chew and swallow is improving and the child learns to use utensils effectively to feed himself or herself.

(text continues on page 8)

TABLE 1.3	TODDLER MOTOR SKILL MILESTONES	
Age	Expected Gross Motor Skill	Expected Fine Motor Skills
12–15 months	Walks independently	Feeds self with finger foods Uses index finger to point
18 months	Climbs stairs with assistance Pulls toys while walking	Masters reaching, grasping, and releasing: stacks blocks, puts things in slots Turns book pages (singly with board book, multiple if paper) Removes shoes and socks Stacks four cubes
24 months	Runs Kicks ball Can stand on tiptoe Carries several toys, or a large toy while walking Climbs onto and down from furniture without assistance	Builds tower of six or seven cubes Right- or left-handed Imitates circular and vertical strokes Scribbles and paints Starting to turn knobs Puts round pegs into holes
36 months	Climbs well Pedals tricycle Runs easily Walks up and down stairs with alternate feet Bends over easily without falling	Undresses self Copies circle Builds a tower of 9 or 10 cubes Holds a pencil in writing position Screws/unscrews lids, nuts, bolts Turns book pages one at a time

Adapted from Feigelman, S. (2011b). Preschool years. In R. M. Kliegman, B. F. Stanton, J. W. St. Geme III, N. F. Schor, & R. E. Behrman (Eds.), *Nelson's textbook of pediatrics* (19th ed.). Philadelphia, PA: Elsevier, Saunders; and Feigelman, S. (2011d). The second year. In R. M. Kliegman, B. F. Stanton, J. W. St. Geme III, N. F. Schor, & R. E. Behrman (Eds.), *Nelson's textbook of pediatrics* (19th ed.). Philadelphia, PA: Elsevier, Saunders.

TABLE 1.4   TODDLER LANGUAGE MILESTONES

Age	Receptive Language	Expressive Language
12 months	Understands common words independent of context Follows a one-step command accompanied by gesture	Uses a finger to point to things Imitates or uses gestures such as waving goodbye Communicates desires with word and gesture combinations Vocal imitation First word
15 months	Looks at adult when communicating Follows a one-step command without gesture Understands 100–150 words	Repeats words that he or she hears Babbles in what sound like sentences
18 months	Understands the word "no" Comprehends 200 words Sometimes answers the question, "What's this?"	Uses at least 5–20 words Uses names of familiar object
24 months	Points to named body parts Points to pictures in books Enjoys listening to simple stories Names a variety of objects in the environment Beginning to use "my" or "mine"	Vocabulary of 40–50 words Sentences of two or three words (me up, want cookie) Asks questions (what that?) Uses simple phrases Uses descriptive words (hungry, hot) Two-thirds of what child says should be understandable Repeats overheard words
30 months	Follows a series of two independent commands	Vocabulary of 150–300 words

(continues on page 8)

TODDLER LANGUAGE MILESTONES *continued*		
Age	Receptive Language	Expressive Language
36 months	Understands most sentences Understands physical relationships (on, in, under) Participates in short conversations May follow a three-part command	Speech usually understood by those who know the child, about half understood by those outside family Asks "why?" Three- to four-word sentences Talks about something that happened in the past Vocabulary of 1,000 words Can say name, age, and gender Uses pronouns and plurals

Adapted from Feigelman, S. (2011b). Preschool years. In R. M. Kliegman, B. F. Stanton, J. W. St. Geme III, N. F. Schor, & R. E. Behrman (Eds.), *Nelson's textbook of pediatrics* (19th ed.). Philadelphia, PA: Elsevier, Saunders; Feigelman, S. (2011d). The second year. In R. M. Kliegman, B. F. Stanton, J. W. St. Geme III, N. F. Schor, & R. E. Behrman (Eds.), *Nelson's textbook of pediatrics* (19th ed.). Philadelphia, PA: Elsevier, Saunders; and Goldson, E., & Reynolds, A. (2012). Child development and behavior. In W. W. Hay, Jr., M. J. Levin, R. R. Deterding, M. J. Abzug, & J. M. Sondheimer (Eds.), *Current diagnosis and treatment: Pediatrics* (21st ed.). New York, NY: McGraw-Hill.

In addition to solid food intake, breastfeeding may extend into the toddler years. The formula-fed child should be weaned from the bottle by 12 to 15 months of age as prolonged bottlefeeding and the use of no-spill "sippy cups" is associated with the development of dental caries (American Academy of Pediatric Dentistry [AAPD], 2014). The 12- to 15 month old is developmentally capable of consuming adequate fluid amounts with a cup, and cups with spouts that do not contain valves are acceptable. Cow's milk should be limited to 16 ounces per day, and fruit juice to a few ounces.

Toddlers require a balanced diet but may often assert their autonomy and display food jags, when only a certain food is preferred.

It is important to form healthy eating habits in toddlerhood, so do not make high-calorie, nutrient-poor foods available to the toddler (Gavin, 2014a). Refer to Appendix A for serving sizes and recommended daily food intake.

Preschool Growth and Development

Preschool children, between 3 and 6 years of age, grow much more slowly than earlier years, and the healthy preschooler is slender and agile, with an upright posture. Cognitive, language, and psychosocial development is substantial throughout the preschool period. As cognitive skills increase, magical thinking abounds (Martorell, Papalia, & Feldman, 2014). Many tasks that began during the toddler years are mastered and perfected during the preschool years, particularly fine motor coordination. The child has learned to tolerate separation from parents, has a longer attention span, and continues to learn skills that will lead to later success in the school-age period.

Psychosocial Development

The psychosocial task of the preschool years according to Erikson (1963) is establishing a sense of initiative versus guilt. The preschooler is an inquisitive learner, very enthusiastic about learning new things. Preschoolers feel a sense of accomplishment when succeeding in activities, and feeling pride in one's accomplishment helps the child to use initiative. However, when the child extends himself or herself further than current capabilities allow, he or she may feel a sense of guilt. Activities associated with this period include:

- likes to please parents
- begins to plan activities, make up games
- initiates activities with others
- acts out the roles of other people (real and imaginary)
- develops sexual identity
- develops conscience
- may take frustrations out on siblings
- likes exploring new things
- enjoys sports, shopping, cooking, and working
- feels remorse when makes wrong choice or behaves badly
- cooperates with other children
- negotiates solutions to conflicts.

Motor and Language Skill Development

As the young child continues to develop, motor skills and language ability increase. Refer to Table 1.5 for details.

(text continues on page 12)

TABLE 1.5   PRESCHOOL MOTOR SKILL AND LANGUAGE DEVELOPMENT

Age	Expected Gross Motor Skills	Expected Fine Motor Skills	Expected Communication and Language Development
4 years	• Throws ball overhand • Kicks ball forward • Catches bounced ball • Hops on one foot • Stands on one foot up to 5 seconds • Alternates feet going up and down steps • Moves backward and forward with agility	• Uses scissors successfully • Copies capital letters • Draws circles and squares • Traces a cross or diamond • Draws a person with two to four body parts • Laces shoes	• Speaks in complete sentences using adult-like grammar • Tells a story that is easy to follow • 75% of speech understood by others outside of family • Asks questions with "who," "how," "how many" • Stays on topic in a conversation • Understands the concepts of "same" and "different" • Asks many questions • Knows names of familiar animals • Names common objects in books and magazines • Knows at least one color • Uses language to engage in make-believe • Follows a three-part command • Can count a few numbers • Vocabulary of 1,500 words

Age	Expected Gross Motor Skills	Expected Fine Motor Skills	Expected Communication and Language Development
5 years	• Stands on one foot 10 seconds or longer • Swings and climbs well • May skip • Somersaults • May learn to skate and swim	• Prints some letters • Draws person with body and at least six parts • Dresses/undresses without assistance • Can learn to tie laces • Uses fork, spoon, and knife (supervised) well • Copies triangle and other geometric patterns • Mostly cares for own toileting needs	• Persons outside of the family can understand most of the child's speech • Explains how an item is used • Participates in long, detailed conversations • Talks about past, future, and imaginary events • Answers questions that use "why" and "when" • Can count up to 10 • Recalls part of a story • Speech should be completely intelligible, even if the child has articulation difficulties • Speech is generally grammatically correct • Vocabulary of 2,100 words • Says name and address

Adapted from Feigelman, S. (2011b). Preschool years. In R. M. Kliegman, B. F. Stanton, J. W. Sr. Geme III, N. F. Schor, & R. E. Behrman (Eds.), *Nelson's textbook of pediatrics* (19th ed.). Philadelphia, PA: Elsevier; Saunders; Goldson, E., & Reynolds, A. (2012). Child development and behavior. In W. W. Hay, Jr., M. J. Levin, R. R. Deterding, M. J. Abzug, & J. M. Sondheimer (Eds.), *Current diagnosis and treatment: Pediatrics* (21st ed.). New York, NY: McGraw-Hill; and Martorell, G. Papalia, D., & Feldman, R. (2014). *A child's world: Infancy through adolescence* (13th ed.). New York, NY: McGraw Hill.

Nutritional Guidelines

The preschool child has a full set of primary teeth, is able to chew and swallow competently, and has learned to use utensils fairly effectively to feed himself or herself. A diet high in nutrient-rich foods such as whole grains, vegetables, fruits, appropriate dairy foods, and lean meats is appropriate for the preschooler. Nutrient-poor, high-calorie foods such as sweets and typical fast foods should be offered only in limited amounts. Preschool children may be picky eaters, preferring only a limited variety of foods or foods prepared in certain ways. They may not be very willing to try new things. The 3 or 4 year old may exhibit "food fads," eating only certain foods over a period of several days. As the child gets older, pickiness lessens and the social context of eating meals becomes more important to the child.

Take Note!

Drinking excess amounts of milk may lead to iron deficiency, as the calcium in milk blocks iron absorption.

School-Aged Child Growth and Development

School-aged children, between 6 and 12 years of age, experience a time of slow progressive physical growth, whereas their social and developmental growth accelerates and increases in complexity. They move toward more abstract thinking. The focus of their world expands from family to teachers, peers, and other outside influences (e.g., coaches, media). The child at this stage becomes increasingly more independent while participating in activities outside the home.

Psychosocial Development

The school-aged child is in Erikson's period of industry versus inferiority (Erikson, 1963). The child who is appropriately nurtured and supported throughout this period will successfully develop a sense of industry. Inferiority occurs with repeated failures with little support or trust from those who are important to the child. Activities associated with this period include:

- interested in how things are made and run
- success in personal and social tasks
- increased activities outside home (e.g., clubs, sports)
- increased interactions with peers
- increased interest in knowledge.

Motor and Language Skill Development

Gross motor and fine motor skills continue to mature throughout the school-age years. Language development accelerates. Refer to Table 1.6.

(text continues on page 14)

TABLE 1.6   SCHOOL-AGE MOTOR SKILL AND LANGUAGE DEVELOPMENT

Age	Expected Gross Motor Skill	Expected Fine Motor Skills	Expected Communication and Language Development
6–12 years	Improvement in coordination, balance and rhythm; ability to ride a two-wheeled bicycle, jump rope, dance, skate, swim. The older school-aged child may exhibit awkwardness due to their bodies growing faster than their ability to compensate	Improved hand–eye coordination and balance; increased precision with writing, printing words, sewing, building models and other crafts; ability to play musical instruments	Language skills accelerate; vocabulary expands; begin to use more complex grammar forms, enjoy jokes and riddles

Nutritional Guidelines

In the school-aged child, the amount of needed calories decreases whereas appetite increases. The school-aged child's calorie needs vary on the basis of age, gender, and activity level. In general, children with higher activity levels and male gender have higher calorie needs (U.S. Department of Agriculture [USDA] and U.S. Department of Health and Human Services [USDHHS], 2010).

In preparation for adolescence, the body fat composition of school-aged children increases. Diet preferences established in the preschool years continue during the school-age period. As the child grows older, influences of family, media, and peers can impact the eating habits of this age group. Some of these influences are parents' work schedule, outside activities, and exercise level of the child. Decreased exercise levels and poor nutritional choices lead to the mounting problem of obesity seen in this age group.

School-age children should choose culturally appropriate foods and snacks from the U.S. Department of Agriculture's MyPlate (Appendix B). MyPlate illustrates the five food groups and encourages children to have half of their plate be fruits and vegetables, to have half of their grains to be whole grains, and to choose lean proteins and calcium-rich foods. The website www.choosemyplate.gov/ offers many tools for the child to use, including development of personalized goals and menus, online dieting and physical activity assessment tools, games, activities, and tips for parents. School-aged children need to limit intake of fat and processed sugars. A prudent diet limits the use of fatty meats, high-fat dairy products, eggs, and hydrogenated shortenings and promotes the consumption of fish and the substitution of polyunsaturated vegetable oils and margarines.

Adolescent Growth and Development

Adolescence spans the years of transition from childhood to adulthood, which is usually between 11 and 20 years of age. Adolescence is a time of rapid growth with dramatic changes in body size and proportions. During this time, sexual characteristics develop and reproductive maturity is achieved. Generally, girls enter puberty earlier (at 9 to 10 years of age) than boys (at 10 to 11 years). Refer to Table 1.7 for physiologic changes in adolescence.

Psychosocial Development

The adolescent is in Erikson's (1963) period of identity versus role confusion. The adolescent struggles during this period to determine his or her own identity. Role confusion often occurs during this period

(text continues on page 16)

TABLE 1.7 PHYSIOLOGIC CHANGES OF ADOLESCENCE

Stage of Adolescence	Changes in Females	Changes in Males
Early adolescence (10–13 years)	Pubic hair begins to curl and spread over mons pubis; genitalia pigmentation increases Breast bud and areola continue to enlarge; no separation of breast First menstrual period (average 12.8 years)	Pubic hair spreads laterally, begins to curl; pigmentation increases Growth and enlargement of testes in scrotum (scrotum reddish in color) and continued lengthening of penis Leggy look due to extremities growing faster than the trunk
Middle adolescence (14–16 years)	Pubic hair becomes coarse in texture and continues to curl; amount of hair increases Areola and papilla separate from the contour of the breast to form a secondary mound	Pubic hair becomes coarser in texture and takes on adult distribution Testes and scrotum continue to grow; scrotal skin darkens; penis grows in width, and glans penis develops May experience breast enlargement Voice changes; more masculine due to rapid enlargement of the larynx and pharynx as well as lung changes
Late adolescence (17–20 years)	Mature pubic hair distribution and coarseness	Mature pubic hair distribution and coarseness Breast enlargement disappears Adult size and shape of testes, scrotum, and penis; scrotal skin darkening

Adapted from Cromer, B. (2011). Chapter 104: Adolescent development. In R. M. Kleigman, B. F. Stanton, J. W. St. Geme III, N. F. Schor, & R. E. Behrman (Eds.), *Nelson textbook of pediatrics* (19th ed., pp. 649–659). Philadelphia, PA: Saunders.

15

but resolves as the adolescent determines a healthy identity. Activities associated with stages of adolescence are as follows.

EARLY ADOLESCENCE (10 TO 13 YEARS)
- Focuses on bodily changes.
- Experiences frequent mood changes.
- Importance placed upon conformity to peer norms and peer acceptance.
- Strives to master skills within peer groups.
- Defining boundaries with parents and authority figures.
- Early stage of emancipation; child struggles to separate from parents while still desiring dependence upon them.
- Identifies with same-sex peers.
- Takes more responsibility for own behaviors.

MIDDLE ADOLESCENCE (14 TO 16 YEARS)
- Continues to adjust to changed body image.
- Tries out different roles within peer groups.
- Need for acceptance by peer group at the highest level.
- Interested in attracting opposite gender.
- Time of greatest conflict with parents or authority figures.

LATE ADOLESCENCE (17 TO 20 YEARS)
- Able to understand implications of behavior and decisions.
- Roles within peer groups established.
- Feels secure with body image.
- Has matured sexual identity.
- Has idealistic career goals.
- Importance of individual friendships emerges.
- Process of emancipation from family almost complete (Erikson, 1963).

Motor and Language Skill Development
During adolescence, gross motor, fine motor, and language skills continue to be developed and refined. Refer to Table 1.8.

Nutritional Guidelines
In adolescence, nutritional needs are increased because of accelerated growth and sexual maturation. Adolescents may appear to be hungry constantly and need regular meals and snacks with adequate nutrients to meet the body's needs.

Adolescents have a need for increased calories, zinc, calcium, and iron for growth. However, the number of calories needed for adolescence depends on the teenager's age and activity level as well as growth patterns. Teenage girls who are moderately active require about 2,000 calories per day (USDA & USDHHS, 2010). Teenage boys who are

(text continues on page 18)

TABLE 1.8   ADOLESCENT MOTOR SKILL AND LANGUAGE DEVELOPMENT

Age	Expected Gross Motor Skill	Expected Fine Motor Skills	Expected Communication and Language Development
Early adolescence (10–13 years); middle adolescence (14–16 years); late adolescence (17–20 years)	Development of endurance; coordination can be a problem due to uneven growth spurts; middle adolescence, speed and accuracy increase and coordination improves; increase in competitiveness	Increased ability to manipulate objects; handwriting is neat; refining finger dexterity and precise eye–hand coordination	Improved communication skills with correct use of grammar and parts of speech; use of slang increases. By late adolescence, language skills comparable with those of adults

TABLE 1.9	SAMPLE DIET FOR THREE CALORIC LEVELS		
	Calories for Three Caloric Levels		
	Lower (About 1,600 Calories)	*Moderate (About 2,200 Calories)*	*Higher (About 2,800 Calories)*
Grain group servings	6	9	11
Vegetable group servings	3	4	5
Fruit group servings	2	3	4
Milk group servings	2–3	2–3	2–3
Meat group (ounces)	5	6	7

Adapted from U.S. Department of Agriculture and U.S. Department of Health and Human Services. (2010). *Dietary guidelines for Americans,* (7th Ed.). Washington, DC: U.S. Government Printing Office.

moderately active require between 2,400 and 2,800 calories per day (see Table 1.9; USDA & USDHHS, 2010).

Adolescents require about 1,300 mg of calcium each day (Gavin, 2014b). Foods high in calcium include milk, white beans, broccoli, cheese, and yogurt. Male adolescents require 11 mg of iron each day and female adolescents require 15 mg each day (Gavin, 2012). Foods high in iron include beef, chicken, fish; liver; peanut butter; nuts and seeds; green peas, lima beans; spinach; strawberries; tomato juice; whole-grain bread; raisins; and watermelon. Protein requirements for adolescent girls between 14 and 18 years of age are 46 g per day, whereas adolescent boys between 14 and 18 years of age require 52 g of protein per day (USDA & USDHHS, 2010). Foods high in protein include meats, fish, poultry, beans, and dairy products.

HEALTH SUPERVISION

Health supervision involves providing services proactively, with the goal of optimizing the child's level of functioning. It ensures the child is growing and developing appropriately, and it promotes the best possible health of the child by teaching parents and children about preventing injury and illness (e.g., proper immunizations and anticipatory guidance). The three components of health supervision include developmental surveillance and screening, injury and disease prevention, and health promotion.

Visit Schedule

Health supervision visits for children without health problems and appropriate growth and development are recommended at birth, within the first week of life, by 1 month, then at 2 months, 4 months, 6 months, 9 months, 12 months, 15 months, 18 months, 24 months, and then yearly until 21 years of age (Bright Futures/American Academy of Pediatrics, 2014). Children with special needs or concerns will have more frequent and intensive visits. Health supervision visits include assessment of physical health along with intellectual and social development and parent–child interaction.

Each health supervision visit will include:

- history and physical assessment, including head circumference (until 2 years of age), height, and weight
- developmental/behavioral assessment
- sensory screening (vision and hearing)
- risk screening (such as anemia screening, lead screening, tuberculin test, hypertension screening, and cholesterol screening)
- immunizations
- health promotion (injury prevention, violence prevention, and nutrition counseling) (Bright Futures/American Academy of Pediatrics, 2014).

Developmental Screening Tools

Developmental surveillance is an ongoing collection of skilled observations made over time during healthcare visits. Components include:

- noting and addressing parental concerns
- obtaining a developmental history
- making accurate observations
- consulting with relevant professionals.

Developmental screenings are brief assessment procedures that identify children who warrant more intensive assessment and testing. Developmental screening assessments may be observational or by caregiver report. A variety of developmental screening tools are available to guide the nurse in assessing development. The pediatric nurse must understand normal growth and development and become proficient at screening for problems related to development. The historical information obtained from the parent or primary caregiver about

(text continues on page 22)

TABLE 1.10	EARLY CHILDHOOD DEVELOPMENTAL WARNING SIGNS
Age	**Warning Sign**
Any age	• No response to environmental stimulus
Any age	• Persistently up on toes (longer than 30 seconds) in supported standing position
Before 3 months	• Rolls over
After 2–3 months	• Persistent fisting
After 4 months	• Persistent head lag
5 months	• Not reaching for toys
6 months	• Lack of tripod sitting • Not smiling • Primitive reflex persistence • Not babbling
9 months	• No reciprocal vocalizations or facial expressions
12 months	• No spoon or crayon use
15–18 months	• Not walking • No first word
Prior to 18 months	• Hand dominance present
By 18 months	• Not walking • Not speaking 15 words • Does not understand function of common household items • No imitative play
After independent walking for several months	• Persistent tiptoe walking • Failure to develop a mature walking pattern
By 2 years	• Does not use two-word sentences • Does not imitate actions • Does not follow basic instructions • Cannot push a toy with wheels • Echolalia (repetitive speech)

EARLY CHILDHOOD DEVELOPMENTAL WARNING SIGNS *continued*

Age	Warning Sign
By 3 years	• Difficulty with stairs • Frequent falling • Cannot build tower of more than four blocks • Difficulty manipulating small objects • Extreme difficulty in separation from parents or caregiver • Cannot copy a circle • Does not engage in make-believe play • Cannot communicate in short phrases • Does not understand simple instructions • Little interest in other children • Unclear speech, persistent drooling
By 4 years	• Cannot jump in place or ride a tricycle • Cannot stack four blocks • Cannot throw ball overhand • Does not grasp crayon with thumb and fingers • Difficulty with scribbling • Cannot copy a circle • Does not use sentences with three or more words • Cannot use the words "me" and "you" appropriately • Ignores other children or does not show interest in interactive games • Will not respond to people outside the family; still clings or cries if parents leave • Resists using toilet, dressing, sleeping • Does not engage in fantasy play
By 5 years	• Unhappy or sad often • Little interest in playing with other children • Unable to separate from parent without major protest • Is extremely aggressive • Is extremely fearful or timid, or unusually passive • Cannot build tower of six to eight blocks • Easily distracted; cannot concentrate on single activity for 5 minutes • Rarely engages in fantasy play • Trouble with eating, sleeping, or using the toilet • Cannot use plurals or past tense • Cannot brush teeth, wash, and dry hands, or undress efficiently

developmental milestones may indicate warning signs or identify risks for developmental delay. Refer to Table 1.10 for developmental warning signs.

Factors placing the infant or toddler at risk for developmental problems include:
- birth weight less than 1,500 g
- gestational age less than 33 weeks
- central nervous system abnormality
- hypoxic ischemic encephalopathy
- maternal prenatal alcohol or drug abuse
- hypertonia
- hypotonia
- hyperbilirubinemia requiring exchange transfusion
- kernicterus
- congenital malformations
- symmetric intrauterine growth deficiency
- perinatal or congenital infection
- suspected sensory impairment
- chronic (greater than 3 months) otitis media with effusion
- inborn error of metabolism
- HIV infection
- lead level above 19 mg/dL
- inappropriate parental concern about developmental issues (e.g., not allowing a 3 year old to feed himself or herself)
- parent with less than high school education
- single parent
- sibling with developmental problems
- parent with developmental disability or mental illness.

Take Note!

Any child who "loses" a developmental milestone—for example, the child able to sit without support who now cannot—needs an immediate full evaluation, as this indicates a significant neurologic problem.

In addition to developmental and behavioral surveillance at every visit, the American Academy of Pediatrics recommends performing a screening test for autism with a standardized developmental tool at 18 and 24 months or at any point that concerns about autism spectrum disorder are raised.

Also, perform a risk assessment for alcohol and drug use at every visit from 11 years to 21 years of age. Refer to thePoint for a list of websites providing these screening tools.

Screening Tests

Screening tests are procedures or laboratory analyses used to identify children with a certain condition. These tests are done to ensure that no person with the disorder is missed. If a screening test gives a positive result, follow-up tests with higher specificity are performed. A risk assessment is performed by the healthcare professional in conjunction with the child and includes objective as well as subjective data to determine the likelihood that the child will develop a condition.

Metabolic Screening

State law determines which metabolic screening tests are mandatory in that state. In addition to screening for hearing loss, the March of Dimes (2015) currently recommends universal newborn metabolic screening tests for 30 disorders for which effective treatment is available.

During the initial health supervision visit, the nurse should confirm that newborn metabolic screening was performed prior to discharge from the birthing unit. If the test was not performed or was performed at <48 hours of age, the screening should be performed at that visit. The metabolic screening results need to be noted in the child's permanent record at the medical home.

Hearing Screening

The AAP recommends hearing screening of all infants. Hearing loss is a common condition in newborns, and even mild hearing loss can cause serious delays in social and emotional development, language acquisition, and cognitive function (Delaney, 2014). Targeted screening based on risk factors will identify only 50% of infants with hearing loss, and with reliable screening tests available, universal screening has been implemented (Delaney, 2014). Screening should be done before discharge from the birthing unit; if not, the newborn needs to be screened before 1 month of age. Behavioral observations of the infant's response to sounds, such as a ringing bell, are not sensitive enough to preclude mild to moderate hearing loss (Delaney, 2014). Accepted methodologies, such as the auditory brain stem response (ABR), should be used.

Screening for hearing loss in older children begins with a history from the primary caregivers. If any problems are noted, audiometry should be performed. When the child is capable of following simple commands reliably, perform some basic procedures to screen for hearing loss. The whisper test is easy to perform but to be valid requires a quiet room that is away from distractions. The Weber and Rinne tests are typically performed together and can be used to screen for sensorineural or conductive hearing loss.

Universal hearing screening with objective testing is recommended at 4, 5, 6, 8, and 10 years of age (Bright Futures/American Academy of Pediatrics, 2014). Appropriate risk assessment should be performed at 7, 9, and 11 through 21 years of age (Bright Futures/American Academy of Pediatrics, 2014). Examples of risk assessment include the following:

- For 3 months to 4 years of age
  - Auditory skill monitoring
  - Developmental surveillance
  - Assessment of parental concerns.
- For older than 4 years of age
  - Difficulty hearing on the telephone
  - Difficulty hearing people in a noisy background
  - Frequent asking of others to repeat themselves
  - Turning the television up too loudly.

More frequent screening is recommended if there is any behavior that indicates the child's hearing may be impaired. Repeated hearing screenings are recommended if a child has risk factors for acquired hearing loss such as:

- family history of hearing loss
- prenatal infection
- anomalies of the head, face, or ears
- low birth weight (less than 1,500 g)
- hyperbilirubinemia requiring exchange transfusion
- ototoxic medications
- low Apgar scores: 4 or lower at 1 minute, or 6 or lower at 5 minutes
- mechanical ventilation lasting 5 days
- syndrome associated with hearing loss
- bacterial meningitis
- neurodegenerative disorders
- persistent pulmonary hypertension
- otitis media with effusion for 3 months (Delaney, 2014).

Vision Screening

Perform vision screening at every scheduled health supervision visit. The screening procedures for children younger than 3 years or for nonverbal children involve evaluating the child's ability to fixate on and follow objects. The neonate should be able to fixate on an object 10 to 12 inches from the face. After fixation, the infant should be able to follow the object to the midline. By 2 months of age, the infant should be able to follow the object to 180 degrees. The technique of photo screening can help identify problems such as ocular malalignment, refractive error, and lens and retinal problems.

> *Take Note!*
> Use objects with black and white patterns when perform-
> ing vision screening on an infant younger than 6 months. The
> infant's vision at this age is more attuned to high-contrast patterns
> than to colors. Try checkerboard patterns or concentric circles. Animal
> figures such as pandas and dalmatians also work well.

After 3 years of age, a variety of standardized age-appropriate vision screening charts are available. These charts include the "tumbling E" and Allen figures. By 5 or 6 years of age, most children know the alphabet well enough to use the traditional Snellen chart for vision screening.

Perform screenings when children are alert, as fatigue and lack of interest can mimic poor vision. When using any vision-screening chart, follow several simple steps:

• Place the chart at the child's eye level.
• Place a mark on the floor 20 ft from the chart.
• Align the child's heels on the mark.
• Have the child read each line with one eye covered and then with the other eye covered.
• Have the child read each line with both eyes.

In addition to visual acuity screening, screen children for color discrimination. Any child with eye abnormalities or who has failed visual screening needs to be evaluated by a specialist appropriately trained to treat children.

Iron Deficiency Anemia Screening

Infants, young children and teenage girls are at a higher risk for iron deficiency (National Institutes of Health, 2015). Iron deficiency can cause cognitive and motor deficits resulting in developmental delays and behavioral disturbances.

The American Academy of Pediatrics recommends assessing for risk factors related to iron-deficiency anemia at 4, 15, 18, 30 months and then annually and performing a hematocrit or hemoglobin at 12 months (Bright Futures/American Academy of Pediatrics, 2014). It is important for the nurse to assess for risk factors related to iron deficiency anemia at each health supervision visit.

Children at high risk for iron deficiency anemia include:

• those from low-income families
• those eligible for the Special Supplemental Nutrition Program for Women, Infants, and Children (WIC)
• migrants or recently arrived refugees (Baker, Greer, & The Committee on Nutrition, 2010).

Other risk factors for iron deficiency anemia include:

- periods of rapid growth
- low birth weight or preterm infants
- low dietary intake of meat, fish, poultry, and ascorbic acid
- macrobiotic diets
- inappropriate consumption of cow's milk
- use of infant formula not fortified with iron
- exclusive breastfeeding after 6 months of age without iron-fortified supplemental foods
- meal skipping, frequent dieting
- pregnancy or recent pregnancy
- intensive physical training
- recent blood loss, heavy/lengthy menstrual periods
- long-term use of aspirin or nonsteroidal anti-inflammatory drugs (NSAIDs)
- parasitic infections.

Lead Screening

Blood lead levels greater than 5 mcg/dL can lead to a wide variety of symptoms and problems, such as headaches, stomach pain, inattentiveness, irritability, hyperactivity, decreased bone and muscle growth, poor muscle coordination, problems with language and speech, cognitive impairments, hearing problems, and seizures (Centers for Disease Control and Prevention, 2013b; Vyas, 2015). It has also been found that even low blood lead levels can harm children and result in IQ deficits, attention-related behavior problems, and poor academic achievement (Centers for Disease Control and Prevention, 2012a). Studies have also shown that these effects cannot be reversed (Centers for Disease Control and Prevention, 2012a). Therefore a shift to primary prevention is essential. Ensuring that no children spend time or live in homes, buildings, or environments where they are exposed to lead hazards is key. Educate parents on lead hazards and encourage them to avoid exposure of their children. Lead hazards include homes or buildings built before 1978; contaminated soil and dust; water that flows through old lead pipes or faucets; foods stored in containers that are painted with lead paint (such as lead glazed pottery or lead crystal); canned food imported from other countries which may be sealed with lead; toys or toy jewelry which may be painted with lead paint or have lead components; and folk remedies which may contain lead, such as greta and azarcon (United States Environmental Protection Agency, 2015). The Advisory Committee on Childhood Lead Poisoning Prevention recommends that healthcare providers follow local and state lead screening guidelines (Centers for Disease Control and Prevention, 2012a). The American Academy of Pediatrics Bright Future guidelines recommends performing a risk assessment and if positive screen at 6, 9, 12, 18, and 24 months and at 3, 4, 5, and 6 years (Bright Futures/American Academy of Pediatrics, 2014).

> ### Take Note!
>
> Many cases of elevated blood lead levels have been reported in children who are recent immigrants, refugees, or international adoptees. The CDC recommends blood lead testing for these children upon entering the United States and a repeat test 3 to 6 months after placement in permanent residence (Centers for Disease Control and Prevention, 2013a).

Hypertension Screening

Obesity and resulting hypertension has been on the rise in children and can lead to adult cardiovascular disease. Universal hypertension screening for children beginning at 3 years of age is recommended (Bright Futures/American Academy of Pediatrics, 2014). If the child has risk factors for systemic hypertension, such as preterm birth, very low birth weight, renal disease, organ transplant, congenital heart disease, or other illnesses associated with hypertension, then screening begins when the risk factor becomes apparent (Bright Futures/American Academy of Pediatrics, 2014).

The guidelines for determining hypertension in children and adolescents utilize body size to be more precise. Gender, age, and sex are used to determine specific systolic and diastolic blood pressure percentiles. Refer to Appendix C for Blood Pressure Charts for Children and Adolescents. Auscultation is the preferred method of measuring blood pressure in children and an elevated blood pressure level must be confirmed on repeated visits before a diagnosis of hypertension is given. Refer to Box 1.1 for hypertension guidelines.

Hyperlipidemia Screening

Atherosclerosis has been documented in children, and a link exists between high lipid levels and the development of these lesions. Bright Futures Guidelines recommend universal screening for dyslipidemia between 9 and 11 years of age and again between 18 and 21 years of age (Bright Futures/American Academy of Pediatrics, 2014). Performing a risk assessment screening at 24 months and at 4, 6, 8, and 12 through 17 years of age is also recommended. Selectively screening children at high risk for hyperlipidemia can reduce their lifelong risk of coronary artery disease.

BOX 1.1

CHILDHOOD HYPERTENSION GUIDELINES

Optimal/normal	<90th percentile for sex, age, and height
Prehypertension	BP at or above 120/80 mm Hg but <95th percentile for sex, age, and height
Stage 1 Hypertension	≥95th percentile <99th percentile + 5 mm Hg for sex, age, and height on three separate occasions
Stage 2 Hypertension	≥99th percentile + 5 mm Hg for sex, age, and height on three separate occasions

---

Adapted from National Heart, Lung, and Blood Institute. (2012). *Expert panel on integrated guidelines for cardiovascular health and risk reduction in children and adolescents. Summary report (NIH Publication No. 12–7486).* Washington, DC: U.S. Department of Health and Human Services.

The risk assessment focuses on the child's family history (National Heart, Lung, and Blood Institute, 2012).

- Screen if parents, grandparents, aunts/uncles, and/or siblings, have or had documented:
  - Coronary atherosclerosis
  - Myocardial infarction
  - Angina pectoris
  - Peripheral vascular disease
  - Cerebrovascular disease/stroke
  - Coronary artery bypass graft/stent/angioplasty at younger than 55 years in males and younger than 65 years in females
  - Sudden cardiac death
- Screen if a parent's blood cholesterol level is 240 mg/dL or higher.
- Screen at healthcare provider's discretion if:
  - Parental history is unobtainable.
  - Child has diabetes or hypertension.
  - Child has the following lifestyle risk factors:
    - Cigarette smoking
    - Obesity
    - Sedentary lifestyle
    - High-fat dietary intake.

> **Take Note!**
>
> To increase cooperation from young children during screen-
> ings, set up a reward system. Easy-to-do rewards include the
> following:
>
> - Stamping the back of the child's hand with a "smiley face."
> - Making an eye cover by placing two stickers back to back over
>   a tongue blade and letting the child keep the cover after the
>   screening.
> - Copying a design onto a sheet of paper and letting the child
>   take it home to color.
> - Letting the child play with a simple device such as a penlight
>   or stethoscope.

Immunization Schedule

The Advisory Committee on Immunization Practices (ACIP), a branch of the CDC, reviews the recommended immunization schedule yearly and updates the schedules to ensure that it accurately reflects current best practice. Go to this link http://www.cdc.gov/vaccines/schedules/hcp/index.html for up-to-date immunizations schedules.

Health Promotion

Health promotion focuses on maintaining or enhancing the physical and mental health of clients. The principal components of health promotion are identifying risk factors for a disease, facilitating lifestyle changes to eliminate or reduce those risk factors, and empowering clients at the individual and community levels to develop resources to optimize their health. The nurse implements health promotion through education and anticipatory guidance.

Anticipatory guidance is primary prevention. The "skeleton" of the guidance provided involves common childhood health problems. The nurse fleshes out this information using the results of risk assessments and screening tests, health concerns unique to the child, and the interests and concerns of the parents. Age-related anticipatory guidance along with topics such as oral health, healthy weight, activity, personal hygiene, and safe sun exposure are examples of important anticipatory guidance topics.

HEALTH ASSESSMENT

Obtaining a thorough and accurate health assessment is the basis for sound nursing care. The health assessment of a child should include a complete health history and physical examination.

Health History

Assess the child and family for the following:

Demographics

Include the child's name, age, gender, and other pertinent demographic information.

Chief Complaint

Record the complaint in the child's or parent's own words.

History of Present Illness

For each concern, determine:
- onset
- duration
- characteristics course
- previous episodes
- previous testing or therapies
- what makes it better and what makes it worse
- what the concern means to the child and family.

Exposure to Infectious Agents

Past Health History

Include:
- prenatal history
- perinatal history (any problems with labor and delivery)
- past illnesses, or any other health or developmental problems
- child's history of illnesses (recurrent, chronic, or serious)
- any accidents or injuries in the past
- operations or hospitalizations
- diet
- allergies to foods, medications, animals, environmental or contact agents, or latex products (note reaction and severity)
- immunization status
- medications (dosage and schedule, when the last dose was given)
- menstrual history (in female preadolescents and female adolescents).

Family Health History

Include age and health status of parents, siblings, and other family members.

Review of Systems

Inquire about history (both current and past), of problems related to:
- growth and development
- skin
- head and neck
- eyes and vision

- ears and hearing
- mouth, teeth, and throat
- respiratory system and breasts
- cardiovascular system
- gastrointestinal system
- genitourinary system
- musculoskeletal system
- neurologic system
- endocrine system
- hematologic system.

Developmental History

Inquire about:

- landmarks in gross motor control
- attained fine motor skills
- self-care ability
- toilet training
- feeding skills
- social skills
- comfort articles
- habits
- daycare attendance and preschool or school adjustment and achievements.

Functional History

Ask questions related to:

- safety measures
- routine health care and dental care
- nutrition
- physical activity and organized sports, play, and recreation
- television and computer habits
- sleep behavior and bedtime
- elimination patterns and any concerns
- hearing or vision problems (dates of last screenings and results)
- relationships with other family members and friends, coping and temperament, discipline strategies, attention, or school behavior problems
- religious involvement and other spiritual practices
- use of adaptive and assistive devices such as eyeglasses or contact lenses, hearing aids, walkers, braces, or wheelchairs; and
- sexual practices. (Burns, Dunn, Brady, Starr, & Blosser, 2013).

Family Composition, Resources, and Home Environment

Note whom the child lives with and in what type of home, as well as note financial resources including health insurance.

Physical Examination

The physical examination should include general appearance, vital signs, body measurements, and skin, hair, nails, head, neck, eyes, ears, nose, sinuses, mouth, throat, thorax, lungs, breasts, heart, peripheral perfusion, abdomen, genitalia, anus, musculoskeletal, and neurologic assessments.

Vital Signs

Note the child's vital signs. Include the temperature route and ensure the child is quiet when the blood pressure is taken. Refer to Table 1.11 for heart rate and respiratory ranges by age group. Note if the child's vital signs fall outside of the recommended ranges. At times, hospitalized children may be observed on a cardiac apnea monitor (Fig. 1.1). Always manually check the heart rate and respiratory rate to correlate with the numbers displayed on the monitor. In many institutions, oxygen saturation via pulse oximetry and pain assessment are evaluated when the vital signs are obtained.

Body Measurements

Determine the child's weight, length/height, and head circumference. Plot the weight, length, head circumference, and weight for stature on the gender-appropriate growth chart for birth to 36 months. Plot the weight, height, and body mass index (BMI) on the gender-appropriate growth chart for 2 to 20 years. Refer to Appendix D for the growth charts.

Use the sample physical assessment provided in Box 1.2 as a quick guide to assessing the child in the clinical setting.

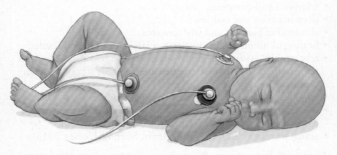

FIGURE 1.1 Placement of cardiac apnea monitor leads: white on the right upper chest, black on the left upper chest, and green or red on the abdomen (not over bone).

TABLE 1.11 HEART RATE AND RESPIRATORY RATE RANGES BY AGE GROUP

	Infant	Toddler	Preschooler	School-Age	Adolescent
Heart rate	80–150	70–120	65–110	60–100	55–95
Respiratory rate	25–55	20–30	20–25	14–22	12–18

Adapted from Schaider, J., Barkin, R. M., Hayden, S. R., Wolfe, R. E., Barkin, A. Z., Shayne, P., & Rosen, P. (2014). *Rosen & Barkin's 5-minute emergency medicine consult* (5th ed.). Philadelphia, PA: Lippincott Williams & Wilkins.

BOX 1.2

SAMPLE PHYSICAL ASSESSMENT

Vital Signs: T _____ **P** _____ **R** _____ **B/P** _____
(note if NOT w/in normal range age)

Oxygen Saturation: _____ **Pain Assessment** _____
(note type of pain scale used)

Growth *(use growth charts):*

Weight: _____ pounds _____ kg _____ percentile
for age

Height or Length: _____ inches _____ cm _____
percentile for age

Weight for Length: _____ percentile for age **OR**
BMI _____ percentile for age

Head Circumference (<2 years): _____ cm _____
percentile for age

General:
*Alert, interactive, developmentally appropriate for age. Oriented ×3
(older children). State where the child is (in bed or crib with SR up,
on mom's lap, etc.). Include any tubes, oxygen, or IVs attached to the
child.*

Skin, Hair, Nails:
*Skin pink, warm, dry, intact without lesions or rashes (if present,
describe). Briefly describe hair and nails (note alopecia, shaving, nail
abnormalities).*

Head/Neck:
*Normocephalic, atraumatic. Neck supple with full ROM. Note
lymphadenopathy if present. Describe abnormalities.*

Eyes:
*Eyes symmetric, without redness or drainage (describe abnormali-
ties). PERRLA. Younger infants: follows. Older infants and children:
vision appears grossly intact. Describe abnormalities.*

Ears:
*Ears symmetric, appropriately positioned, no drainage or preauricu-
lar pits/tags. Hearing grossly intact. Describe abnormalities.*

Nose, Sinuses, Mouth, Throat:
*Nose midline, without drainage. No sinus tenderness upon palpa-
tion. Oral mucosa moist and pink. Note number and condition of
teeth. Pharynx pink, note tonsil size. Describe abnormalities.*

SAMPLE PHYSICAL ASSESSMENT *continued*

Respiratory:
Respirations easy with symmetric chest rise. Breath sounds clear throughout with adequate aeration. Note adventitious or diminished breath sounds. If increased WOB, describe location and severity of retractions.

Cardiovascular:
Heart rate regular without murmur (or irregular with respirations [sinus arrhythmia]). Color pink. No edema. Pulses strong and equal throughout. Describe abnormalities.

Abdomen:
Abdomen soft, nontender, nondistended, no masses or organomegaly. Positive bowel sounds x4 quadrants. Describe abnormalities.

Genitalia/Anus:
Normal male or female genitalia. Boys: both testes down, circumcised or noncircumcised. Preadolescents and adolescents: Tanner staging. Describe abnormalities.

Musculoskeletal:
Moves all extremities through full range of motion. Adequate strength. Normotonic. Describe abnormalities.

Neurologic:
Lusty cry (if infant). Level of consciousness. Interactivity with parents and environment. Appropriate responses. Perform additional neurologic tests if indicated. Describe abnormalities.

PAIN ASSESSMENT AND MANAGEMENT

History and Physical Assessment

Assessment of pain in children consists of both subjective and objective data collection. The acronym QUESTT is an excellent way to remember the key principles of pain assessment (Baker & Wong, 1987):

- Question the child.
- Use a reliable and valid pain scale.
- Evaluate the child's behavior and physiologic changes to establish a baseline and determine the effectiveness of the intervention. The child's behavior and motor activity may include irritability and protection as well as withdrawal of the affected painful area.

- Secure the parent's involvement.
- Take the cause of pain into account when intervening.
- Take action.

History

When assessing pain in children, tailor the assessment to the child's developmental level and ask questions geared to the child's cognitive ability.

QUESTIONING THE CHILD

When questioning the child, phrase the questions in a manner that the child will be able to understand on the basis of his or her developmental level. Some input from the child's family might be helpful in determining where best to focus the questions. When questioning the child, inquire about the following:

- Ask the child what pain means to him or her.
- Attempt to determine what word the child uses to denote pain. Some children may not understand the term "pain" but do understand terms such as "hurt," "ouchie," or "boo-boo."
- Inquire about similar experiences in the past and how he or she responded. Determine whether the child let others know that he or she was hurting and how this message was conveyed (e.g., crying, acting out, or pointing to the hurting area).
- Review the history of the pain and various influences such as cultural aspects, caregiver attitudes or expectations, previous experiences, and any education or teaching related to pain management.
- Determine the child's previous exposure to pain, if any, and how the child responded.
- Question about location, quality, severity, and onset of the pain, as well as the circumstances in which the child experiences the pain. Have the child point to the area where it hurts, or identify the location on a diagram or doll.
- Inquire about conditions, if any, that preceded the onset of pain and the conditions that followed the onset of pain.
- Find out about any associated symptoms, such as weight loss, fever, vomiting, or diarrhea, which may indicate a current illness.
- Ask about any recent trauma, including any interventions that were used in an attempt to relieve the pain.
- Inquire what the child wants others, including the nurse, to do when the child is hurting.
- Question the child about measures that seem to be most effective in relieving the pain. Ask whether there is anything special the child wants to tell the nurse, such as a special pain relief technique or a specific comfort object.

If the child is experiencing chronic or recurrent pain, suggest the child and family record information in a symptom diary. Explain that this will be helpful in identifying the best ways to manage the pain.

QUESTIONING THE PARENTS

The questions posed to the parents are similar in focus to those posed to the child. When questioning the parents, use the following examples as a guide for assessing the child's pain:

- Has your child ever been in pain before? If so, what was the cause of the pain? How long did he or she have the pain? Where was the pain located?
- How did your child react to the pain? What did you do to lessen the pain?
- Did your child let you know that he or she was in pain? Did he or she tell you or did you notice something?
- Are there any special signs that let you know that your child is hurting? If so, what are they?
- Is there anything that your child does or that you do when he or she is hurting that helps relieve the pain?
- Does one thing work better than another when your child is hurting?
- Is there any special information that you want to tell me about your child?

Physical Assessment

Physical examination of the child for pain primarily involves the skills of observation and inspection. Auscultation also may be used to assess for changes in vital signs, specifically heart rate and blood pressure.

Observe for physical signs and symptoms of pain, keeping in mind the child's developmental level, including the following:

- Facial expressions of discomfort, grimacing, or crying.
- Movements that may suggest pain. For example, an infant or toddler may pull on the ear when experiencing ear pain. The child may move the head from side to side, suggesting head pain. Typically, children with abdominal pain will lie on one side and draw their knees up to the abdomen.
- The child's gait: A limp or avoidance of weight bearing may suggest leg pain.
- Immobility, guarding of a particular body area, or refusal to move an area may be observed.
- Inspect the skin for flushing or diaphoresis, possible indicators of pain.
- Monitor vital signs for changes. Pulse or heart rate, respiratory rate, and blood pressure may increase.
- Other physiologic parameters suggesting pain may include elevated intracranial pressure and pulmonary vascular resistance and decreased oxygen saturation levels.

Take Note!

The body responds to acute pain via the sympathetic nervous system, leading to stimulation and subsequently an increase in vital signs. However, if the child has persistent or chronic pain, the body adapts and these changes may be less noticeable (Oakes, 2011).

The child also may exhibit behavioral changes indicating pain including
- irritability and restlessness
- clenching of teeth or fists, body stiffening, or increased muscle tension; and
- changes in the child's behavior—for example, a child who previously was talkative and playful who becomes quiet and almost withdrawn.

Each child is an individual with unique responses to pain, so it is important to ensure that observations of behavior do indeed reflect the child's pain level. To help ensure the accuracy of observations, several pain rating scales, including self-report tools and physiologic and behavioral assessment tools, have been developed to help quantify the observations. The most common are discussed as follows.

Take Note!

Pay close attention to the child's cultural background and how these beliefs may be affecting the behavioral response to pain.

Pain Rating Scales

Various pain assessment or pain rating scales are available. These scales allow the child to report his or her pain, and the pain level is quantified. Many healthcare facilities have specific policies and procedures related to pain assessment, including the frequency of assessment, the rating tool to use, and nursing interventions to be instituted on the basis of the rating.

Take Note!

Typically, different pain rating scales are appropriate for different developmental levels. However, children may regress when in pain, so a simpler tool may be needed to make sure that the child understands what is being asked. Regardless of the tool used, nurses need to be consistent in using the same tool so that appropriate comparisons can be made and effective interventions can be planned and implemented. Using the most appropriate tool consistently allows the most accurate assessment of the child's pain.

Self-Report Tools

Use self-report measures in conjunction with observation and discussion with the child and family, especially in children younger than 5 or children with cognitive impairments (AAP and the American Pain Society, 2001; von Baeyer, 2014). Several self-report tools are available for clinical use. The most common are discussed as follows.

FACES PAIN RATING SCALE

The FACES pain rating scale is a self-report tool that can be used by children as young as 3 or 4 years of age (Oakes, 2011). See Figure 1.2. Follow these guidelines when using the FACES pain rating scale:
- Ask the child to point to the facial expression that best describes how he or she is feeling.
- Document the number corresponding to the word description and face.

NUMERIC SCALES

The numeric scale can be used with children 8 years or older (von Baeyer, 2014). See Figure 1.3. Follow these guidelines when using the numeric scale:
- Explain the scale to the child.

Wong-Baker FACES Pain Rating Scale

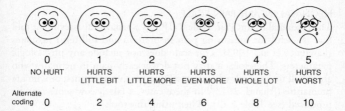

0	1	2	3	4	5
NO HURT	HURTS LITTLE BIT	HURTS LITTLE MORE	HURTS EVEN MORE	HURTS WHOLE LOT	HURTS WORST

Alternate coding

0	2	4	6	8	10

Instructions: Explain to the person that each face is for a person who feels happy because he has no pain (hurt) or sad because he has some or a lot of pain. **Face 0** is very happy because he doesn't hurt at all. **Face 1** hurts just a little bit. **Face 2** hurts a little more. **Face 3** hurts even more. **Face 4** hurts a whole lot. **Face 5** hurts as much as you can imagine, although you don't have to be crying to feel this bad. Ask the person to choose the face that best describes how he is feeling.

FIGURE 1.2 FACES pain rating scale. (From Hockenberry, M. J., & Wilson, D. (2009). *Wong's essentials of pediatric nursing* (8th ed., p. 162). St. Louis, MO: Elsevier Mosby. Used with permission. Copyright, Mosby.)

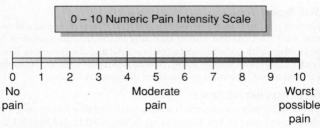

FIGURE 1.3 Numeric pain scale.

- Ask the child to pick the number that best describes his or her level of pain.
- Document this number as the pain score.

Physiologic and Behavioral Pain Assessment Tools

Using physiologic and behavioral pain assessment tools allows measurement of specific parameters and changes that would indicate that the child is experiencing pain. The most common of these tools are discussed as follows.

NEONATAL INFANT PAIN SCALE

The Neonatal Infant Pain Scale (NIPS) is a behavioral assessment tool that is useful for measuring pain in preterm and full-term neonates (Lawrence et al., 1993). This scale does not include any physiologic parameters. Therefore, it may not detect early pain in neonates who are too ill to respond, who are receiving paralyzing agents, or who are premature (Anand, 2013). In these cases, a falsely low score may be produced (see Table 1.12). When using this tool:
- observe the infant and score each parameter.
- total the scores; the maximum score that can be achieved is 7. A higher score indicates increased pain.

r-FLACC BEHAVIORAL SCALE FOR PAIN IN NONVERBAL YOUNG CHILDREN AND CHILDREN WITH COGNITIVE IMPAIRMENT

The revised FLACC (r-FLACC) is used in the same manner as the original FLACC but it includes additional descriptors of behaviors most commonly associated with pain that have been validated in children with cognitive impairment (Hauer & Jones, 2015). It has been demonstrated to be a reliable tool for children from 2 months to 7 years of age (Oakes, 2011) see Table 1.13. When using this tool:

TABLE 1.12 — THE NEONATAL INFANT PAIN SCALE

Parameter	Finding	Score
Facial expression	Relaxed (restful face; neutral expression)	0
	Grimace (tight facial muscles; furrowed brow, chin, or jaw; negative facial expression)	1
Cry	No cry (quiet; not crying)	0
	Whimper (mild intermittent moaning)	1
	Vigorous crying (loud screaming, shrill, continuous)	2
Breathing patterns	Relaxed	0
	Change in breathing (irregular; faster than usual; gagging; breath holding)	1
Arms	Relaxed (no muscular rigidity; occasional random movements of arm)	0
	Flexed/extended (tense, straight, rigid, or rapid flexion or extension)	1
Legs	Relaxed (no muscular rigidity; occasional random movements of leg)	0
	Flexed/extended (tense, straight, rigid, or rapid flexion or extension)	1
State of arousal	Sleeping/awake (quiet, peaceful; settled)	0
	Fussy (alert, restless, thrashing)	1

Used with permission from Lawrence, J., Alcock, D., McGrath, P., Kay, J., MacMurray, S. B., & Dulberg, C. (1993). The development of a tool to assess neonatal pain. *Neonatal Network, 12*(6), 59–66.

- observe the child with the legs and body uncovered. If the child is awake, observe him or her for 1 to 2 minutes; if sleeping, observe the child for 2 minutes or longer.
- total the scores; the maximum score that can be achieved is 10. The higher the total score, the more intense the pain.

Nonpharmacologic Pain Management

Various techniques may be available to assist in managing mild pain in children or to augment the effectiveness of medications for moderate or severe pain. Two types of techniques are behavior/cognitive strategies and biophysical strategies. When using these techniques with children, it is important for the parents to be involved in the process.

TABLE 1.13 r-FLACC BEHAVIORAL SCALE

Category	Scoring		
	0	1	2
Face	No particular expression or smile	Occasional grimace or frown, withdrawn, disinterested; **appears sad or worried**[a]	Frequent to constant frown, clenched jaw, quivering chin; **distress-looking face: expression of fright or panic**[a]
Legs	Normal position or relaxed	Uneasy, restless, tense; **occasional tremors**[a]	Kicking, or legs drawn up; **marked increase in spasticity, constant tremors or jerking**[a]
Activity	Lying quietly, normal position, moves easily	Squirming, shifting back and forth, tense; **mildly agitated (e.g., head back and forth, aggression); shallow, splinting respirations intermittent sighs**[a]	Arched, rigid, or jerking; **severe agitation, head banging, shivering (not rigors); breath-holding, gasping or sharp intake of breath; severe splinting**[a]
Cry	No cry (awake or asleep)	Moans or whimpers, occasional complaint; **occasional verbal outburst or grunt**[a]	Crying steadily, screams or sobs, frequent complaints; **repeated outbursts, constant grunting**[a]
Consolability	Content, relaxed	Reassured by occasional touching, hugging, or being talked to, distractible	Difficult to console or comfort; **pushing away caregiver, resisting care or comfort measures**[a]

Each of the five categories is scored from 0 to 2, which results in a total score between 0 and 10. © 2002, The Regents of the University of Michigan. All rights reserved.

[a]Revised descriptors shown in bold.

The nurse plays a major role in teaching the child and family about nonpharmacologic pain interventions. It is important to help the child and family choose the most appropriate and most effective methods and to ensure that the child and parents use the method before pain occurs as well as before the pain increases (see Teaching Guidelines 1.1).

Teaching Guidelines 1.1
TEACHING TO MANAGE PAIN WITHOUT DRUGS

- Review the methods available and choose the method(s) that your child and you find best for your situation.
- Learn to identify the ways in which your child shows pain or demonstrates he or she is anxious about the possibility of pain. For example, does he or she get restless, make a face, or get flushed in the face?
- Begin using the technique chosen before your child experiences pain or when your child first indicates he or she is anxious about, or beginning to experience, pain.
- Practice the technique with your child and encourage the child to use the technique when he or she feels anxious about pain or anticipates that a procedure or experience will be painful.
- Perform the technique with your child. For example, take the deep breath in and out or blow bubbles with him or her; listen to the music; or play the computer game with your child.
- Avoid using terms such as "hurt" or "pain" that suggest or cause your child to expect pain.
- Use descriptive terms such as pushing, pulling, pinching, or heat.
- Avoid overly descriptive or judgmental statements, such as "this will really hurt a lot" or "this will be terrible."
- Stay with your child as much as possible; speak softly and gently stroke or cuddle your child.
- Offer praise, positive reinforcement, hugs, and support for using the technique even when it was not effective.

Behavioral-Cognitive Strategies

Behavioral-cognitive strategies for pain management involve measures that require the child to focus on a specific area rather than the pain. These strategies help to change the interpretation of the painful stimuli, reducing pain perception or making pain more tolerable. Typically, these interventions work well with older children, but younger children also benefit from these techniques if they are adapted to the child's age and developmental level. Common behavioral-cognitive strategies include the following:

- Relaxation
- Distraction: Various methods can be used for distraction, including
  - counting
  - repetition of specific phrases or words, such as "ouch"
  - listening to music or singing
  - playing games, including computer and video games
  - blowing bubbles or blowing pinwheels or party favors
  - listening to favorite stories
  - watching cartoons, television shows, or movies
  - visiting with friends
  - humor
- Imagery
- Biofeedback
- Thought stopping
- Positive self-talk.

Biophysical Interventions

Biophysical interventions focus on interfering with the transmission of pain impulses reaching the brain. Examples of biophysical interventions include:

- application of heat and cold
- massage and pressure
- nonnutritive sucking in newborns (including the use of sucrose solution)
- transcutaneous electrical nerve stimulation (TENS).

Pharmacologic Pain Management

Pharmacologic interventions involve the administration of drugs for pain relief. The selection of the method is determined by the drug being administered, the child's status, the type, intensity, and location of the pain, and any factors that may be influencing the child's pain.

Analgesics (medications for pain relief) typically fall into one of two categories: nonopioid analgesics and opioid analgesics. Anesthetics may also be used. Drugs such as sedatives and hypnotics may be used as adjuvant medications to help minimize anxiety or provide or assist with pain relief when typical analgesics are ineffective.

Nonopioid Analgesics

Nonopioid analgesics are used to treat mild to moderate pain and are often combined with opioids for more effective pain relief. Nonopioid analgesics include:

- acetaminophen
- NSAIDs such as ibuprofen, ketorolac, naproxen, indomethacin, diclofenac, and piroxicam.

Take Note!

Aspirin should not be used in infants or children for analgesic and antipyretic purposes because of the high risk of Reye syndrome.

Opioid Analgesics

Opioid analgesics are typically used for moderate to severe pain. Opioid agents include:

- morphine
- fentanyl
- meperidine
- hydromorphone
- oxycodone
- hydrocodone
- pentazocine
- butorphanol
- nalbuphine.

Take Note!

When administering parenteral or epidural opioids, always have naloxone readily available to reverse the opioid's effects should respiratory depression occur.

Adjuvant Drugs

Adjuvant drugs are drugs that are used to promote more effective pain relief, either alone or in combination with nonopioids or opioids. Their primary indication is for diagnoses other than pain. These agents are not classified as analgesics but may provide a coanalgesic effect or may treat side effects. Benzodiazepines, such as diazepam and midazolam, help to relieve anxiety. Midazolam also produces amnesia. Anticonvulsants, such as gabapentin, and tricyclic antidepressants, such as amitriptyline and nortriptyline, are used to treat neuropathic pain.

Drug Administration Methods

There are various methods for administering pain medications to children. The preferred methods are the oral, rectal, intravenous (IV), topical, or local nerve block routes. Epidural administration and moderate sedation can also be used.

In patient-controlled analgesia (PCA), a computerized pump is programmed to deliver an infusion of analgesics via a catheter inserted intravenously, epidurally, or subcutaneously. The analgesic may be given as a continuous infusion, as a continuous infusion supplemented by patient-delivered bolus doses, or as patient-delivered bolus doses only. Typically, the child presses a button to administer a bolus dose. In some cases, agent-activated PCA is used.

Serious adverse events, such as oversedation, respiratory depression, and even death can occur when family members, caregivers, or clinicians who are not authorized administer PCA doses "by proxy" (The Joint Commission, 2004; Cooney et al., 2013). The Institute for Safe Medication Practices (ISMP) recommends developing specific criteria in any situation where authorized agent-activated PCA is being used (D'Arcy, 2011; Cooney et al., 2013). Proper education and instruction is crucial in any situation where someone other than the child may be administering PCA doses. Thorough assessment is necessary to ensure the child's pain is neither undertreated nor overtreated.

PCA has been used to control postoperative pain and the pain associated with trauma, cancer, and sickle cell crisis. It can be used in acute care settings or in the home. Most commonly, morphine, hydromorphone, and fentanyl are the drugs used with PCA. The dosage is based on the child's response.

Local Anesthetic Application

A local anesthetic may sometimes be used to alleviate the pain associated with procedures such as venipuncture, injections, wound repair, lumbar puncture, or accessing of implanted ports. Local anesthesia is a type of regional analgesia that blocks or numbs specific nerves in a region of the body.

Local anesthetics include topical forms, such as creams, agents delivered by iontophoresis, vapocoolants, and skin refrigerants, and injectable forms.

TOPICAL FORMS
- EMLA (eutectic mixture of local anesthetics [lidocaine and prilocaine])
- TAC (tetracaine, epinephrine, cocaine) and LET (lidocaine, epinephrine, tetracaine)
- liposomal lidocaine ELA-max or LMX4 (lidocaine 4%)
- Needle-free powder lidocaine
- Iontophoretic lidocaine (Numby Stuff)
- Vapocoolant spray.

INJECTABLE FORMS
Injectable forms of lidocaine or procaine can be administered subcutaneously or intradermally around the procedural area approximately 5 to 10 minutes before the procedure. Common problems with this form of anesthetic include the pain associated with the subcutaneous (SC) injection and some burning associated with lidocaine administration, as well as blanching of the skin.

Epidural Analgesia

Epidural analgesia is typically used postoperatively, providing analgesia to the lower body for approximately 12 to 14 hours. The small amount of medication used with this type of analgesia causes less sedation, thereby allowing the child to participate more actively in postoperative care activities.

Frequent assessment, ranging from every 1 to 2 to 2 to 4 hours, is imperative and includes:
- heart rate
- respiratory rate
- depth of sedation
- blood pressure
- pain level
- motor function
- adverse reactions (e.g., nausea, vomiting, and pruritus)
- catheter site (including ensuring the occlusive dressing is intact)
- dermatome level (Fig. 1.4) (Oakes, 2011).

Moderate (Conscious) Sedation

Moderate sedation used to be labeled conscious sedation, but the term conscious has been replaced because it can be misleading (Coté, Wilson, & the Work Group on Sedation, 2011). It is a medically controlled state of depressed consciousness that allows protective reflexes to be maintained so that the child has the ability to maintain a patent airway and respond to physical or verbal stimulation.

Moderate sedation is used for procedures that are painful and stressful. For example, moderate sedation is suggested instead of restraints, especially for toddlers and preschool children who are undergoing frightening or invasive procedures and who are manifesting extreme anxiety and behavioral upset. Other indications include situations involving
- evidence that the child is experiencing a heightened stress reaction—attempting to flee, crying inconsolably, or flailing;
- verbalization by the child that he or she is frightened and does not want to be touched;
- inability to remain immobilized, such as during laceration repair or computed tomography (CT); and
- any procedure that is painful and fear-provoking.

The route of administering the medications for sedation should follow the guidelines of atraumatic care. Oral, topical, or an existing IV route should be used. Personnel administering moderate sedation must be specially trained, with strong resuscitation and advanced pediatric life support skills, and emergency equipment and medications must be readily available (Coté, et al., 2011).

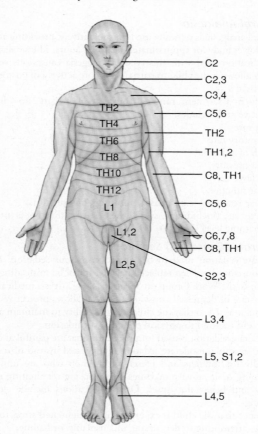

FIGURE 1.4 Diagram of dermatomes. The level of anesthesia should not go higher than T4, the nipple line, in children.

Nurse's Role in Pharmacologic Pain Management

The nurse plays a major role in providing pharmacologic pain relief. As with any medication, the nurse is responsible for adhering to the rights of medication administration. It is also important to have a solid knowledge base about the medications used for pain relief.

Assessment is crucial when pharmacologic pain interventions are used. An initial assessment of pain provides a baseline from which

TABLE 1.14	INTERVENTIONS FOR COMMON OPIOID-INDUCED ADVERSE EFFECTS
Adverse Effect	**Nursing Interventions**
Constipation	Encourage fluid intake unless contraindicated. Ensure intake of high-fiber foods, including fruits, if allowed. Encourage activity, including ambulation if possible. Obtain order for stool softener. Administer laxative as ordered.
Pruritus	Apply cool compresses and lotions. Administer antihistamine as ordered.
Nausea and vomiting	Inform child and parents that these symptoms usually subside in 1–2 days. Encourage small frequent meals with bland foods. Administer antiemetic if ordered.

options for relief can be chosen. Factors that can affect the choice of analgesic, such as the child's age, pain intensity, physiologic status, or previous experiences with pain, also need to be considered. It is important to act as an advocate for the child and the family to ensure that the most appropriate pharmacologic agent is chosen for the situation.

Assessment is ongoing once the agent is administered. Monitor physiologic parameters such as level of consciousness, vital signs, oxygen saturation levels, and urinary output for changes that might indicate an adverse reaction to the agent. More intensive monitoring is needed when agents are administered intravenously or epidurally or by moderate sedation.

Monitor the child closely for evidence of adverse effects (Table 1.14).

Pain Management for Procedures
Use behavioral and pharmacologic approaches to significantly reduce the pain and distress of procedures. Implement the guiding principles of atraumatic care, which include the following:
• Prepare the child and parents ahead of time about the procedure.
• Use topical EMLA, iontophoretic lidocaine, vapocoolant spray, or buffered lidocaine at the intended site of a skin or vessel puncture.

- Keep all equipment out of site until it is ready to be used.
- Use therapeutic hugging to secure the child (see Fig. 1.11).
- Use the smallest gauge needle possible or an automated lancet device to puncture the skin.
- Use an intermittent infusion device or peripherally inserted central catheter (PICC) if multiple or repeated blood samples are necessary. Coordinate care so that several tests can be performed from one sample if possible.
- Opt for venipuncture in newborns instead of heel sticks if the amount of blood needed would require much squeezing.
- Use kangaroo care (skin-to-skin contact) for newborns before and after heel stick.
- Provide nonnutritive sucking, with sucrose solution, if appropriate, pacifier, or breastfeeding for newborns several minutes before the procedure.

PEDIATRIC MEDICATION ADMINISTRATION

Medication administration in children requires particular attention to safety due to the physiologic, psychological, and cognitive differences inherent in children. Adapt medication administration principles and techniques to meet the child's needs. Always adhere to the "rights" of medication administration. These rights were developed to ensure patient safety by decreasing the occurrence of medication errors. Some experts have added additional rights, such as right documentation, right to be educated, right to refuse, right form, and right approach. These additional rights are important to consider to increase patient safety and satisfaction.

Rights of Medication Administration

Right Medication
- Check order and expiration dates.
- Know action of medication and potential side effects (use pharmacy, drug formulary).
- Ensure that the medication provided is the medication that is ordered.

Right Patient
- Confirm patient identity two ways. Children may deny their identity in attempt to avoid an unpleasant situation, may play in another child's bed, or may remove the ID bracelet.
- Confirm identity each time medication is given.

- Verify child's name with caregiver to provide additional verification.
- Use technology when available (i.e., bar code systems).

Right Time
- Give within 20 to 30 minutes of the ordered time.
- For a medication given on an as-needed basis, know when it was last given and how much was given during the past 24 hours.

Right Route of Administration
- Check ordered route and ensure this is the most effective and safe route for this child; clarify any order that is confusing or unclear.
- Give the medication by the route ordered. If there is a need to change route, always check with the prescriber (e.g., if a child is vomiting and has an order for an oral medication, the medication may need to be given via the IV or rectal route).

Right Dose
- Calculate the recommended dose according to child's weight and double check your calculations.
- Always question the pharmacist and/or the prescriber if the ordered dose falls outside the recommended dose range.

Take Note!

If a parent, caregiver, or patient questions whether a medication should be given, listen attentively, answer their questions, and double check the order.

Developmental Issues and Concerns
Always give developmentally appropriate, truthful explanations before administering medications to children. Include why the drug is needed, what the child will experience, what is expected of the child, and how the parents can participate and support their child. Use a positive, firm approach with the child. Assess the child's previous experience with medication administration.

Atraumatic Care
Enlist the help of a child life specialist when possible.

Refer to the following examples for nursing interventions based on developmental stage.

Infant
- Involve parents in medication administration to reduce stress for infant.
- Ensure that parents hold and comfort infant during intervention.

Toddler
- Follow routines and rituals from home in giving medications if these are safe and positive approaches.
- Involve parents in medication administration.
- Offer simple choices (e.g., "Do you want Mom or me to give you your medicine?").
- Allow child to touch or handle equipment as appropriate.

Atraumatic Care

Use positions that are comforting to the child, such as therapeutic hugging during injections (see Fig. 1.11). Have the child sit on the caregiver's lap with the caregiver holding the child's arms and legs to his or her body. After administration, encourage the parents or caregivers to hold and cuddle the child and offer praise.

Preschool
- Provide an opportunity to play with the equipment and allow a positive response to explanations and comforting.
- Provide choices that are possible and keep them simple (e.g., "Do you want juice or water with your medication?" or "Which medication do you want to take first?").
- Do not ask, "Will you take your medicine now?"
- Involve parents in medication administration.
- Be aware that giving suppositories is particularly upsetting to children in this age group because of their fears of bodily intrusion and mutilation.

School Age
- Explain, in simple terms, the purpose of the medication.
- Seek the child's assistance, such as putting pills in cup or opening the packet, and allow a broader range of choices.
- Establish a reward system to enhance cooperation, if necessary.

Adolescent
- Approach in the same manner as adults, with respect and sensitivity to their needs.
- Maintain the adolescent's privacy as much as possible.

A traumatic Care

Encourage the child to participate in care and provide the child with developmentally appropriate options, such as which fluid to drink with the medication or which flavor of ice pop to suck on before or after the administration.

Dosage Calculation

Dose Determination by Body Weight

Determine appropriate dosing based on the child's weight. The recommended dosage is usually expressed as the amount of drug to be given over a 24-hour period (mg/kg/day) or as a single dose (mg/kg/dose). Differentiate between the 24-hour dosage and the single dose.

1. Check the child's weight.
2. If the child's weight is in pounds, convert it to kilograms (divide the child's weight in pounds by 2.2).
3. Check a drug reference for the safe dose range (e.g., 10 to 20 mg/kg of body weight).
4. Calculate the low safe dose.
5. Calculate the high safe dose.
6. Determine if the dose ordered is within this range.

Take Note!

Pay close attention to ensure if the safe range dose is for 24 hours (mg/day) or a single dose period (mg/dose)

The following is an example:
- Calculate the low safe dose range (e.g., 50 to 100 mg/kg and the child weighs 25 kg):
  - Set up a proportion using the low safe dose range
    $50 \text{ mg}/1 \text{ kg} = x \text{ mg}/25 \text{ kg}$
- Solve for x by cross-multiplying:
    $1 \times x = 50 \times 25$
    $x = 1,250 \text{ mg}$
- Calculate the high safe dose range:
  - Set up a proportion using the high safe dose range
    $100 \text{ mg}/1 \text{ kg} = x \text{ mg}/25 \text{ kg}$
  - Solve for x by cross-multiplying:
    $1 \times x = 100 \times 25$
    $x = 2,500$
- Compare the safe dose range (for this example, 1,250 to 2,500 mg) with the ordered dose. If the dose falls within the range, the dose is safe.

> *Take Note!*
>
> The pediatric dosage should not exceed the minimum recommended adult dosage. Generally, once a child or adolescent weighs ≥40 to 50 kg, the adult dose is often prescribed (Bowden & Greenberg, 2012).

Dose Determination by Body Surface Area

Calculating the dosage based on body surface area (BSA) takes into account the child's metabolic rate and growth. It is commonly used for chemotherapeutic agents. Some recommended medication doses may read "mg/BSA/dose." To determine the dose using BSA, you will need to know the child's height and weight, which will be plotted on a nomogram (Fig. 1.5). Use the following guidelines to determine BSA:

- Check the child's weight and height.
- Using the nomogram, draw a line to connect the height measurement in the left column and the weight measurement in the right column.
- Determine the point where this line intersects the line in the surface area column. This is the BSA, expressed in meters squared (m^2).

Once the BSA is determined, use the recommended dosage range to calculate the safe dosage.

Routes of Administration

> *Take Note!*
>
> Prior to administration of any medication wash hands and don gloves if necessary. Adhere to the rights of medication administration.

Oral Administration

Oral medications are supplied in many forms, such as liquids (elixirs, syrups, or suspensions), powders, tablets, and capsules. Generally, children younger than 5 to 6 years are at risk for aspiration because they have difficulty swallowing tablets or capsules. Therefore, if a tablet or capsule is the only oral form available, it needs to be crushed or opened and mixed with a pleasant tasting liquid or a small amount (generally no more than a tablespoon) of a nonessential food such as applesauce. The crushed tablet or inside of a capsule may taste bitter, so never mix it with formula or other essential foods. Otherwise, the child may associate the bitter taste with the food and later refuse to eat it.

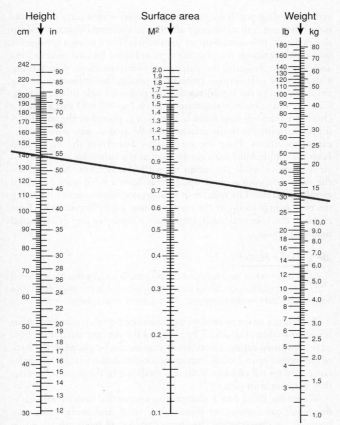

FIGURE 1.5 Nomogram to determine body surface area.

Take Note!

Before crushing a pill or opening a capsule, always check that this will not alter the intended effects of the drug. Certain drug formulations should not be crushed. Never crush or open an enteric coated or time-release tablet or capsule.

Always shake liquid medications to ensure even drug distribution. The key to administering liquid forms of oral medications is to use calibrated equipment such as a medicine cup, spoon, plastic oral syringe, or dropper. If a dropper is packaged with a certain medication, never use it to administer another medication because the drop size may vary from one dropper to another. When using a syringe for oral administration, use only the type intended for oral medications and not one designed for parenteral administration. When using a dropper or oral syringe (without a needle) for infants or young children, direct the liquid toward the posterior side of the mouth. Give the drug slowly in small amounts (0.2 to 0.5 mL) and allow the child to swallow before more medication is placed in the mouth. A nipple without the bottle attached can be used to administer medication to infants. Place the medication directly in the nipple and keep the nipple filled with medication as the infant sucks so that no air is taken in while the infant takes the medication. Always place the infant or young child upright (at least a 45-degree angle) to avoid aspiration. The toddler or young preschooler may enjoy using the oral syringe to squirt the medicine into his or her mouth. Older children can take oral medication from a medicine cup or measured medicine spoon.

Take Note!

Never force an oral medication into a child's mouth or pinch the child's nose. Doing so increases the risk for aspiration and interferes with the development of a trusting relationship.

As children adapt to swallowing tablets or capsules, administration is similar to that of adults. When helping the younger child learn how to swallow medication, the tablet or capsule can be placed at the back of the tongue or in a small amount of food such as ice cream or applesauce. Always tell children if there is medicine in the food; otherwise, they may not trust you.

When the child has a nasogastric, orogastric, nasojejunal, nasoduodenal, gastrostomy, or jejunostomy tube, oral medications may be given via these devices. Be aware that not all medications can be placed directly into the duodenum or jejunum. Medication must be supplied in a liquid form, or a crushed tablet or opened capsule can be mixed with a liquid. Mix powdered medications or crushed tablets with warm water to dissolve contents and prevent tube occlusion.

Always check tube placement before administering the medication. After administration, flush the tube to maintain patency.

Take Note!

Parental involvement in medication administration, when possible, helps decrease stress on the child and provides an opportunity for teaching and evaluating parental techniques.

Rectal Administration

The rectal route is not a preferred route for medication administration in children. However, the rectal route may be used when the child is vomiting or receiving nothing by mouth (NPO). Use age-appropriate explanations and reassurance. Helping the child to maintain the correct position may be necessary to ensure proper insertion and safety.

Lubricate the suppository well with a water-soluble lubricant. With the child in the side-lying position, insert the suppository into the rectum quickly but gently. Use a gloved finger or a finger cot to insert the suppository. Insert the suppository above the anal sphincter. For an infant or child younger than 3 years, use the fifth finger for insertion. For an older child, use the index finger. To prevent expulsion of the suppository, hold the buttocks together for several minutes or until the child loses the urge to defecate. If the child has a bowel movement within 10 to 30 minutes after administration of the medication, examine the stool for the presence of the suppository. If it is observed, notify the physician or nurse practitioner to determine whether the drug needs to be administered again.

Ophthalmic Administration

Ophthalmic medications are typically supplied in the form of drops or ointment. Ensure that the medication is at room temperature. Proper positioning of the child is necessary to control the child's head; keep the child's hands from interfering and prevent injury to the eye. Attempt to administer the medication when the child is not crying to ensure that the medication reaches its intended target area.

Place the child in the supine position, slightly hyperextending the neck with the head lower than the body so that the medication will be dispersed over the cornea. Rest the heel of your hand on the child's forehead to stabilize it. Retract the lower eyelid and place the medication in the conjunctival sac; maintain sterile technique by being careful not to touch the tip of the tube or dropper to the sac (Fig. 1.6). For eye drops, place the prescribed number of drops into the lower conjunctival sac. For ointment, apply the medication in a thin ribbon from the inner canthus outward without touching the eye or eyelashes. If the child is old enough to cooperate, instruct the child to gently close the eyes to allow the medication to be dispersed.

If a child is uncooperative, he or she may need to be immobilized in order to administer the eye drops. Alternatively, one or two drops on the inner canthus of the closed eye can be administered while the child is lying supine. When the child opens his or her eye, the drop enters the eye. Always ensure that excess medication is wiped from the skin to prevent systemic absorption. Punctal occlusion after application is

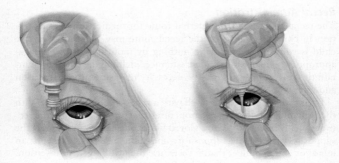

FIGURE 1.6 Administering eye medication: Gently press the lower lid down and have the child look up as the medication is instilled into the lower conjunctival sac.

also important to slow systemic absorption and ensure the medicine stays in the eye.

Otic Administration

Medications for otic administration are typically in the form of eardrops. Reinforce the need for the child to keep the head still. Younger children may require assistance to do so. Be sure that the eardrops are at room temperature. If necessary, roll the container between the palms of your hands to help warm the drops.

Take Note!

Using cold eardrops can cause pain and possibly vertigo or vomiting when they reach the eardrum (Bowden & Greenberg, 2012).

Place the child in a supine or side-lying position with the affected ear exposed. Pull the pinna downward and back in children younger than 3 years and upward and back in older children (Fig. 1.7). Instill the prescribed amount of medication using a dropper being careful not to contaminate the tip of the dropper. Then have the child remain in the same position for several minutes to ensure that the medication stays in the ear canal. Soothe, comfort, and distract the child to allow medication to instill. Massage the area anterior to the affected ear to promote passage of the medication into the ear canal. If necessary, place a piece of cotton or a cotton ball loosely in the ear canal to prevent the medication from leaking.

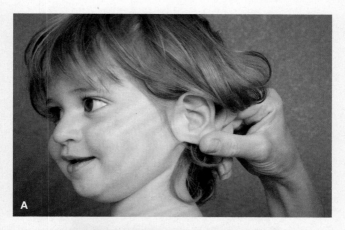

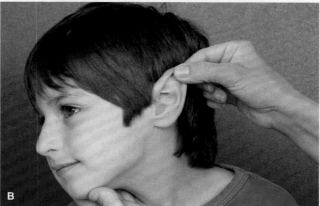

FIGURE 1.7 Administering eardrops. **A:** For the child younger than 3 years, the nurse pulls the pinna of the ear down and back. **B:** For a child older than 3 years, the nurse pulls the pinna of the affected ear up and back.

Nasal Administration

Nasally administered medications are typically drops and sprays. Administering nose drops to infants and young children may be difficult, and additional help may be needed to help maintain the child's position. Ensure medication is at room temperature. Have the child blow his nose

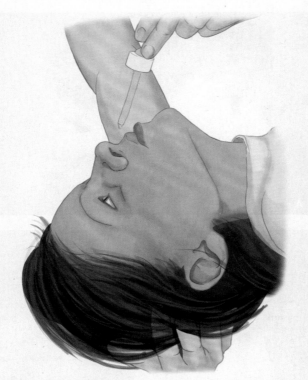

FIGURE 1.8 Administering nose drops. Tilt the head down and back to instill nose drops.

or use a bulb syringe to clear nasal passage of secretions. For nose drops, position the child supine with the head hyperextended to ensure that the drops will flow back into the nares (Fig. 1.8). A pillow or folded towel can be used to facilitate this hyperextension. Place the tip of the dropper just at or inside the nasal opening, taking care not to touch the nares with the dropper. Doing so might stimulate the child to sneeze and therefore contaminating the drop solution. Once the drops are instilled, maintain the child's head in hyperextension for at least 1 minute to ensure that the drops have come in contact with the nasal membranes.

For nasal sprays, position the child upright with the head tilted slightly back and place the tip of the spray bottle just inside the nasal opening and tilted toward the back. Hold one nostril closed (or have the child do this, as appropriate) and instruct the child to take a deep breath through the nostril while the medication is being administered. Squeeze the container, providing just enough force for the spray to be expelled from the container. Using too great a force can push the spray solution and secretions into the sinuses or eustachian tube.

Atraumatic Care

In young infants, instill the medication in one naris at a time because they are obligate nose breathers.

Intramuscular Administration

Intramuscular (IM) administration delivers medication to the muscle. Muscle development and the amount of fluid to be injected determine IM injection sites in children (Fig. 1.9). Determine needle size (gauge and length) by the size of the muscle and the viscosity of the medication. For example, more viscous medications often require a larger gauge needle. In addition, the needle must be long enough to ensure that the medication reaches the muscle.

The preferred injection site for infants less than 7 months is the vastus lateralis muscle (Immunization Action Coalition [IAC], 2012; Bowden & Greenberg, 2012). In infants and children older than 7 months, the ventrogluteal site should be considered (Bowden & Greenberg, 2012). The deltoid muscle is used as an IM injection site in children older than 3 years and may be used in toddlers if the muscle mass is sufficient (IAC, 2012). The dorsogluteal site, often used in adults, is not recommended in children younger than 5 years (Bowden & Greenberg, 2012).

Take Note!

Many experts no longer recommend use of the dorsogluteal site at any age due to the risk of damaging the sciatic nerve (Aschenbrenner & Venable, 2012).

Select the needle size and gauge based on the size of the child's muscle. The goal is to use the smallest length and gauge that will deposit the medication in the muscle (see Table 1.15). Insert the needle into the skin at a 90-degree angle. If the child is a very small infant or has a small muscle mass, use a 45-degree angle. Aspirating and, if no blood was present, injecting the medication was the traditional procedure. Recent research has led to the CDC and the ACIP no longer recommend aspiration before injection of vaccines, heparin and insulin (CDC, 2012b; Kroger, Sumaya, Pickering, & Atkinson, 2011).

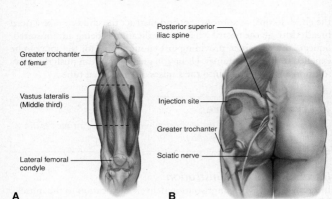

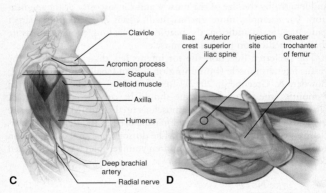

FIGURE 1.9 Locating IM injections sites. **A:** Vastus lateralis: Identify the greater trochanter and the lateral femoral condyle; inject in the middle third and anterior lateral aspects. **B:** Dorsogluteal: Place hand on iliac crest and locate the posterosuperior iliac spine; inject in the outer quadrant formed when an imaginary line is drawn between the trochanter and the iliac spine. **C:** Deltoid: Locate the lateral side of the humerus, one to two finger widths below the acromion process. Inject into upper third of muscle. **D.** Ventrogluteal: Place palm of the left hand on right greater trochanter so that the index finger points toward anterosuperior iliac spine, spread the middle finger to form a V, and inject in the middle of the V.

Subcutaneous and Intradermal Administration

Subcutaneous (SC/SQ) administration distributes medication into the fatty layers of the body. The preferred sites for SC/SQ administration include the anterior thigh, lateral upper arms, and abdomen (Bowden & Greenberg, 2012; IAC, 2012). Use a 3/8- or 5/8-inches, 23- to 25-gauge needle. With the nondominant hand, pinch up the skin to isolate the tissue from the muscle or pull it taut, depending on the amount of adipose tissue present and the length of needle. Insert the needle at a 45- to 90-degree angle, release the skin if pinched, and inject the medication. Remove the needle at the same angle it was inserted.

Intradermal (ID) administration deposits medication just under the epidermis. The forearm is the usual site for administration. ID administration is used primarily for tuberculosis screening and allergy testing. A 1-mL syringe with a 5/8-inches, 25- or 27-gauge needle is commonly used to administer the medication. Insert the needle, with the bevel up, beneath the skin at a 5- to 15-degree angle. Keep fingers and thumb resting on the sides of the syringe to ensure the proper angle.

Intravenous Administration

Use of the IV route requires that the child have an IV device inserted either peripherally or centrally. Most medications given by the IV route must be given at a specified rate and diluted properly to prevent overdose or toxicity due to the rapid onset of action that occurs with this route. It is important to have a thorough knowledge of the drug to be used before administering any IV medication, including the amount of drug to be administered, the minimum dilution of the drug, the type of solution for dilution or infusion, the compatibility or various solutions and medications, the length of time for infusion, and the rate of infusion. Maintain the IV site carefully to prevent complications.

The primary method for IV medication administration is a syringe pump. Refer to Section III, Common Laboratory and Diagnostic Tests and Nursing Procedures (pg 327). If a pump is unavailable, the medication may be administered via a volume control device. The medication is added to the device with a specified amount of compatible fluid and then infused at the ordered rate.

Take Note!

Some facilities have reduced or eliminated the use of volume control devices, especially for medication administration. Be familiar with your facilities policies and procedures and when using a volume control device ensure to label the chamber when medications are added and to check for incompatibilities and potential interaction when multiple medications are given (ISMP, 2009).

TABLE 1.15 GUIDELINES FOR SOLUTION AMOUNT, NEEDLE LENGTH, AND NEEDLE GAUGE FOR INTRAMUSCULAR INJECTIONS[a]

	Solution Amount				Needle Length	Needle Gauge
	Vastus Lateralis	Dorsogluteal	Ventrogluteal	Deltoid		
Infant	0.5–1 mL	Not recommended	Not recommended	Not recommended	5/8 inches	25–27
Toddler	1 mL	Not recommended	1 mL	0.5 mL	5/8–1 inches	22–23
Preschooler	1.5 mL	1.5 mL	1.5 mL	0.5 mL	5/8–1 inches	22–23
School age	1.5–2 mL	1.5–2 mL	1.5–2 mL	0.5 mL	5/8–1.5 inches	22–23
Adolescent	2–2.5 mL	2–2.5 mL	2–2.5 mL	1 mL	5/8–1.5 inches	22–23

[a]Needle size and site needs to be individualized on the basis of the size of the muscle, the amount of adipose tissue, and the amount of solution to be administered.

Adapted from Centers for Disease Control and Prevention. (2012b). Appendix D: Vaccine administration. In W. Atkinson, S. Wolfe, & J. Hamborsky (Eds.), *Epidemiology and prevention of vaccine-preventable diseases* (12th ed., second printing). Washington, DC: Public Health Foundation; Bowden, V. R., & Greenberg, C. S. (2012). *Pediatric nursing procedures* (3rd ed.). Philadelphia, PA: Lippincott Williams & Wilkins.

Direct IV push medication typically is reserved for emergency situations and when therapeutic blood levels must be reached quickly to achieve the desired effect. Direct IV push administration requires that the drug be diluted appropriately and given at a specified rate, such as over 2 to 3 minutes.

Educating the Child and Parents

Teaching the child and parents or caregivers about medication administration is key. Assess the child's and caregiver's understanding of the medication and procedure. The parent and the child need to be aware of what medication is given and why, how it is given, and what to expect from the drug, including adverse effects. When a child is to go home while still taking medications, ensure thorough instruction, including the following:

• Give the proper name of the medication.
• Explain why this medicine is given.
• Clarify the route of administration.
• Describe intended effects and potential adverse effects and when to call the physician or nurse practitioner.
• Provide details about the frequency of the medication.
• Clarify when the next dose is due.
• Describe the length of time medication is to be given. Emphasize the importance of completing the prescribed dose.
• Demonstrate use with the actual syringe that will be used at home, if possible.
• Have parent or caregiver return demonstration of medication administration.
• Advise against use of home measuring devices (e.g., spoon) and emphasize the importance of always using the calibrated dispensing device that was given with the medication.
• Encourage questions or concerns from parents or caregivers.

Preventing Medication Errors

Ways to prevent medication errors include the following:
• Confirm the child's identity.
• Confirm that the child's weight is accurate.
• Always weigh the child in kilograms.
• Double check medication calculations, utilizing another healthcare provider when possible, especially for high-risk medications.
• If a dose seems unusually small or large, verify the order.
• Utilize medication ordering and dispensing systems if available.
• Always report medication errors or near miss errors to help prevent future mistakes.

Take Note!
If a parent, caregiver, or child questions whether a medication should be given, listen attentively, answer his or her questions, and double check the order.

Intravenous Therapy

IV therapy is commonly used to administer medications and fluids to children because it is the quickest, and often the most effective, method of administration. When administering IV therapy, safety is crucial. The nurse must have a solid knowledge base about the fluids or medications to be given as well as a thorough understanding of the child's physical and emotional development.

IV therapy may be administered via a peripheral vein or a central vein. Peripheral IV therapy sites commonly include the hands, feet, and forearms (Fig. 1.10). Use the nondominant extremity for insertion, if possible.

Take Note!
When selecting an IV site in an extremity, always choose the most distal site. Doing so prevents injury to the veins superior to the site and allows additional access sites should complications develop in the most distal site.

Central IV therapy usually is administered through a large vein, such as the subclavian, femoral, or jugular vein or the vena cava. The tip of the device lies in the superior vena cava just at the entrance to the right atrium. The device is inserted surgically or percutaneously and exits the body typically in the chest area, just below the clavicle. A device can be inserted via a peripheral vein, such as the median, cephalic, or basilic vein, and then threaded into the superior vena cava.

Peripheral Access Devices

Devices used for peripheral venous access in a child include over-the-needle catheters or winged infusion sets, commonly referred to as "butterflies" or scalp vein needles. Needle size on the device varies. Typically, the needle ranges from 21- to 25-gauge, depending on the child's size. The rule of thumb is to use the smallest gauge catheter with the shortest length possible to prevent traumatizing the child's fragile veins. Typically, peripheral IV devices are used for short-term therapy, usually averaging 3 to 5 days (O'Grady et al., 2011). Midline catheters are also available, and the CDC recommends the use of midline catheters if therapy is to exceed 6 days (O'Grady et al., 2011). Midline catheters can stay in for up to 2 months (Bowden & Greenberg, 2012).

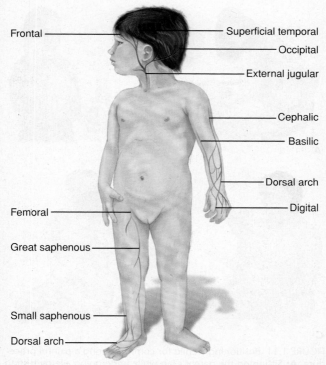

FIGURE 1.10 Preferred peripheral sites for IV insertion. In infants up to about 9 months of age, the scalp veins may be used.

The procedure for inserting peripheral IV access devices in children is very similar to inserting peripheral IV access devices in adults. Special considerations in children include the following:
• Insertion of an IV therapy device is traumatic. Follow the principles of atraumatic care. (See Fig. 1.11.)

Atraumatic Care

Use therapeutic play to assist the child in preparation and coping for the procedure. Enlist help from a child life specialist when possible.

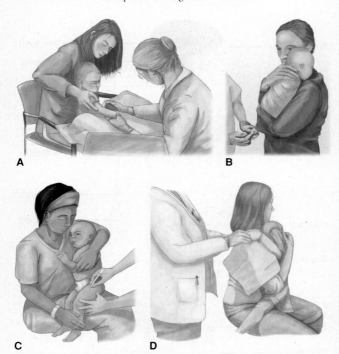

FIGURE 1.11 Positioning a child for comfort during a painful procedure. **A:** Sitting on the parent's lap while undergoing allergy testing provides this toddler with a sense of comfort. **B:** Position the infant cuddled over the parent's (preferable) or the nurse's shoulder when obtaining a heel stick. **C:** Use "therapeutic hugging" to position a child while the child is receiving an IM injection. **D:** Use "therapeutic hugging" to position a child while the child is having an IV line inserted.

- Establish rapport with the child and parents. Inform them about IV therapy and what to expect. Be honest with the child.
- Explain that the venipuncture will hurt but only for a short time. Provide the child with a time frame that he or she can understand, such as the time it takes to brush his or her teeth or eat a snack.
- If possible, select a site using hand veins rather than wrist or upper arm veins to reduce the risk of phlebitis. Avoid using lower

extremity veins and areas of joint flexion if possible because these are associated with an increased risk of thrombophlebitis and other complications (Bowden & Greenberg, 2012).

- Ensure adequate pain relief using pharmacologic and nonpharmacologic methods prior to insertion of the device (see section on Pain Management for Procedures, above, for more information about management of pain related to procedures).
- Allow the antiseptic used to prepare the site to dry completely before attempting insertion.
- Use a barrier such as a gauze or washcloth or the sleeve of the child's gown under the tourniquet to avoid pinching or damaging the skin.
- If the child's veins are difficult to locate, use a device to transilluminate the vein.
- Make only two attempts to gain access; if you are unsuccessful after two attempts, allow another individual two attempts to access a site. If still unsuccessful, evaluate the need for insertion of another device.

Take Note!

Some facilities have policies in place allowing only one stick per nurse with a maximum of two sticks. After this, it is important to notify the physician or nurse practitioner unless the situation is an emergency.

- Encourage parental participation as appropriate in helping to position the child or to provide comfort positioning, such as therapeutic hugging.
- Protect the site from bumping by using a security device such as the I.V. House dressing (Fig. 1.12)

Central Access Devices

Central venous access devices are indicated when the child lacks suitable peripheral access, requires IV fluid or medication for a prolonged period of time, or is to receive specific treatments, such as the administration of highly concentrated solutions or irritating drugs that require rapid dilution like chemotherapeutic agents, parenteral nutrition, or blood and blood products. Typically, chest radiography is performed after a central venous access device is inserted to verify proper placement. No fluids are administered until correct placement is confirmed.

Fluid Administration

Administering IV fluids to an infant or child requires close attention to the child's fluid status. Typically, the amount of fluid to be

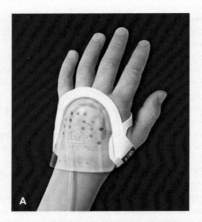

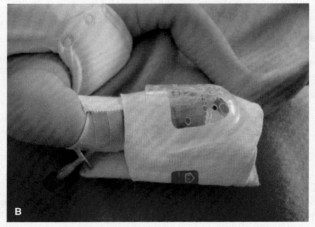

FIGURE 1.12 **A:** I.V. House dressing over the IV site on a child's hand. **B:** I.V. House dressing over the site on an infant's foot.

administered in a day (24 hours) is determined by the child's weight (in kg) using the following formula:
- 100 mL per kg of body weight for the first 10 kg
- 50 mL per kg of body weight for the next 10 kg
- 20 mL per kg of body weight for the remainder of body weight in kg. See Table 1.16.

TABLE 1.16	INTRAVENOUS MAINTENANCE FLUID CALCULATIONS BY BODY WEIGHT EXAMPLES
<10 kg in weight	100 mL per kg of weight = # mL for 24 hours Example: A child weighs 7.4 kg. 7.4 × 100 = 740 mL (daily requirement) 740/24 = 30.8 or 31 mL/hour
11–20 kg in weight	100 mL per kg of weight for the first 10 kg + 50 mL/kg for the next 10 kg = # mL for 24 hours Example: A child weighs 16 kg. (10 × 100 = 1,000) plus (6 × 50 = 300) Total = 1,300 mL (daily requirement) 1,300(24 = 54 mL/hour
>20 kg in weight	100 mL/kg for the first 10 kg + 50 mL/kg for the next 10 kg + 20 mL/kg for each kg >20 kg = # mL for 24 hours Example: A child weighs 30 kg. (10 × 100 = 1,000) plus (10 × 50 = 500) plus (10 × 20 = 200) Total = 1,700 mL (daily requirement) 1,700/24 = 70.8 or 71 mL/hour

Infants and young children are at increased risk for fluid volume overload compared with adults. Throughout the course of therapy, monitor the fluid infusion rate and volume closely, as often as every hour. If a volume control set is used to administer the IV infusion, fill the device with the allotted amount of fluid that the child is to receive in 1 hour. Inspect the insertion site every 1 to 2 hours for inflammation or infiltration. Note signs of inflammation such as warmth, redness, induration, or tender skin. Check closely for signs of infiltration such as cool, blanched, or puffy skin. In addition to monitoring the fluid infusion, closely monitor the child's output. Expected urine output for children and adolescents is 1 to 2 mL/kg/hour.

Take Note!

When measuring the output of an infant or child who is not toilet-trained or who is incontinent, weigh the diaper to determine the output. Remember that 1 g of weight is equal to 1 mL of fluid.

Flushing the IV catheter when the device is used intermittently may be necessary to maintain patency, such as before and/or after medication is administered and after obtaining blood specimens. Always follow your agency's policy for flushing IV catheters.

Take Note!

When flushing or administering medications through a PICC, follow the manufacturer's recommended syringe size, because PICCs are fragile. Using a larger volume syringe (i.e., 5 mL or larger) exerts less pressure on the PICC, thereby reducing the risk of rupture (Bowden & Greenberg, 2012).

If the child is receiving IV therapy via a central venous access device, provide site care using sterile technique and flush the device according to agency policy. Note the exit site for the device and inspect it frequently for signs of infection. If the device has multiple lumens, label each lumen with its use (i.e., blood specimen, medication, or fluid). Always check the compatibilities of solutions and medications being given simultaneously.

Discontinuing the IV Device

Prepare the child for removal of the IV device in much the same manner as for insertion. Many children may fear the removal of the device to the same extent that they feared its insertion. Explain what is to occur and enlist the child's help in the removal.

Atraumatic Care

If appropriate, allow the child to assist in removing the tape or dressing. This gives the child a sense of control over the situation and also encourages his or her cooperation.

In addition, practice atraumatic care by doing the following:
- Use water or adhesive remover to help loosen the tape.
- If a transparent dressing is in place, gently lift off the dressing by pulling up opposite corners using a motion parallel to the skin surface.
- Avoid using scissors to cut the tape, but if cutting the tape is necessary, be sure that the child's fingers are clear of the tape and scissors.
- Turn off the infusion solution and pump.
- Once all tape and dressings are removed, gently slide the IV device out using a motion opposite to that used for the insertion.
- Apply pressure to the site with a dry gauze dressing and then cover with a small adhesive bandage. If possible, allow the child to choose the bandage.

MANAGING EMERGENCIES

Health History

Obtain the health history rapidly while evaluating the child and providing life-saving interventions. A brief history is needed initially, followed by a more thorough history after the child is stabilized. Determine the child's mechanism of injury or the caregiver's description of the events that led to the emergency situation.

Physical Examination and Intervention

In an emergency, perform a rapid cardiopulmonary assessment and intervene immediately if alterations are noted. As the brief history is being obtained, begin the rapid cardiopulmonary assessment. Most pediatric arrests are related primarily to airway and breathing and usually only secondarily to the heart. Supported breathing may be all that is needed if the child has a strong, adequate pulse. Always perform the assessment and interventions in that order.

Take Note!

Assessment and management of the airway of a prearresting or arresting child is ALWAYS the first intervention in a pediatric emergency. Intervene if there is an airway problem before moving on to assessment of breathing. If an intervention for breathing is required, start it before proceeding to assessment of circulation.

Airway Evaluation and Management

Assess airway patency, positioning the airway in a manner that promotes good airflow. If secretions are obstructing the airway, suction the airway to remove them. If the child is unconscious or has just been injured, open the airway using the head tilt-chin lift maneuver (Fig. 1.13).

Take Note!

If cervical spine injury is a possibility, do not use the head tilt-chin lift maneuver; use only the jaw-thrust technique for opening the airway.

Breathing Evaluation and Management

After establishing an open airway, turn your head and place your ear over the child's mouth to determine spontaneous respirations. Look to see whether the child's chest is rising, listen for air escaping, and note if you feel any air coming out of the child's nose or mouth. If the child is not breathing, begin rescue breathing. Otherwise, count the respiratory rate. Observe the child's color. Note depth of respiration,

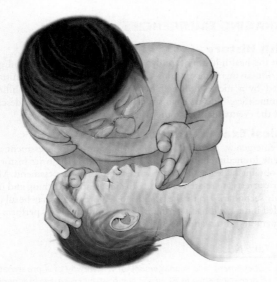

FIGURE 1.13 Head tilt-chin lift maneuver in a child.

chest rise, adequacy of airflow in all lung fields, and the presence of adventitious sounds. Evaluate for increased work of breathing and the use of accessory muscles. When signs of respiratory distress are noted, immediately place the child on oxygen at 100% and apply a pulse oximeter to monitor oxygen saturation levels. For the child receiving 100% oxygen who does not improve with repositioning, begin assisted ventilation with a bag–valve–mask (BVM) device.

Circulation Evaluation and Management

Next evaluate circulation. Note the heart rate, quality of pulses and perfusion, skin color and temperature, blood pressure, cardiac rhythm, and level of consciousness. Determine the heart rate via direct auscultation or palpation of central pulses.

 Take Note!

ALWAYS evaluate the presence of a heart rate by auscultation of the heart or by palpation of central pulses. NEVER use the cardiac monitor to determine whether the child has a heart rate. The presence of a cardiac rhythm is not a reliable method for evaluation of the ability to perfuse the body. In certain circumstances, a rhythm continues but there is no pulse (pulseless electrical activity).

The minimum acceptable blood pressure of a child experiencing an emergency is systolic blood pressure of 70 + (2 times the age in years). For example, a 4 year old should have a minimal systolic blood pressure of 78: 70 + (2 × 4) = 78. Place the child on a cardiac monitor to evaluate the cardiac rhythm.

If assessment reveals that the child has no heart rate (pulse) despite adequate respiratory interventions, begin cardiac compressions. High-quality chest compressions of adequate rate and depth are essential (Kleinman et al., 2010).

If the circulation or perfusion is compromised, then fluid resuscitation is necessary. Establish large-bore IV access immediately and administer isotonic fluid rapidly. Provide 20 mL/kg of normal saline (NS) or lactated Ringer's (LR) as an IV bolus (if the infant is younger than 1 month, administer 10 mL/kg). Limit peripheral IV access in the child with altered perfusion to three attempts or 90 seconds and then assist with insertion of an intraosseous needle for fluid administration.

Additional Physical Examination Components

Quickly evaluate the sensorium in an older child. If the child is an infant, evaluate his or her interest in the environment and response to parents. An infant who is not interested in the environment or seems unable to recognize his or her parents is a cause for concern. Evaluate the child's head. In the infant or young toddler, palpate the anterior fontanel to determine whether it is normal (soft and flat), depressed, or full. Next assess eye opening and pupillary reactivity.

Take Note!

A nonreactive pupil is an ominous sign indicating a need for immediate relief of increased intracranial pressure.

Evaluate for spontaneous movement of the extremities. The Pediatric Glasgow Coma Scale may also be used to evaluate the neurologic status in children (American Heart Association, 2011). See Figure 1.14. Remove the child's clothing and thoroughly examine the skin for bruising, lesions, or rashes. Note obvious extremity deformity or abdominal distention. Determine level of pain. If the child is awake and verbal, use an age-appropriate pain assessment scale to determine the child's pain level. If the child is sedated or unconscious, assess pain with a standardized scale.

Laboratory and Diagnostic Testing

Laboratory tests can help to distinguish the cause of the emergency or additional problems that need to be treated. These tests may include the following:

- Arterial blood gases (ABGs), obtained initially and then serially to assess for changes.

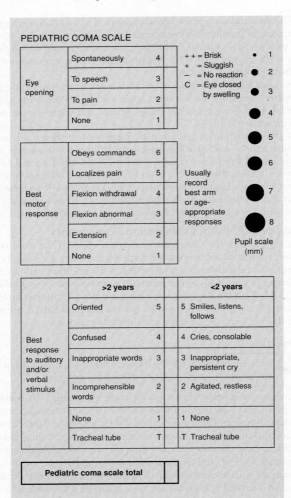

PEDIATRIC COMA SCALE

Eye opening	Spontaneously	4
	To speech	3
	To pain	2
	None	1

+ + = Brisk
+ = Sluggish
− = No reaction
C = Eye closed by swelling

Best motor response	Obeys commands	6
	Localizes pain	5
	Flexion withdrawal	4
	Flexion abnormal	3
	Extension	2
	None	1

Usually record best arm or age-appropriate responses

Pupil scale (mm)

Best response to auditory and/or verbal stimulus	>2 years		<2 years	
	Oriented	5	5 Smiles, listens, follows	
	Confused	4	4 Cries, consolable	
	Inappropriate words	3	3 Inappropriate, persistent cry	
	Incomprehensible words	2	2 Agitated, restless	
	None	1	1 None	
	Tracheal tube	T	T Tracheal tube	

Pediatric coma scale total	

FIGURE 1.14 Pediatric Glasgow Coma Scale (GCS). The Pediatric GCS provides for developmentally appropriate cues to assess level of consciousness (LOC) in infants and children. Numeric values are assigned to the levels of response and the sum provides an overall picture, as well as an objective measure, of the child's LOC. The lower the score, the less responsive the child.

- Electrolytes and glucose levels.
- Complete blood cell (CBC) count.
- Blood cultures.
- Urinalysis.
- Toxicology panel.
- Erythrocyte sedimentation rate (ESR), C-reactive protein (CRP).
- Urine and spinal fluid cultures.
- For the trauma victim: amylase, liver enzymes, and blood type and cross-match.
- Radiography, CT scanning, or magnetic resonance imaging (MRI).

Additional Nursing Interventions

Provide cardiopulmonary resuscitation as needed (refer to Table 1.17). Assist with defibrillation or synchronized cardioversion as needed. For defibrillation, use 2 joules/kg initially, increasing to 4 joules/kg as needed. Energy for cardioversion is delivered at 0.5 to 1 joule/kg. Utilize the Broselow tape or the child's individualized emergency sheet to determine equipment sizes and medication doses. Medications commonly used in a pediatric arrest situation are discussed in Table 1.18.

TABLE 1.17	RATIOS OF BREATHS TO COMPRESSIONS	
Age	**One-Person CPR**	**Two-Person CPR**
Infant	• 30 compressions to two breaths • Hand placement: two fingers, placed one fingerbreadth below the nipple line	• 15 compressions to two breaths • Hand placement: two thumbs encircling the chest at the nipple line
Child	• 30 compressions to two breaths • Hand placement: heel of hand or two hands (adult position in larger child), pressing on the sternum at the nipple line	• 15 compressions to two breaths • Hand placement: heel of one hand or two hands (adult position in larger child), pressing on the sternum at the nipple line

CPR, cardiopulmonary resuscitation.
Adapted from Berg, M. D., Schexnayder, S. M., Chameides, L., Terry, M., Donoghue, A., Hickey, R. W., ..., Hazinski, M. F. (2010). Part 13: Pediatric basic life support—2010 American Heart Association guidelines for cardiopulmonary resuscitation and emergency cardiovascular care. *Circulation, 122*, S862–S875.

TABLE 1.18 PEDIATRIC EMERGENCY MEDICATIONS

Medication	Action/Indication	Nursing Implications
Adenosine (antiarrhythmic)	Slows conduction through AV node, restoring normal sinus rhythm Supraventricular tachycardia	• Administer via IV route at a dose ranging from 0.05 to 0.1 mg/kg. • Administer very rapidly (1–2 seconds) followed by a rapid, generous saline flush. • Repeat every 1–2 minutes, increasing by 0.05–0.1 mg/kg with each dose (maximum dose 0.3 mg/kg). • Monitor for shortness of breath, dyspnea, worsening of asthma.
Atropine (anticholinergic)	Increases cardiac output, dries secretions, inhibits serotonin and histamine Sinus bradycardia, asystole, pulseless electrical activity	• Administer via IV, IO, or ET route at a dose of 0.02 mg/kg (child: maximum dose 0.5 mg; adolescent: 1 mg). • Repeat every 5 minutes as needed. • Give undiluted over 30 seconds for IV or IO route. • Dilute with 3–5 mL NS for ET route; follow with five positive pressure ventilations. • Do not mix with sodium bicarbonate (incompatible).
Epinephrine (adrenergic)	Stimulates - and -adrenergic receptors, increasing heart rate and systemic vascular resistance Bradycardia, anaphylaxis	• A dose of 0.01 mg/kg (0.1 mL/kg of 1:10,000 solution) or via ET route at 0.1 mg/kg (0.1 mL/kg of 1:1,000 solution). • During CPR, repeat every 3–5 minutes. • Monitor for ventricular arrhythmias. • High doses may cause tachycardia in newborns. • Because of risk of extravasation and subsequent tissue necrosis, give through a central catheter if possible. • May also be used as a bronchodilator IV or via inhalation (racemic epinephrine)

Medication	Action/Indication	Nursing Implications
Glucose	Increases blood glucose level Hypoglycemia	• Administer via IV or IO route at a dose of 1 to 2 mL/kg (D50%); maximum dose 2–4 mL/kg. • When administering via a peripheral IV catheter, dilute 1:1 with sterile water to make D25%. Monitor IV site for infiltration and tissue extravasation. • Monitor blood glucose levels closely.
Lidocaine (antidysrhythmic)	Decreases automaticity of conduction tissues of the heart Ventricular arrhythmias	• Administer via IV or IO route at a dose of 1 mg/kg; administer via ET route at dose two times IV dose diluted with 3–5 mL NS, followed by positive pressure ventilation. Maximum dose 5 mg/kg or 100 mg/dose. • Monitor ECG continuously. • Contraindicated in complete heart block. • With larger than normal doses, monitor for hypotension or seizures.
Naloxone (opioid antagonist)	Antagonizes action of narcotic agents Reversal of respiratory depression related to narcotic effects	• Administer via IV, IO, SC, or ET route at a dose of 0.01–0.1 mg/kg in children <5 years or <20 kg or at a dose of 2 mg in children >5 years or >20 kg. Onset of action is within 2–5 minutes. • May repeat dose as necessary; narcotic effects outlast therapeutic effects of naloxone.

AV, atrioventricular; IO, intraosseous; ET, endotracheal; ECG, electrocardiogram.

Adapted from Kleinman, M. E., Chameides, L., Schexnayder, S. M., Samson, R. A., Hazinski, M. F., Atkins, D. L., ... Zaritsky, A. L. (2010). Part 14: Pediatric advanced life support—2010 American Heart Association guidelines for cardiopulmonary resuscitation and emergency cardiovascular care. *Circulation, 122,* S876–S908; Taketomo, C. K., Hodding, J. H., & Kraus, D. M. (2013). *Pediatric & neonatal dosage handbook* (20th ed.). Hudson, OH: Lexicomp.

REFERENCES AND RECOMMENDED READINGS

American Academy of Pediatric Dentistry. (2014). *Guideline on infant oral health care.* Retrieved October 6, 2015, from http://www.aapd.org/media/Policies_Guidelines/G_InfantOralHealthCare.pdf

American Academy of Pediatrics. (2012). Breastfeeding and the use of human milk. *Pediatrics,* 129(3), e827–e841. doi: 10.1542/peds.2011–3552.

American Academy of Pediatrics and the American Pain Society. (2001). Policy statement: The assessment and management of acute pain in infants, children, and adolescents. *Pediatrics,* 108(3), 793–797.

American Heart Association. (2011). Pediatric advanced life support provider manual. Dallas, TX: Author.

Anand, K. J. S. (2013). *Assessment of neonatal pain.* UpToDate. Retrieved October 6, 2015, from http://www.uptodate.com/contents/assessment-of-neonatal-pain

Aschenbrenner, D. S., & Venable, S. J. (2012). *Drug therapy in nursing* (4th ed.). Philadelphia, PA: Lippincott Williams & Wilkins.

Baker, C. M., & Wong, D. L. (1987). Q.U.E.S.T.: A process of pain assessment in children. *Orthopaedic Nursing,* 6(1), 11–21.

Baker, R. D., Greer, F. R., & The Committee on Nutrition. (2010). Clinical report. Diagnosis and prevention of iron deficiency and iron-deficiency anemia in infants and young children (0–3 years of age). *Pediatrics,* 126(5), 1040–1050.

Berg, M. D., Schexnayder, S. M., Chameides, L., Terry, M., Donoghue, A., Hickey, R. W., …, Hazinski, M. F. (2010). Part 13: Pediatric basic life support—2010 American Heart Association guidelines for cardiopulmonary resuscitation and emergency cardiovascular care. *Circulation,* 122, S862–S875.

Bickley, L. (2013). *Bates' guide to physical examination and history taking* (11th ed.). Philadelphia, PA: Lippincott Williams & Wilkins.

Bowden, V. R., & Greenberg, C. S. (2012). *Pediatric nursing procedures* (3rd ed.). Philadelphia, PA: Lippincott Williams & Wilkins.

Bright Futures/American Academy of Pediatrics. (2014). *Recommendations for preventive pediatric health care.* Retrieved on October 6, 2015, from http://www.aap.org/en-us/professional-resources/practice-support/Periodicity/Periodicity%20Schedule_FINAL.pdf

Burns, C. E., Dunn, A. M., Brady, M. A., Starr, N. B., & Blosser, C. G. (2013). *Pediatric primary care* (5th ed.). Philadelphia, PA: Saunders.

Centers for Disease Control and Prevention. (2010). *Growth charts.* Retrieved October 6, 2015, from http://www.cdc.gov/growthcharts

Centers for Disease Control and Prevention. (2012a). *CDC response to Advisory Committee on Childhood Lead Poisoning Prevention recommendations in "low level lead exposure harms children: A renewed call of primary prevention".* Retrieved October 6, 2015, from http://www.cdc.gov/nceh/lead/ACCLPP/CDC_Response_Lead_Exposure_Recs.pdf

Centers for Disease Control and Prevention. (2012b). Appendix D: Vaccine administration. In W. Atkinson, S. Wolfe, & J. Hamborsky (Eds.), *Epidemiology and prevention of vaccine-preventable diseases* (12th ed., second printing). Washington, DC: Public Health Foundation.

Centers for Disease Control and Prevention. (2013a). *Screening for lead during the domestic medical examination for newly arrived refugees.* Retrieved October 6, 2015, from http://www.cdc.gov/immigrantrefugeehealth/guidelines/lead-guidelines.html

Centers for Disease Control and Prevention. (2013b). *Use and interpretation of the WHO and CDC growth charts for children from birth to 20 years in the United States.* Retrieved October 6, 2015, from http://www.cdc.gov/nccdphp/dnpa/growthcharts/resources/growthchart.pdf

Centers for Disease Control and Prevention. (2015a). *Birth-18 years & "catch-up" immunization schedules.* Retrieved October 6, 2015, from http://www.cdc.gov/vaccines/schedules/hcp/child-adolescent.html

Centers for Disease Control and Prevention. (2015b). *Body mass index.* Retrieved October 6, 2015, from http://www.cdc.gov/healthyweight/assessing/bmi/index.html

Centers for Disease Control and Prevention. (2015c). *Catch-up immunization schedule for persons aged 4 months through 18 years who start late or who are more than 1 month behind.* Retrieved October 6, 2015, from http://www.cdc.gov/vaccines/schedules/downloads/child/catchup-schedule-pr.pdf

Centers for Disease Control and Prevention. (2015d). *Lead.* Retrieved October 6, 2015, from http://www.cdc.gov/nceh/lead/

Cooney M. F., Czarnecki M., Dunwoody C., Eksterowicz N., Merkel S., Oakes L., & Wuhrman E. (2013). American Society for Pain Management Nursing position statement with clinical practice guidelines: Authorized agent controlled analgesia. *Pain Management Nursing,* 14(3), 176–181.

Coté, C. J., Wilson, S., & the Work Group on Sedation. (2011). *Guidelines for monitoring and management of pediatric patients during and after sedation for diagnostic and therapeutic procedures: An update.* Retrieved October 6, 2015, from http://pediatrics.aappublications.org/content/118/6/2587.long

Cromer, B. (2011). Chapter 104: Adolescent development. In R. M. Kleigman, B. F. Stanton, J. W. St. Geme III, N. F. Schor, & R. E. Behrman (Eds.), *Nelson textbook of pediatrics* (19th ed., pp. 649–659). Philadelphia, PA: Saunders.

D'Arcy, Y. (2011). New thinking about postoperative pain management. *OR Nurse,* 5(6), 28–36.

Delaney, A. M. (2014). *Newborn hearing screening.* Retrieved October 6, 2015, from http://emedicine.medscape.com/article/836646-overview#a1

Dietz, W. H., & Stern, L. (2012). *Nutrition: What every parent needs to know* (2nd ed.). Elk Grove Village, IL: American Academy of Pediatrics.

Erikson, E. H. (1963). *Childhood and society* (2nd ed.). New York, NY: W. W. Norton & Company.

Feigelman, S. (2011a). Middle childhood. In R. M. Kliegman, B. F. Stanton, J. W. St. Geme III, N. F. Schor, & R. E. Behrman (Eds.), (*Nelson's textbook of pediatrics* (19th ed.). Philadelphia, PA: Saunders.

Feigelman, S. (2011b). Preschool years. In R. M. Kliegman, B. F. Stanton, J. W. St. Geme III, N. F. Schor, & R. E. Behrman (Eds.), (*Nelson's textbook of pediatrics* (19th ed.). Philadelphia, PA: Elsevier, Saunders.

Feigelman, S. (2011c). The first year. In R. M. Kliegman, B. F. Stanton, J. W. St. Geme III, N. F. Schor, & R. E. Behrman (Eds.), (*Nelson's textbook of pediatrics* (19th ed.). Philadelphia, PA: Elsevier, Saunders.

Feigelman, S. (2011d). The second year. In R. M. Kliegman, B. F. Stanton, J. W. St. Geme III, N. F. Schor, & R. E. Behrman (Eds.), (*Nelson's textbook of pediatrics* (19th ed.). Philadelphia, PA: Elsevier, Saunders.

Gavin, M. L. (2012). *Iron and your child.* Retrieved October 6, 2015, from http://kidshealth.org/parent/growth/feeding/iron.html#

Gavin, M. (2014a). *Toddlers at the table: Avoiding power struggles.* Retrieved October 6, 2015 from http://kidshealth.org/parent/nutrition_center/healthy_eating/toddler_meals.html?tracking=P_RelatedArticle#

Gavin, M. L. (2014b). *Calcium.* Retrieved October 6, 2015, from http://kidshealth.org/teen/food_fitness/nutrition/calcium.html#

Goldson, E., & Reynolds, A. (2012). Child development and behavior. In W. W. Hay, Jr., M. J. Levin, R. R. Deterding, M. J. Abzug, & J. M. Sondheimer (Eds.), *Current diagnosis and treatment: Pediatrics* (21st ed.). New York, NY: McGraw-Hill.

Gupta, R. C. (2014). *All about sleep.* Retrieved October 6, 2015, from http://kidshealth.org/parent/general/sleep/sleep.html

Haemer, M., Primark, L. E., & Krebs, N. R. (2012). Normal childhood nutrition and its disorders. In W. W. Hay, M. J. Levin, R. R. Deterding, et al. (Eds.) *Current diagnosis & treatment: Pediatrics* (21st ed.). New York, NY: McGraw Hill.

Hauer, J., & Jones, B. L. (2015). *Evaluation and management of pain in children.* Retrieved October 6, 2015 from http://www.uptodate.com/contents/evaluation-and-management-of-pain-in-children

Hockenberry, M. J., & Wilson, D. (2009). *Wong's essentials of pediatric nursing* (8th ed., p. 162). St. Louis, MO: Elsevier Mosby.

Immunization Action Coalition. (2012). *How to administer intramuscular (IM) and how to administer subcutaneous (SC) injections.* Retrieved June 1, 2015, from http://www.immunize.org/catg.d/p2020.pdf

Institute for Safe Medication Practices. (2009). *Medication safety alert! Safety briefs,* 14(11), Retrieved October 6, 2015, from http://www.ismp.org/newsletters/acutecare/issues/20090604.pdf

Kleinman, M. E., Chameides, L., Schexnayder, S. M., Samson, R. A., Hazinski, M. F., Atkins, D. L., …, Zaritsky, A. L. (2010). Part 14: Pediatric advanced life support—2010 American Heart Association guidelines for cardiopulmonary resuscitation and emergency cardiovascular care. *Circulation,* 122, S876–S908.

Kliegman, R. M., Stanton, B., St. Geme, J., Schor, N. & Behrman, R. E. (2011). *Nelson's textbook of pediatrics* (19th ed.). Philadelphia, PA: Saunders.

Kroger, A. T., Sumaya, C. V., Pickering, L. K., & Atkinson, W. L. (2011). General recommendations on immunization recommendations of the Advisory Committee on Immunization Practices (ACIP). *Morbidity and Mortality Weekly Report,* 60(RR02), 1–60. Retrieved June 1, 2015, from http://www.cdc.gov/mmwr/preview/mmwrhtml/rr6002a1.htm?s_cid = rr6002a1_e

Lawrence, J., Alcock, D., McGrath, P., Kay, J., MacMurray, S. B., & Dulberg, C. (1993). The development of a tool to assess neonatal pain. *Neonatal Network,* 12(6), 59–66.

March of Dimes. (2015). *Newborn screening tests for your baby.* Retrieved October 6, 2015, from http://www.marchofdimes.com/baby/newborn-screening-tests-for-your-baby.aspx

Martorell, G., Papalia, D., & Feldman, R. (2014). *A child's world: Infancy through adolescence* (13th ed.). New York, NY: McGraw Hill.

Merkel, S. I., Voepel-Lewis, T., Shayevitz, J. R., & Malviya, S. (1997). The FLACC: A behavioral scale for scoring postoperative pain in young children. *Pediatric Nursing,* 23(3), 293–297.

National Heart, Lung, and Blood Institute. (2012). *Expert panel on integrated guidelines for cardiovascular health and risk reduction in children and adolescents. Summary report (NIH Publication No. 12–7486).* Washington, DC: U.S. Department of Health and Human Services. Retrieved March 27, 2014, from http://www.nhlbi.nih.gov/guidelines/cvd_ped/peds_guidelines_sum.pdf

National Institutes of Health (2015). *Iron: Dietary Supplemental Fact Sheet.* Retrieved on October 7, 2015 from https://ods.od.nih.gov/factsheets/Iron-HealthProfessional/

Oakes, L. (2011). *Compact clinical guide to infant and child pain management. An evidence-based approach for nurses.* D'Arcy, Y (Series Ed.). New York, NY: Springer Publishing Company, LLC.

O'Grady, N. P., Alexander, M., Burns, L. A., Dellinger, E. P., Garland, J., Heard, S. O., & the Healthcare Infection Control Practices Advisory Committee (HICPAC). (2011). Guidelines for the prevention of intravascular catheter-related infections. *Clinical Infectious Diseases,* 52, e1–e32.

Schaider, J., Barkin, R. M., Hayden, S. R., Wolfe, R. E., Barkin, A. Z., Shayne, P., & Rosen, P. (2014). *Rosen & Barkin's 5-minute emergency medicine consult* (5th ed.). Philadelphia, PA: Lippincott Williams & Wilkins.

Stettler, N., Bhatia, J., Parish, A., & Stallings, V. A. (2011). Feeding healthy infants, children, and adolescents. In R. M. Kliegman, B. F. Stanton, J. W. St. Geme III, N. F. Schor, & R. E. Behrman (Eds.), (*Nelson's textbook of pediatrics* (19th ed.). Philadelphia, PA: Elsevier, Saunders.

Taketomo, C. K., Hodding, J. H., & Kraus, D. M. (2013). *Pediatric & neonatal dosage handbook* (20th ed.). Hudson, OH: Lexicomp.

The Joint Commission. (2004). *Sentinel event alert. Patient controlled analgesia by proxy.* Retrieved October 6, 2015 from http://www.jointcommission.org/assets/1/18/SEA_33.PDF

U.S. Department of Agriculture. (n. d.). *Daily food plan for preschoolers.* Retrieved June 1, 2015 from http://www.choosemyplate.gov/PRESCHOOLERS/Plan/index.html

U.S. Department of Agriculture and U.S. Department of Health and Human Services. (2010). *Dietary guidelines for Americans* (7th Ed.). Washington, DC: U.S. Government Printing Office.

U.S. Department of Agriculture Food and Nutrition Service. (2012). *Healthy eating for preschoolers.* Retrieved on October 6, 2015 from http://www.choosemyplate.gov/sites/default/files/audiences/HealthyEatingForPreschoolers-MiniPoster.pdf

United States Environmental Protection Agency. (2015). *Lead.* Retrieved on October 6, 2015 from http://www2.epa.gov/lead

von Baeyer, C. L. (2014). Chapter 36: Self report: The primary source of assessment after infancy. In P. J. McGrath, B. J. Stevens, S. M. Walker, & W. T. Zempsky (Eds.), *Oxford textbook of paediatric pain* (pp. 370–378). Oxford, UK: Oxford University Press.

Vyas, S. T. (2015). *Lead poisoning.* Retrieved on October 6, 2015 from http://kidshealth.org/parent/medical/brain/lead_poisoning.html#

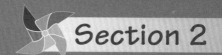

Section 2

Nursing Care for Children with Common Health Disorders

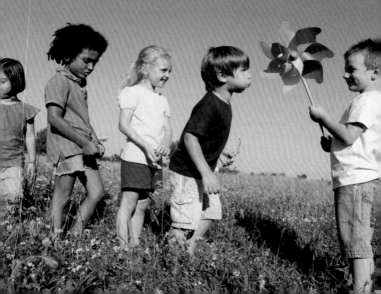

ABUSE AND VIOLENCE

Description

- Physical abuse refers to injuries that are intentionally inflicted and that result in morbidity or mortality.
- Sexual abuse refers to involvement of the child in any activity meant to provide sexual gratification to an adult.
- Emotional abuse may be verbal denigration of the child or may occur as a result of the child witnessing domestic violence.
- Neglect is defined as failure to provide a child with appropriate food, clothing, shelter, medical care, and schooling (Chiesa & Sirotnak, 2014).
- Despite the lack of adequate statistics, it is well known that the problem of abuse and violence is widespread. Parents or caregivers are the most frequent perpetrators of abuse against children (Chiesa & Sirotnak, 2014).
- Long-term sequelae of abuse and violence include mood and anxiety disorders, posttraumatic stress disorder, reactive attachment disorder, later substance abuse, perpetuation of the violence cycle, and unknown neurobiologic effects.

Pathophysiology

- The abusive perpetrator usually forces the victim into silence, making cases of abuse difficult to determine.
- Children usually do not want to admit that their parent or relative has hurt them, partly from feelings of guilt and partly because they do not want to lose that parent.
- Abuse and violence occur across all socioeconomic levels but are more prevalent among the poor (Chiesa & Sirotnak, 2014).
- Being a victim of abuse places children at risk for low self-esteem, poor academic achievement, poor emotional health, and social difficulties.

Therapeutic Management

- Physical treatment of the injury
- Palliative care in some cases
- Intervention to preserve or restore the child's mental well-being as well as family functioning
- All states require by law that healthcare professionals report suspected cases of abuse or neglect to protect children (Child Welfare Information Gateway, 2014).

Assessment Findings

Health History

- History of hurting self or others (e.g., cutting)
- Running away

BOX 2.1

QUESTIONS TO USE IN IDENTIFYING ABUSE AND VIOLENCE

- **Ask the child:**
  - Are you afraid of anyone at home?
  - Who could you tell if someone hurt you or touched you in a way that made you uncomfortable?
  - Has anyone hurt you or touched you in that way?
- **Ask parents:**
  - Are you afraid of anyone at home?
  - Do you ever feel like you may hit or hurt your child when frustrated?

- Attempting suicide
- Being involved in high-risk behaviors
- Indications of sexual abuse may include inappropriate sexual behavior for developmental age, such as seductiveness.
- When obtaining the health history, pay particular attention to statements made by the child's parent or caretaker. Is the history given consistent with the injury?
- Identify abuse and violence by screening all children and families (Box 2.1).

Risk Factors
- Risk factors for being abused in children include:
  - poverty
  - prematurity
  - cerebral palsy
  - chronic illness and
  - intellectual disability.
- Risk factors for abusing in parents or caretakers include:
  - a history of being abused themselves
  - alcohol or substance abuse or
  - extreme stress.

Physical Examination
- Fear or excessive desire to please the parent
- Lower level of consciousness (LOC) in the infant
- Oropharyngeal inflammation
- Anal/penile/vaginal bleeding or discharge
- Bruises (especially on the chest, head, neck, or abdomen)
- Burns (particularly in a stocking or glove pattern, or only on the soles or palms)

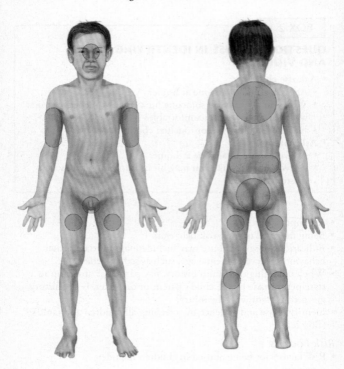

 Common nonaccidental injury sites

FIGURE 2.1 Injury sites that are suspicious for abuse.

- Cuts, abrasions, contusions, scars, or any other unusual or suspicious marks, particularly those in various stages of healing
- Figure 2.1 shows injury sites usually indicative of abuse
- Figure 2.2 is a photograph of a child who was beaten with an electric cord.

Take Note!

A delay in seeking medical treatment, a history that changes over time, or a history of trauma that is inconsistent with the observed injury all suggest child abuse.

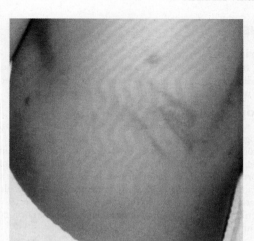

FIGURE 2.2 Note the mark left from a looped electric cord.

Laboratory and Diagnostic Tests
- Radiographic skeletal survey or bone scan may show current or past fractures.
- Computed tomographic (CT) scan of the head might demonstrate intracranial hemorrhage.
- Rectal, oral, vaginal, or urethral specimens may reveal sexually transmitted infections such as gonorrhea or *Chlamydia* infection.

Nursing Interventions
- Refer suspected cases of neglect or abuse to the local child protection agency. In the hospital, contact the social worker.
- Provide consistent care to the abused child by assigning a core group of nurses.
- Role-model appropriate caretaking activities to the parent or caregiver. Call attention to normal growth and development activities noted in the infant or child, as sometimes parents have expectations of child behavior that may be unrealistic based on the child's age, leading to the abuse. Praise parents and caretakers for taking appropriate steps toward getting help and for providing appropriate care to the child.
- Refer parents to Parents Anonymous, an organization dedicated to the prevention of child abuse through strengthening of the family (parentsanonymous.org).

ACNE

Description
- Acne, the most common skin condition occurring in childhood (Morelli & Prok, 2014), is a disorder that affects the pilosebaceous unit.
- Acne most commonly affects infants and adolescents.

Pathophysiology
- Acne neonatorum occurs as a response to the presence of maternal androgens.
- Androgenous hormones stimulate sebaceous gland proliferation and sebum production in adolescents between 12 and 16 years of age.
- Abnormal shedding of the outermost layer of the skin (the stratum corneum) occurs at the level of the follicular opening, resulting in a keratin plug that fills the follicle.
- Bacterial overgrowth of *Propionibacterium acnes* then occurs, and inflammatory lesions and clogged pores occur.

Therapeutic Management
- Acne neonatorum usually does not require any treatment.
- Acne vulgaris treatment often includes gentle skin cleansing and medication therapy such as benzoyl peroxide, salicylic acid, retinoids, and topical or oral antibiotics. Isotretinoin (Accutane) may be used in severe cases.

Assessment Findings

Health History
- Oily face or scalp
- Acne lesion development
- Family history of acne
- Medication use (corticosteroids, androgens, lithium, phenytoin, isoniazid)
- History of an endocrine disorder
- Increase in lesions before menstrual periods.

Risk Factors
- Preadolescent or adolescent age
- Male gender
- An oily complexion
- Cushing syndrome, or other disease process resulting in increased androgen production.

Physical Examination
- Open and closed comedones, inflammatory papules, pustules, nodules, or cysts

- Hypertrophic scarring
- Oily skin and oily hair.

Nursing Interventions

- Acne neonatorum:
  - Instruct parents to avoid picking or squeezing the pimples.
  - Teach parents to wash the affected areas daily with clear water, avoiding use of fragranced soaps or lotions on the area with acne.
- Acne vulgaris:
  - Avoid oil-based cosmetics and hair product.
  - Administer medications as ordered, and teach teens how to use them.
  - Encourage the child to use a humectant moisturizer.
  - Teach teens to cleanse skin twice daily with mild soap and water.
  - Teach teens to avoid picking or squeezing the lesions and to use a noncomedogenic sunscreen with an SPF of 30.
  - Teach adolescents that the prescribed topical medications must be used daily and that it may take 4 to 6 weeks to see results.
  - Teach boys to shave gently and avoid using dull razors so as not to further irritate the condition.
  - Explain the importance of being on a pregnancy prevention program to all adolescent girls taking isotretinoin who are sexually active; the drug causes defects in fetal development (Vernon, Brady, Starr, & Petersen-Smith, 2013).
  - Provide emotional support to adolescents undergoing acne therapy. Refer teens for counseling if necessary.

Take Note!

Chocolate, skim milk, and French fries have not been proven to contribute to the incidence or severity of acne. However, advise teens to wash their hands after eating greasy finger foods to avoid spreading additional oil to the surface of the face (Morelli & Prok, 2014).

ACUTE GLOMERULONEPHRITIS

Description

- Acute glomerulonephritis is a condition in which immune processes injure the glomeruli.
- It can progress to uremia and renal failure (either acute or chronic; Gaylord & Petersen-Smith, 2013).

Pathophysiology

- Immune mechanisms cause inflammation, which results in altered glomerular structure and function in both kidneys. It often occurs following an infection, usually an upper respiratory or skin infection.

- The most common form is acute poststreptococcal glomerulone-phritis (APSGN). APSGN is caused by an antibody–antigen reaction secondary to an infection with a nephritogenic strain of group A beta-hemolytic streptococci.

Therapeutic Management

- There is no specific medical treatment of APSGN. Treatment is aimed at maintaining fluid volume and managing hypertension. If renal involvement progresses, dialysis may become necessary.
- If there is evidence of a current streptococcal infection, antibiotic therapy will be necessary.

Assessment Findings

Health History

- Fever
- Lethargy
- Headache
- Decreased urine output
- Abdominal pain
- Vomiting or anorexia.

Risk Factors

- Recent episode of pharyngitis or other streptococcal infection
- Age >2 years
- Male sex.

Physical Examination

- Increased blood pressure (common)
- Mild edema
- Increased work of breathing, cough, crackles, and gallop (from cardiopulmonary congestion)
- Gross hematuria (urine is tea-colored, cola-colored, or even a dirty green color).

Laboratory and Diagnostic Tests

- Urine dipstick: proteinuria, hematuria
- Serum creatinine and blood urea nitrogen (BUN): may be normal or elevated
- Serum complement level: depressed
- Erythrocyte sedimentation rate (ESR): elevated
- Anti-streptolysin (ASO) and DNase B antigen titer: elevated (if streptococcal infection is the cause).

Nursing Interventions

- Administer antihypertensives such as labetalol or nifedipine and diuretics as ordered.

- Monitor blood pressure frequently.
- Maintain sodium and fluid restrictions as prescribed during the initial edematous phase.
- Weigh the child daily on the same scale wearing the same amount of clothing.
- Monitor increasing urine output and note improvement in the urine color.
- Document resolution of edema.
- Provide careful neurologic evaluation, as hypertension may cause encephalopathy and seizures.
- Provide the child with age-appropriate activities and cluster care to allow rest periods.
- For home management, teach the family to monitor urine output and color, take blood pressure measurements, restrict the diet as prescribed, and encourage rest.

Take Note!

Avoid use of nonsteroidal anti-inflammatory drugs (NSAIDs) in children with questionable renal function, as the antiprostaglandin action of NSAIDs may cause a further decrease in the glomerular filtration rate (Solomon, 2014).

ACUTE LYMPHOBLASTIC LEUKEMIA

Description

- Acute lymphoblastic leukemia (ALL) is the most common form of cancer in children and is classified according to the type of cells involved: T cell, B cell, early pre-B cell, or pre-B cell. Most children will achieve initial remission if appropriate treatment is given.
- Prognosis is based upon the white blood cell (WBC) count at diagnosis, the type of cytogenetic factors and immunophenotype, the age at diagnosis, and the extent of extramedullary involvement.
- Complications include infection, hemorrhage, poor growth, and central nervous system (CNS), bone, or testicular involvement.

Pathophysiology

- In ALL, abnormal fragile lymphoblasts abound in the blood-forming tissues. These lymphoblasts lack the infection-fighting capabilities of the normal WBCs, grow excessively, and replace the normal cells in the bone marrow.
- The proliferating leukemic cells demonstrate massive metabolic needs, depriving normal body cells of needed nutrients, and resulting in fatigue, weight loss or growth arrest, and muscle wasting.

- The bone marrow becomes unable to maintain normal levels of red blood cells (RBCs), WBCs, and platelets, so anemia, neutropenia, and thrombocytopenia result. With leukemic cell infiltration into the bone, joint and bone pain may occur. The leukemic cells may permeate the lymph nodes, causing diffuse lymphadenopathy, or the liver and spleen, resulting in hepatosplenomegaly. With spread to the CNS, vomiting, headache, seizures, coma, vision alterations, or cranial nerve palsies may occur (Zupanec & Tomlinson, 2010).

Therapeutic Management

- Therapeutic management of the child with ALL focuses on giving chemotherapy to eradicate the leukemic cells and restore normal bone marrow function.
- Treatment is divided into three stages, with CNS prophylaxis given at each stage (Table 2.1).

Assessment Findings

Health History

- Fever (may be persistent or recurrent, with unknown cause)
- Recurrent infection
- Fatigue
- Malaise or listlessness
- Pallor
- Unusual bleeding or bruising
- Abdominal pain, nausea, or vomiting
- Bone pain
- Headache (Zupanec & Tomlinson, 2010).

Risk Factors

- Male gender, age 2 to 5 years
- Caucasian race
- Down syndrome
- Shwachman syndrome
- Ataxia-telangiectasia
- X-ray exposure in utero
- Previous radiation-treated cancer (Zupanec & Tomlinson, 2010).

Physical Examination

- Fever
- Petechiae
- Purpura or unusual bruising
- Signs of skin infection
- Adventitious breath sounds
- Enlarged lymph nodes

(text continues on page 96)

TABLE 2.1   THREE-STAGE TREATMENT OF THE CHILD WITH ALL

Stage	Purpose	Length	Usual Medications
Induction	Rapid induction of complete remission	3–4 weeks	Oral steroids, IV vincristine, IM L-asparaginase, daunomycin (high-risk)
Consolidation (intensification)	Strengthen remission, reduce leukemic cell burden	Varies	High-dose methotrexate, 6-mercaptopurine; possibly cyclophosphamide, cytarabine, asparaginase, thioguanine, epipodophyllotoxins
Maintenance	Eliminate all residual leukemic cells	2–3 years	Low-dose: daily 6-mercaptopurine, weekly methotrexate, intermittent IV vincristine and oral steroids
CNS prophylaxis	Reduce risk of development of CNS disease	Given periodically in all stages	Intrathecal chemotherapy; cranial radiation is used infrequently

IM, intramuscular.
Adapted from Graham, D. K., Craddock, J. A., Quinones, R. R., Keating, A. K., Maloney, K. Foreman, N. K., Giller, R. H., Greffe, B. S. (2014). Neoplastic disease. In W. W. Hay, M. J. Levin, R. R. Deterding, & M. J. Abzug (Eds.), *Current pediatric diagnosis and treatment* (22nd ed.). New York, NY: McGraw-Hill; Zupanec, S., & Tomlinson, D. (2010). Leukemia. In D. Tomlinson, & N. E. Kline (Eds.), *Pediatric oncology nursing*. New York, NY: Springer.

- Liver or spleen enlargement
- Abdominal tenderness.

> **Take Note!**
>
> Changes in behavior or personality, headache, irritability, dizziness, persistent nausea or vomiting, seizures, gait changes, lethargy, or altered level of consciousness may indicate CNS infiltration with leukemic cells. Immediately report these findings to the pediatric oncologist.

Laboratory and Diagnostic Tests

- Abnormal complete blood cell (CBC) counts: low hemoglobin and hematocrit, decreased RBC count, decreased platelet count, and elevated, normal, or decreased WBC count.
- Peripheral blood smear may reveal blasts.
- Stained smear from bone marrow aspiration will show >25% lymphoblasts. Bone marrow aspirate is also examined for immunophenotyping (lymphoid vs. myeloid, and level of cancer cell maturity) and cytogenetic analysis (determines abnormalities in chromosome number and structure). Immunophenotyping and cytogenetic analysis are used in the classification of the leukemia, which helps guide treatment.
- Lumbar puncture will reveal whether leukemic cells have infiltrated the CNS.
- Liver function tests and BUN and creatinine levels determine liver and renal function, which if abnormal may preclude treatment with certain chemotherapeutic agents.
- Chest x-ray may reveal pneumonia or a mediastinal mass.

Nursing Interventions

- Administer chemotherapy as ordered, utilizing personal protective equipment as indicated. Dispose of all equipment used in chemotherapy preparation and administration in a puncture-resistant container.
- Calculate the chemotherapy dose correctly based on the child's body surface area (BSA). To use a nomogram to calculate BSA, draw a straight line between the child's height on the left and the child's weight on the right. The point at which the straight line crosses the center is the child's BSA expressed in meters squared (Fig. 2.3). Or, use this formula to calculate BSA: BSA (m^2) = the square root of (height [in cm] × weight [in kg] divided by 3,600). For example, for a child 140 cm tall and weighing 30 kg: 140 × 30 = 4,200; 4,200/3,600 = 1.167; and the square root of 1.167 is 1.08. The BSA would be 1.08.
- Administer blood product transfusion as ordered.

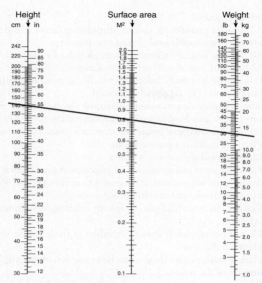

Height	Surface area	Weight
cm in	M²	lb kg

FIGURE 2.3 Body surface area.

Take Note!

Blood products administered to children with any type of leukemia should be irradiated, cytomegalovirus (CMV) negative, and leukodepleted. This treatment of blood products before transfusion will decrease the amount of antibodies in the blood, an important factor in preventing graft-versus-host disease should hematopoietic stem cell transplantation (HSCT) become necessary at a later date (Nixon, 2010).

- Manage side effects of chemotherapy.
  - Prevent hemorrhage:
    - Assess for petechiae, purpura, bruising, or bleeding.
    - Encourage quiet activities or play to avoid trauma.
    - Avoid rectal temperatures and examinations to prevent rectal mucosal damage that results in bleeding. Post a sign at the head of the bed stating "no rectal temperatures or medications."
    - Avoid intramuscular injections and lumbar puncture if possible.
    - For active or uncontrolled bleeding, transfuse platelets as ordered to control bleeding.

- Prevent infection:
  - Administer granulocyte colony-stimulating factor as ordered to promote neutrophil growth and maturation.
  - Administer varicella zoster immunoglobulin (VZIG) within 72 hours of exposure to active chickenpox.
  - If the child is actively infected with chickenpox, administer intravenous (IV) acyclovir as ordered.
- Follow neutropenic precautions when the absolute neutrophil count is very low. Neutropenic precautions include the following:
  - Perform hand hygiene before and after each contact with the child.
  - Place the child in a private room.
  - Monitor vital signs every 4 hours.
  - Assess for signs and symptoms of infection at least every 8 hours.
  - Avoid rectal suppositories, enemas, or examinations; urinary catheterization; and invasive procedures.
  - Restrict visitors with fever, cough, or other signs/symptoms of infection.
  - Do not permit raw fruits or vegetables or fresh flowers or live plants in the room.
  - Place a mask on the child when he or she is being transported outside of the room.
  - Perform dental care with a soft toothbrush if the platelet count is adequate.
  - Children with neutropenia and fever must be started on IV broad-spectrum antibiotics without delay to avoid overwhelming sepsis.
  - Administer prophylactic antibiotics as ordered and teach the parents to administer them at home.
  - Teaching Guidelines 2.1 gives further information about infection prevention at home.

Teaching Guidelines 2.1
PREVENTION OF INFECTION IN CHILDREN RECEIVING CHEMOTHERAPY FOR CANCER

- Practice meticulous hygiene (oral, personal, perianal).
- Avoid known ill contacts, especially persons with chickenpox.
- Immediately notify physician if exposed to chickenpox.
- Avoid crowded areas.
- Do not let the child receive live vaccines.
- Do not take the child's temperature rectally or give medications by the rectal route.
- Administer twice-daily trimethoprim-sulfamethoxazole for 3 consecutive days each week as ordered for the prevention of *Pneumocystis* pneumonia.

- Reduce pain:
  - Use distraction techniques such as listening to music, watching TV, or playing games.
  - Administrate mild analgesics such as acetaminophen for acute episodes of pain, utilization of EMLA cream prior to venipuncture, port access, lumbar puncture, and bone marrow aspiration, application of heat or cold to the painful area, and narcotic analgesic administration for episodes of acute severe pain or for palliation of chronic pain (Simon, 2010).

ANOREXIA NERVOSA AND BULIMIA NERVOSA

Description
- Anorexia nervosa and bulimia are common eating disorders affecting primarily adolescents, though younger children may also be affected.
- Anorexia nervosa is characterized by dramatic weight loss as a result of decreased food intake and sharply increased physical exercise.
- Bulimia refers to a cycle of normal food intake, followed by binge eating and then purging; the adolescent remains at a near-normal weight (Garzon, 2013).

Pathophysiology
- In American society, being thin is highly valued, compounding the problem. The adolescent may have low self-esteem, leading to increased need for acceptance.

Therapeutic Management
- Most children with eating disorders can be treated successfully on an outpatient basis.
- Those with anorexia who display severe weight loss, unstable vital signs, food refusal, or arrested pubertal development or who require enteral nutrition will need to be hospitalized.
- Refeeding syndrome (cardiovascular, hematologic, and neurologic complications) may occur in the severely malnourished patient if rapid nutritional replacement is given, so slow refeeding is essential to avoid complications.

Assessment Findings

Health History
- Weight loss
- Depression
- Family history
- Female gender

- Caucasian race
- Preoccupation with appearance
- Obsessive traits
- Low self-esteem; history of constipation
- Syncope
- Secondary amenorrhea
- Abdominal pain
- Periodic episodes of cold hands and feet
- History of multiple fears
- High need for acceptance
- Disordered body image
- Perfectionism.

Risk Factors
- Adolescent age
- Female gender
- Caucasian race.

Physical Examination
- Anorexia
  - Severely underweight, with a body mass index of less than 17
  - Cachetic appearance
  - Dry sallow skin
  - Thinning scalp hair
  - Soft sparse body hair
  - Nail pitting
  - Low temperature
  - Bradycardia
  - Hypotension
  - Murmur (mitral valve prolapse occurs in about one third of children)
- Bulimia
  - Normal weight or slightly overweight (bulimic)
  - Calluses on the backs of the knuckles
  - Eroded dental enamel
  - Red gums
  - Inflamed throat (from self-induced vomiting).

Laboratory and Diagnostic Tests
- Serum electrolytes may reveal mild to severe disturbances.
- Electrocardiogram may indicate cardiac dysrhythmias.

Nursing Interventions
- Assess vital signs frequently for orthostatic hypotension, irregular and decreased pulse, or hypothermia.
- Give phosphorus supplements as ordered.

- Consult the nutritionist for assistance with calculating caloric needs and determining an appropriate diet. Aim for a weight gain goal of 0.5 to 2 pounds per week.
- Instruct the child and family to keep a daily journal of intake, binging (excessive consumption) and purging (forced vomiting) behaviors, mood, and exercise.
- Assist the child and family to plan a suitably structured routine for the child that includes meals, snacks, and appropriate physical activity.
- Use the physical findings associated with anorexia to educate the child about the consequences of malnutrition and how they can be remedied with adequate nutrient intake.
- Assess the child's need for intervention for concomitant depression or anxiety, as well as therapy.
- Provide emotional support and positive reinforcement to the child and family.
- Refer the family to local support groups or online resources such as the Academy for Eating Disorders (www.aedweb.org) or the National Eating Disorders Association (www.nationaleatingdisorders.org).

ASTHMA

Description

- Asthma is a chronic inflammatory airway disorder characterized by airway hyperresponsiveness, airway edema, and mucous production. Airway obstruction resulting from asthma might be partially or completely reversed. Severity ranges from long periods of control with infrequent acute exacerbations in some children to the presence of persistent daily symptoms in others.
- Air pollution, allergens, family history, and viral infections might all play a role in asthma (John & Brady, 2013a).
- A significant long-term complication, chronic airway remodeling, may result from recurrent asthma exacerbation and inflammation (Sirivimonpan, 2013).
- Children with asthma are more susceptible to serious bacterial and viral respiratory infections (John & Brady, 2013a). Acute complications also include status asthmaticus and respiratory failure.

Take Note!

Teach the child and family that exposure to cigarette smoke increases the need for medications in children with asthma as well as the frequency of asthma exacerbations. Both indoor air quality and environmental pollution contribute to asthma in children (Sirivimonpan, 2013).

Pathophysiology

- Asthma results from a complex variety of responses in relation to a trigger. When trigger exposure occurs, mast cells, T lymphocytes, macrophages, and epithelial cells are involved in the release of inflammatory mediators.
- Eosinophils and neutrophils migrate to the airway, causing injury. Chemical mediators such as leukotrienes, bradykinin, histamine, and platelet-activating factor also contribute to the inflammatory response.
- Airway mucous secretion is increased, mucociliary function changes, and airway smooth muscle responsiveness increases. As a result, acute bronchoconstriction, airway edema, and mucous plugging occur.
- Airway remodeling occurs as a result of chronic inflammation of the airway (Sirivimonpan, 2013). Following the acute response to a trigger, continued allergen response results in a chronic phase. During this phase, the epithelial cells are denuded and the influx of inflammatory cells into the airway continues. This results in structural changes of the airway that are irreversible, and further loss of pulmonary function might occur.
- The irreversible changes include thickening of the sub-basement membrane, subepithelial fibrosis, airway smooth muscle hypertrophy and hyperplasia, blood vessel proliferation and dilation, and mucous gland hyperplasia and hypersecretion (Sirivimonpan, 2013).
- In some individuals with poorly controlled asthma, these changes may be permanent, resulting in decreased responsiveness to therapy.

Therapeutic Management

- Current goals of medical therapy are avoidance of asthma triggers and reduction or control of inflammatory episodes.
- The most recent recommendations by the NAEPP (2007) suggest a stepwise approach to medication management as well as control of environmental factors (allergens) and comorbid conditions that affect asthma.
- The stepwise approach to asthma treatment involves increasing medications as the child's condition worsens and then backing off treatment as he or she improves (Table 2.2).

Assessment Findings

Health History

- Cough (particularly at night)
- Hacking cough initially nonproductive, eventually becoming productive of frothy sputum

TABLE 2.2   STEPWISE APPROACH TO ASTHMA MANAGEMENT

All children: child education, environmental control, and management of comorbidities at each step. Consider referral to asthma specialist at step 3. (Step 2 and above are persistent asthma.)

Step 1 (intermittent asthma)
  Preferred: short-acting β_2-agonist PRN

Step 2
  Preferred: low-dose inhaled corticosteroid
  Alternative: cromolyn or leukotriene modifier

Step 3
  Preferred: medium-dose inhaled corticosteroid (all ages) OR low-dose inhaled corticosteroid and leukotriene modifier or long-acting β_2-agonist (children older than 4 years)

Step 4
  Preferred: medium-dose inhaled corticosteroids and long-acting β_2-agonist (can use leukotriene modifier in children younger than 4 years)

Step 5
  Preferred: high-dose inhaled corticosteroids and long-acting β_2-agonist (or leukotriene modifier or theophylline)

Step 6
  Preferred: high-dose inhaled corticosteroids, long-acting β_2-agonist, and oral systemic corticosteroids

Adapted from National Asthma Education and Prevention Program. (2007). Expert panel report 3: Guidelines for the diagnosis and management of asthma (NIH Publication No. 07–4051). Bethesda, MD: National Institutes of Health, National Heart, Lung and Blood Institute.
These recommendations are intended to be used as a guide in individualized asthma care.

- Difficulty breathing (shortness of breath, chest tightness or pain, dyspnea with exercise)
- Wheezing.

Risk Factors
- History of allergic rhinitis or atopic dermatitis
- Family history of atopy
- Recurrent episodes of wheezing
- Known allergies
- Seasonal response to environmental pollen, tobacco smoke exposure, or poverty.

Physical Examination
- Cyanosis

- Variable work of breathing (retractions, accessory muscle use, head bobbing)
- Anxious or fearful appearance, lethargy, or irritability
- Cough, audible wheeze might be present
- Wheezing, coarseness, and/or decreased aeration upon auscultation.

Laboratory and Diagnostic Tests

- Oxygen saturation may be normal or significantly decreased (via pulse oximetry).
- Chest x-ray usually reveals hyperinflation.
- Blood gases may reveal carbon dioxide retention and hypoxemia.
- Peak expiratory flow rate is decreased during an exacerbation.

Nursing Interventions

- Frequently assess the child's respiratory and neurologic status.
- Administer supplemental oxygen and medications as ordered.
- Provide family/child education about the lifelong management of asthma.
- Ensure each child/family is in receipt of a written action plan related to routine and illness asthma management (Fig. 2.4).
- Ensure the child has relief medication available at all times (even at school).
- Educate families and children on the appropriate use of nebulizers, metered-dose inhalers, spacers, dry-powder inhalers, and Diskus, as

Yellow Zone: Getting Worse **Contact Physician if using quick relief more than 2 times per week.**

Symptoms
- Some problems breathing
- Cough, wheeze or chest tight
- Problems working or playing
- Wake at night

Peak Flow Meter
Between 50 to 80% of personal best or
________ to ________

Continue control medicines and add:

Medicine	How Much to Take	When To Take It

IF your symptoms (and peak flow, if used) return to Green Zone after one hour of the quick relief treatment, THEN
- ○ Take quick-relief medication every 4 hours for 1 to 2 days
- ○ Change your long-term control medicines by ________
- ○ Contact your physician for follow-up care

IF your symptoms (and peak flow, if used) DO NOT return to the GREEN ZONE after 1 hour of the quick relief treatment, THEN
- ○ Take quick-relief treatment again
- ○ Change your long-term control medicines by ________
- ○ Call your physician/Health Care Provider within _____ hours of modifying your medication routine

Red Zone: Medical Alert **Ambulance/Emergency Phone Number:**

Symptoms
- Lots of problems breathing
- Cannot work or play
- Getting worse instead of better
- Medicine is not helping

Peak Flow Meter
Between 0 to 50% of personal best or
________ to ________

Continue control medicines and add:

Medicine	How Much to Take	When To Take It

Go to the hospital or call for an ambulance if
- ○ Still in the red zone after 15 minutes
- ○ If you have not been able to reach your physician/health care provider for help
- ○ ________

Call an ambulance immediately if the following danger signs are present
- ○ Trouble walking/talking due to shortness of breath
- ○ Lips or fingernails are blue

FIGURE 2.4 Asthma action plan (Used with permission from American Academy of Allergy Asthma & Immunology, www.aaaai.org).

well as the purposes, functions, and side effects of the medications they deliver. Require return demonstrations of equipment use to ensure that children and families can use the equipment properly (Teaching Guidelines 2.2).
- Instruct in and require return demonstration of peak flow meter.
- Teach families about allergen avoidance (Teaching Guidelines 2.3).
- Transfer care and management to the child as developmentally able.
- Offer support and refer families to local and national groups as needed.

Take Note!

The NAEPP (2007) recommends use of a spacer or holding chamber with metered-dose inhalers to increase the bioavailability of medication in the lungs.

Teaching Guidelines 2.2
USING ASTHMA MEDICATION DELIVERY DEVICES

Nebulizer
1. Plug in the nebulizer and connect the air compressor tubing.

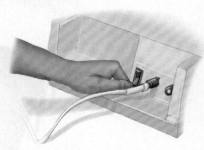

2. Add the medication to the medicine cup.

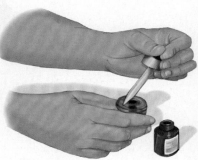

3. Attach the mask or the mouthpiece and hose to the medicine cup.

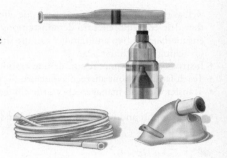

4. Place the mask on the child *or*

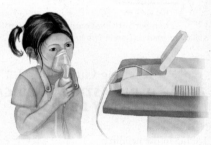

5. Instruct the child to close the lips around the mouthpiece and breathe through the mouth.

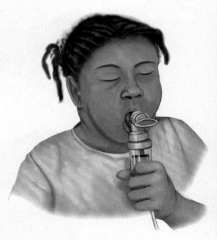

6. After use, wash the mouthpiece and medicine cup with water and allow to air dry.

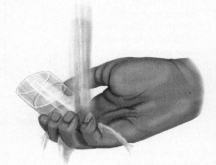

Metered-Dose Inhaler
1. Shake the inhaler and take off the cap.

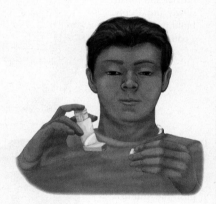

2. Attach the inhaler to the spacer or holding chamber.
3. Breathe out completely.

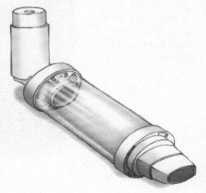

4. Put the spacer mouthpiece in the mouth (or place the mask over the child's nose and mouth, ensuring a good seal).

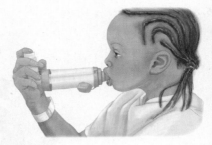

5. Compress the inhaler and inhale slowly and deeply. Hold the breath for a count of 10.

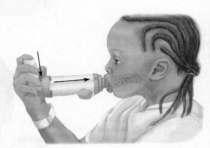

Diskus
1. Hold the Diskus in a horizontal position in one hand and push the thumb grip with the thumb of your other hand away from you until mouthpiece is exposed.

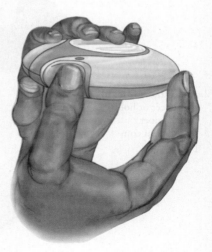

2. Push the lever until it clicks (the dose is now loaded).
3. Breathe out fully.

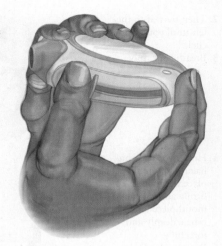

4. Place your mouth securely around the mouthpiece and breathe in fully and quickly through your mouth.
5. Remove the Diskus, hold the breath for 10 seconds, and then breathe out.

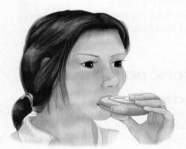

Turbuhaler

1. Hold the Turbuhaler upright. Load the dose by twisting the brown grip fully to the right.

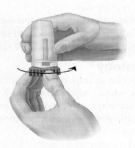

2. Then twist it to the left until you hear it click.
3. Breathe out fully.

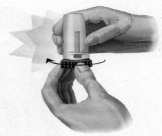

4. Holding the Turbu-haler horizontally, place the mouth firmly around the mouthpiece and inhale deeply and forcefully.
5. Remove the Turbu-haler from the mouth and then breathe out.

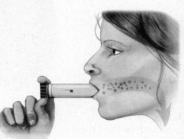

ATOPIC DERMATITIS

Description

- Atopic dermatitis (eczema) is one of the disorders in the atopy family (along with asthma and allergic rhinitis).
- Atopic dermatitis is a chronic disorder with a relapsing and remitting nature, characterized by extreme itching and inflamed, reddened, and swollen skin.
- The chronic itching associated with atopic dermatitis causes a great deal of psychological distress, and the child's self-image may be affected.
- Difficulty sleeping may occur because of the itching.

Pathophysiology

- Skin reaction occurs in response to specific allergens, usually food (especially eggs, wheat, milk, and peanuts), environmental triggers (e.g., molds, dust mites, and cat dander), or other factors such as high or low ambient temperatures, perspiring, scratching, skin irritants, or stress.
- When the child encounters a triggering antigen, antigen-present-ing cells stimulate interleukins to begin the inflammatory process.

(text continues on page 112)

Teaching Guidelines 2.3
CONTROLLING EXPOSURE TO ALLERGENS

Tobacco
- Avoid all exposure to tobacco smoke.
- If parents cannot quit, they must not smoke inside the home or car.

Dust Mites
- Use pillow and mattress covers.
- Wash sheets, pillowcases, and comforters once a week in 130°F water.
- Use blinds rather than curtains in bedroom.
- Remove stuffed animals from bedroom.
- Reduce indoor humidity to <50%.
- Remove carpet from bedroom.
- Clean solid-surface floors with wet mop each week.

Pet Dander
- Remove pets from home permanently.
- If unable to remove them, keep them out of bedroom and off carpet and upholstered furniture.

Cockroaches
- Keep kitchen very clean.
- Avoiding leaving food or drinks out.
- Use pesticides if necessary, but ensure that the asthmatic child is not inside the home when the pesticide is sprayed.

Indoor Molds
- Repair water leaks.
- Use dehumidifier to keep basement dry.
- Reduce indoor humidity to <50%.

Outdoor Molds, Pollen, and Air Pollution
- Avoid going outdoors when mold and pollen counts are high.
- Avoid outdoor activity when pollution levels are high.

Adapted from National Asthma Education and Prevention Program. (2007). Expert panel report 3: Guidelines for the diagnosis and management of asthma (NIH Publication No. 07–4051). Bethesda, MD: National Institutes of Health, National Heart, Lung and Blood Institute; John, R. M. & Brady, M. A. (2013b). Respiratory disorders. In C. E. Burns, A. M. Dunn., M. A. Brady, N. B. Starr, & C. G. Blosser (Eds.), *Pediatric primary care* (5th ed.). Philadelphia, PA: Elsevier Saunders.

The skin begins to feel pruritic and the child starts to scratch. The sensation of itchiness comes first and then the rash becomes apparent. The scratching causes the rash to appear.

Therapeutic Management

- Good skin hydration
- Application of topical corticosteroids or immunomodulators
- Oral antihistamines for sedative effects
- Antibiotics if secondary infection occurs.

Assessment Findings

Health History

- Wiggling or scratching
- Dry skin
- Scratch marks noticed by the parents
- Disrupted sleep
- Irritability.

Risk Factors

- Family history of atopic dermatitis, allergic rhinitis, or asthma
- Child's history of asthma or allergic rhinitis
- Food or environmental allergies.

Physical Examination

- Wiggling or active scratching
- Dry, scaly, or flaky skin, hypertrophy, or lichenification (Fig. 2.5)
- Dry lesions or weepy papules or vesicles

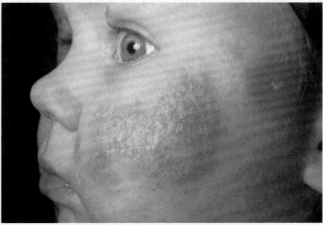

FIGURE 2.5 Atopic dermatitis rash is red, dry, and scaly.

- Rash distribution in children younger than 2 years: face, scalp, wrists, and extensor surfaces of the arms or legs; in older children: most common in flexor areas but can occur anywhere on the skin
- Erythema or warmth (secondary bacterial infection)
- Areas of hyperpigmentation or hypopigmentation
- Symptoms of allergic rhinitis
- Wheezing (with associated asthma).

Laboratory and Diagnostic Tests
- Serum immunoglobulin (Ig) E levels: may be elevated in the child with atopic dermatitis.
- Skin prick allergy testing: may determine the food or environmental allergen to which the child is sensitive.

Nursing Interventions
- Avoid hot water and any skin or hair product containing perfumes, dyes, or fragrance.
- Bathe the child twice daily in warm (not hot) water, using a mild soap to clean only the dirty areas.
- Slightly pat the child dry after the bath, but do not rub with the towel, leaving the child moist.
- Apply topical ointments or creams as prescribed to the affected area.
- Apply fragrance-free moisturizer over the prescribed topical medication and all over the child's body. Apply moisture multiple times throughout the day.
- Teach parents to avoid clothing made of synthetic fabrics or wool and to avoid known triggers.
- Cut the child's fingernails short and keep them clean.
- Prevent the child from scratching (may require antihistamines at bedtime).
- Behavior modification may be helpful with scratching.

Take Note!

Vaseline or generic petrolatum is an inexpensive, readily available moisturizer.

ATTENTION DEFICIT HYPERACTIVITY DISORDER

Description
- Attention deficit hyperactivity disorder (ADHD) is characterized by inattention, impulsivity, distractibility, and hyperactivity.
- Three subtypes of ADHD exist: hyperactive-impulsive, inattentive, and combined.

- The child with ADHD has a disruption in learning ability, socialization, and compliance, thus placing significant demands on the child, parents, teachers, and community.
- Children and teens with ADHD experience frustration, labile moods, emotional outbursts, peer rejection, poor school performance, low self-esteem, poor metacognitive abilities such as poor organization, poor time management, and the inability to break a project down into a series of smaller tasks (Starr, Fookson, Burns, & Bowman-Harvey, 2013).

Pathophysiology
- Although the exact cause of ADHD remains unidentified, current thought includes its etiology as an alteration in the dopamine and norepinephrine neurotransmitter system.
- The symptoms of impulsivity, hyperactivity, and inattention begin before 7 years of age and persist longer than 6 months.

Therapeutic Management
- Medication management of ADHD includes the use of psychostimulants, nonstimulant norepinephrine reuptake inhibitors, and/or alpha-agonist antihypertensive agents, helping to increase the child's ability to pay attention and decrease the level of impulsive behavior.
- Behavior therapy and classroom restructuring may be useful.

Assessment Findings
Health History
- Inattentiveness
- Behavioral issues
- Larger than usual number of accidents
- Family history of ADHD
- School performance problems, including inability to stay on task, poor organizational skills, talking out of turn, leaving his or her desk frequently, and either neglecting to complete or forgetting to turn in in-class and homework assignments.

Risk Factors
- Head trauma
- Lead exposure
- Cigarette smoke exposure
- Prematurity
- Low birth weight.

Physical Examination
- Quickness
- Agility

- Fearlessness
- Desire to touch or explore everything in the room.

Nursing Interventions
- Provide emotional support, allowing enough time for families to air their concerns. Work with the child and family to develop goals such as completion of homework, improved communication, or increasing independence in self-care.
- Flag the child's chart and set up a schedule for systematic communication with the family and the school.
- Teach families and school personnel to use behavioral techniques such as time-out, positive reinforcement, reward or privilege withdrawal, or a token system.
- Refer families to local support groups and the national ADHD support group (www.chadd.org).
- Teach families that stimulant medications should be taken in the morning to decrease the adverse effect of insomnia. Some children may experience decreased appetite, so giving the medication with or after the meal may be beneficial.

AUTISM

Description
- Autism spectrum disorder (ASD), also termed pervasive developmental disorder, has its onset in infancy or early childhood; it can range from mild to severe.
- Autistic behaviors may be first noticed in infancy as developmental delays or between 12 and 36 months of age when the child regresses or loses previously acquired skills. Parental concerns about development may be sensitive indicators of the development of autism.
- Children with ASD display impaired social interactions and communication as well as perseverative or stereotypic behaviors. They may fail to develop interpersonal relationships and experience social isolation. Many children with autism are intellectually disabled, requiring lifelong supervision. However, some are intellectually gifted.

Pathophysiology
- Although the exact etiology of autism is unknown, it may be due to genetic makeup, brain abnormalities, altered chemistry, a virus, or toxic chemicals.

Therapeutic Management
- The goal of therapeutic management is for the child to reach optimal functioning within the limitations of the disorder.

- Each child's treatment is individualized; behavioral and communication therapies are very important. Children with ASD respond very well to highly structured educational environments.
- Stimulants may be used to control hyperactivity, and antipsychotic medications are sometimes helpful in children with repetitive and aggressive behaviors.

Assessment Findings

Health History

- Delay or regression in developmental skills, particularly speech and language abilities
- Mutism
- Utterance of only sounds (not words)
- Repetition of words or phrases over and over
- Repetitive activity (often for hours at a time)
- Bizarre motor and stereotypic behaviors
- Infantile resistance to cuddling
- Lack of eye contact
- Indifference to touch or affection
- Little change in facial expression
- Toddler hyperactivity, aggression, temper tantrums, or self-injurious behaviors, such as head-banging or hand-biting
- Hypersensitivity to touch
- Hyposensitivity to pain.

Physical Examination

- Lack of eye contact
- Failure to look at objects pointed to by the examiner
- Failure to point to himself
- Failure to let his or her needs be known
- Perseverative play activities
- Unusual behavior such as hand-flapping or spinning
- Macrocephaly or microcephaly
- Large, prominent, or posteriorly rotated ears
- Hypo- or hyperpigmented skin lesions
- Asymmetry of nerve function or palsy
- Hypertonia
- Hypotonia
- Alterations in deep tendon reflexes
- Toe-walking
- Loose gait
- Poor coordination.

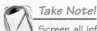

Take Note!

Screen all infants and toddlers for the following warning signs of autism:
- Not babbling by 12 months
- Not pointing or using gestures by 12 months
- No single words by 16 months
- No two-word utterances by 24 months
- Losing language or social skills at any age (Starr et al., 2013).

Nursing Interventions

- At initial diagnosis, provide extensive emotional support, professional guidance, and education about the disorder to the parents.
- Assess the fit between the child's developmental needs and the treatment plan.
- Help parents overcome barriers to obtain appropriate educational, developmental, and behavioral treatment programs.
- Ensure that children younger than 36 months receive services via the local early intervention program and children 3 years and older have an Individualized Education Program (IEP) in place if enrolled in the public school system.
- Stress the importance of rigid, unchanging routines, as children with ASD often act out when their routine changes (which is likely to occur if the child must be hospitalized for another condition).
- Assess the parents' need for respite care and make referrals accordingly.
- Provide positive feedback to parents for their perseverance in working with their child.

BACTERIAL SKIN INFECTIONS

Description

- Bacterial infections of the skin include bullous and nonbullous impetigo, folliculitis, cellulitis, and staphylococcal scalded skin syndrome. Impetigo, folliculitis, and cellulitis are usually self-limited disorders that rarely become severe.
- Of particular concern are bacterial skin infections caused by community-acquired methicillin-resistant *Staphylococcus aureus* (CA-MRSA; Baddour, 2015).
- CA-MRSA infection most commonly occurs as a skin or soft tissue infection, such as cellulitis or an abscess.

Pathophysiology

- Bacterial skin infections are often caused by *S. aureus* and group A beta-hemolytic streptococci, which are ordinarily normal flora on the skin.
- Impetigo is a readily recognizable skin rash.
- Nonbullous impetigo generally follows some type of skin trauma or may arise as a secondary bacterial infection.
- Both types of impetigo most often result from toxin production by *S. aureus*.
- Folliculitis, infection of the hair follicle, most often results from occlusion of the hair follicle.
- Cellulitis is a localized infection and inflammation of the skin and subcutaneous tissues and is usually preceded by skin trauma of some sort.
- Staphylococcal scalded skin syndrome results from infection with *S. aureus* that produces a toxin, which then causes exfoliation. It has an abrupt onset and results in diffuse erythema and skin tenderness.

Therapeutic Management

- Appropriate hygiene
- Topical or systemic antibiotics depending upon extent and severity of skin involvement
- Cool compresses to remove crusting with impetigo; warm compresses for folliculitis

Assessment Findings

Health History

- History of skin disruption such as a cut, scrape, insect/spider bite, or body piercing.

Risk Factors

- Poor hygiene
- For *CA-MRSA infection:*
  - Turf burns
  - Towel sharing
  - Participation in team sports
  - Attendance at daycare or outdoor camps
- For *folliculitis:*
  - Prolonged contact with contaminated water
  - Maceration
  - A moist environment
  - Use of occlusive emollient products.

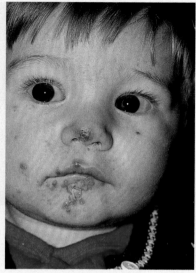

FIGURE 2.6 Impetigo.

Physical Examination

- *Nonbullous impetigo*
  - Papules progressing to vesicles and then painless pustules with a narrow erythematous border
  - Honey-colored exudate when lesions rupture, forming a crust on the ulcer-like base (Fig. 2.6)
  - Regional lymphadenopathy
- *Bullous impetigo*
  - Fever
  - Red macules and bullous eruptions on an erythematous base
  - Regional lymphadenopathy
- *Folliculitis*
  - Red, raised hair follicles
- *Cellulitis*
  - Fever
  - Erythema
  - Pain
  - Edema
  - Warmth at the site of skin disruption (Fig. 2.7)
  - Regional lymphadenopathy.

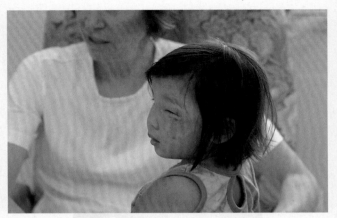

FIGURE 2.7 Cellulitis.

- *Staphylococcal scalded skin syndrome*
  - Fever
  - Flattish bullae that rupture within hours, leaving a red, weeping surface.

Laboratory and Diagnostic Tests
- Blood cultures are indicated in the child with cellulitis with lymphangitic streaking and in all cases of periorbital or orbital cellulitis.

Nursing Interventions
- Administer antibiotics topically or systemically as prescribed.
- Soak impetiginous lesions with cool compresses or Burow solution to remove crusts before applying topical antibiotics.
- Teach the family about antibiotic administration, care of the lesions or rash, and the importance of cleanliness, hygiene, and keeping fingernails short and clean.
- For impetigo, removal from school or daycare is not necessary unless the condition is widespread or actively weeping.
- Prevent transmission of nosocomial MRSA by appropriately isolating children according to the institution's policy when the child is hospitalized.
- In children with scalded skin syndrome, decrease the risk of scarring by handling minimally, applying soothing ointments as the skin heals, and avoiding corticosteroids.

BACTERIAL MENINGITIS

Description
- Bacterial meningitis is an infection of the meninges, the lining that surrounds the brain and the spinal cord.
- It can lead to brain damage, nerve damage, deafness, stroke, and even death.

Pathophysiology
- Bacterial meningitis causes inflammation, swelling, purulent exudates, and tissue damage to the brain.
- It can occur as a secondary infection to upper respiratory infections (URIs), sinus infections, or ear infections and can also be the result of direct introduction through lumbar puncture; skull fracture or severe head injury; neurosurgical intervention; congenital structural abnormalities, such as spina bifida; or the presence of foreign bodies, such as a ventricular shunt or cochlear implant (Table 2.3).

Therapeutic Management
- Bacterial meningitis is a medical emergency and requires prompt hospitalization and treatment.

TABLE 2.3	COMMON CAUSES OF MENINGITIS IN DIFFERENT AGE GROUPS
Age Affected	**Causative Organism**
Newborns and infants (birth to 3 months)	*Escherichia coli;* Streptococcus group B; *Listeria monocytogenes; Pseudomonas aerug*inosa; staphylococuus species
Infants and children (3 months to 6 years)	*Streptococcus pneumoniae; Neisseria meningitides* (meningococcal meningitis); *Haemophilus influenzae* type B
Older children and adolescents (6 years to 16 years)	*Streptococcus pneumoniae; N. meningitides* (meningococcal meningitis); *Mycobacterium tuberculosis*

Adapted from Zak, M., & Chan, V. W. (2014). Chapter 46: Pediatric neurologic disorders. In S. M. Nettina (Ed.), *Lippincott manual of nursing practice* (10th ed., pp. 1545–1575). Philadelphia, PA: Wolters/Kluwer Health: Lippincott Williams & Wilkins; Centers for Disease Control and Prevention. (2014a). Meningitis: Bacterial Meningiti. Retrieved October 10, 2015 from http://www.cdc.gov/meningitis/bacterial.html

- IV antibiotics will be started immediately after the lumbar puncture and blood cultures have been obtained if bacterial meningitis is suspected.
- The length of therapy and specific antibiotic will be determined on the basis of the analysis and the culture and sensitivity of the cerebrospinal fluid (CSF).
- Corticosteroids may be ordered to help reduce the inflammatory process.
- Specific medical treatment varies on the basis of the suspected causative organism and will be determined by the physician or nurse practitioner.

Assessment Findings

Health History

- Sudden onset of symptoms
- Preceding respiratory illness or sore throat
- Presence of fever and chills
- Headache
- Vomiting
- Photophobia
- Stiff neck
- Rash
- Irritability
- Drowsiness
- Lethargy
- Muscle rigidity
- Seizures
- Symptoms in infants can be more subtle and atypical and include poor sucking and feeding, weak cry, lethargy, and vomiting.

Risk Factors

- Young age: 1 month to 5 years, with most cases in children younger than 1 year and adolescents and young adults 15 to 24 years of age
- Any fever or illness during pregnancy or around delivery (for infants younger than 3 months)
- Exposure to ill people
- Exposure to tuberculosis
- Recent travel
- History of maternal illness
- Recent neurosurgical procedure or head trauma
- Presence of a foreign body, such as a shunt or a cochlear implant
- Immunocompromised status
- Close-contact living spaces such as dormitories or military bases
- Daycare attendance.

Physical Examination
- The infant with bacterial meningitis may rest in the opisthotonic position.
- The older child may complain of neck pain.
- In the infant, a bulging fontanel may be present (which is often a late sign).
- The infant may be consolable when lying still as opposed to being held.
- Positive Kernig sign and Brudzinski signs may be present.
- Petechial, vesicular, or macular rash may be present.

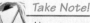

Take Note!
Abrupt eruption of a petechial or purplish rash can be indicative of meningococcemia (infection with *Neisseria meningitides*). Immediate medical attention is warranted.

Laboratory and Diagnostic Tests
- Lumbar puncture: Fluid pressure will be measured and a sample is obtained for analysis and culture. CSF will reveal increased WBCs and protein and low glucose levels (the bacteria present feed on the glucose).
- CBC count: WBCs will be elevated.
- Blood, urine, and nasopharyngeal culture—Performed to look for source of infection and to rule out sepsis. Blood culture will be positive in cases of septicemia.

Nursing Interventions
- Administer prescribed antibiotics as soon as possible after obtaining cultures
- Initiate supportive measures to ensure proper ventilation, reduce the inflammatory response, and help prevent injury to the brain.
- Interventions are aimed at reducing intracranial pressure (ICP) and maintaining cerebral perfusion along with treating fluid volume deficit, controlling seizures, and preventing injury that may result from altered LOC or seizure activity.
- Initiate appropriate isolation precautions. In addition to standard precautions, infants and children with a diagnosis of bacterial meningitis will be placed on droplet isolation until 24 hours of antibiotics have been received to help prevent transmission to others.
- Manage and reduce fever.
- Administer antipyretics such as acetaminophen and NSAIDS such as ibuprofen, per order. Institute nonpharmacologic measures if needed.

- Teach the family that early recognition of the signs and symptoms of meningitis is essential in preventing morbidity and mortality.
- Teach the parents about the ways to prevent bacterial meningitis including the following:
  - Minimize contact with anyone suspected of having meningitis. Most at risk are those living with the child or anyone with whom the child played or was in close contact.
  - Postexposure prophylaxis and postexposure immunization may be effective.
  - Control measures should be initiated in environments where risk exists. Disinfect toys and other shared objects to decrease transmission of the microorganisms to others.
  - To reduce group B streptococcal infection in neonates, screen pregnant women; if the screening results are positive, administer intrapartum antibiotics.
  - Vaccines are available for some specific causative organisms, but complete vaccination prevention is not possible at this time. The *Haemophilus influenzae* type B (Hib) vaccine is routine starting at 2 months of age and all children should be immunized to continue the reduction of bacterial meningitis caused by *H. influenzae* type B. The pneumococcal vaccine is also routine for all children starting at 2 months of age and should be considered for preschoolers who are at risk. Children at risk include those with immunodeficiency; sickle cell disease; asplenia; chronic pulmonary, cardiac, or renal disease; diabetes mellitus (DM); cochlear implants; cerebrospinal leaks; and organ transplants.
  - Administer the meningococcal vaccination to all children aged 11 to 12 years with a booster at age 16; adolescents who receive their first dose at 13 to 15 years need a booster between 16 and 18 years; vaccination of certain at-risk groups such as all college freshmen living in dormitories; and children who are at high risk, such as children with chronic conditions or immune suppression or those who travel to high-risk areas or live in crowded conditions (American Academy of Pediatrics, 2015; MacNeil & Cohn, 2011).

BONE TUMORS (OSTEOSARCOMA AND EWING SARCOMA)

Description
- Common bone tumors in children are osteosarcoma and Ewing sarcoma (Hendershot, 2010).
- They are most often diagnosed in adolescence.

- Frequently, the tumor is diagnosed when an adolescent seeks care for pain related to a traumatic event (thus, the tumor is incidentally discovered).

Pathophysiology

- Osteosarcoma presumably arises from the embryonic mesenchymal tissue that forms the bones.
- The most common sites for osteosarcoma are in the long bones, particularly the proximal humerus, proximal tibia, and distal femur.
- Complications of osteosarcoma include metastasis and recurrence of disease within 3 years (Graham et al., 2014).
- Ewing sarcoma is a highly malignant bone tumor occurring most frequently in the pelvis, chest wall, vertebrae, and long bone diaphyses (midshaft).
- About 25% of children with Ewing sarcoma demonstrate metastasis, and the prognosis depends on the extent of metastasis (Graham et al., 2014).

Therapeutic Management

- Chemotherapy may be used before surgery to decrease the size of the tumor.
- Surgical removal of the tumor may involve radical amputation or limb salvage surgery (Abed & Grimer, 2010).
- Radiation may also be used.
- Postsurgical chemotherapy treats/prevents metastasis.

Assessment Findings

Health History

- Pain (often dull, for several months with osteosarcoma; with Ewing sarcoma, pain may become constant and severe)
- Limp
- Limitation of motion
- Possibly fever (Ewing sarcoma).

Physical Examination

- Erythema and swelling of the affected limb.

Laboratory and Diagnostic Tests

- CT scan or magnetic resonance imaging (MRI) reveals the extent of the lesion and, possibly, metastasis.
- Biopsy of the lesion yields tumor type.
- Bone scan determines the extent of metastasis.
- Bone marrow aspiration may also be used to evaluate metastasis.

Nursing Interventions

- Refer to the section on leukemia for information related to care of the child receiving chemotherapy.

- Present preoperative teaching at the adolescent's developmental level and ensure that he or she is included in planning treatment.
- Provide support and encouragement to decrease anxiety and improve self-esteem related to body image changes.
- Provide routine orthopedic postoperative care.
- If amputation is necessary, educate the adolescent and parents on the care of the stump and prosthesis (if ordered), as well as crutch walking.
- Refer the adolescent to another teen who has undergone a similar procedure or to a peer support group if available.

BRAIN TUMOR

Description
- Brain tumors are the most common form of solid tumor and the second most common type of cancer in children (Graham et al., 2014).
- Slightly more than half of brain tumors arise in the posterior fossa (infratentorial); the rest are supratentorial in origin.
- Some tumors are localized (low-grade), whereas others are of higher grade and more invasive. The prognosis depends on the location of the tumor and extent of tumor.
- Complications of brain tumors include hydrocephalus, increased ICP, brain stem herniation, and negative effects of radiation such as neuropsychological, intellectual, and endocrinologic sequelae (Kline & O'Hanlon-Curry, 2010; Graham et al., 2014).

Pathophysiology
- The cause of brain tumors is generally not known, but the effects of brain tumors are predictable. As the tumor grows within the cranium, it exerts pressure on the brain tissues surrounding it.
- The tumor mass may compress vital structures in the brain, block CSF flow, or cause edema in the brain.
- The result is an increase in ICP.

Therapeutic Management
- The tumor may be surgically resected depending upon its location within the brain.
- Ventriculoperitoneal shunting is used for children who have also developed hydrocephalus.
- Chemotherapy may be prescribed and radiation may be used in children older than 2 years (not younger because it can have long-term neurocognitive effects; Graham et al., 2014).

Assessment Findings

Health History

- Nausea or vomiting
- Headache
- Unsteady gait
- Blurred or double vision
- Seizures
- Motor abnormality or hemiparesis
- Weakness
- Swallowing difficulties
- Behavior or personality changes
- Irritability
- Failure to thrive
- Developmental delay (in very young children).

Risk Factors

- History of neurofibromatosis
- History of tuberous sclerosis
- Prior treatment of CNS leukemia.

Physical Examination

- Strabismus or nystagmus
- "Sunsetting" eyes
- Head tilt
- Alterations in coordination
- Gait disturbance
- Alteration in pupillary reaction, sensation, or gag reflex
- Sensation or gag reflex
- Cranial nerve palsy
- Lethargy
- Irritability
- Opisthotonos (Fig. 2.8)
- Blood pressure may decrease with increasing ICP.
- Deep tendon reflexes may be hyperreactive.
- The infant may present with a bulging anterior fontanel.

Take Note!

A fixed and dilated pupil is a neurosurgical emergency.

Laboratory and Diagnostic Tests

- CT, MRI, or positron emission tomography will demonstrate evidence of the tumor and its location within the intracranial cavity.

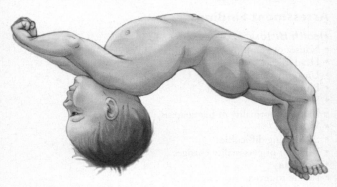

FIGURE 2.8 Opisthotonos.

- Lumbar puncture with CSF cell evaluation may show tumor markers or the presence of alpha-fetoprotein (AFP) or human chorionic gonadotropin, which may assist in the diagnosis.

Nursing Interventions

Preoperative Nursing Interventions
- Monitor for additional increases in ICP.
- Administer dexamethasone as prescribed to decrease intracranial inflammation.
- Prevent straining with bowel movements by the use of a stool softener.
- Assess the child's pain level as well of LOC, vital signs, and pupillary reaction to determine subtle changes as soon as possible.
- Provide a tour of the intensive care unit; instruct the child and family about the possibility of intubation and ventilation in the postoperative period.
- If a ventriculoperitoneal shunt will be placed for the treatment of hydrocephalus caused by the tumor, provide education about shunts to the child and family.
- Shave the portion of the head as determined by the neurosurgeon.

Postoperative Nursing Interventions
- Regulate fluid administration to avoid causing or worsening cerebral edema.
- Administer mannitol or hypertonic dextrose to decrease cerebral edema.

- Assess vital signs frequently, along with checking pupillary reactions and determining LOC (extreme lethargy or coma may be present for several days postoperatively).
- Treat hyperthermia (related to infection of hypothalamic disturbance) with antipyretics such as acetaminophen and with sponge baths, reducing the temperature slowly.
- Monitor for signs of increased ICP.
- Assess pain level (headache is common) and provide analgesics as prescribed.
- Minimize environmental stimuli, providing a calm and quiet atmosphere.
- Check the head dressing for CSF drainage or bleeding.
- Assess for and document the extent of head, face, or neck edema.
- Restrain the child if combative to maintain safety.
- Position the child on the unaffected side with the head of the bed flat or at the level prescribed by the neurosurgeon; maintain head alignment with position changes.

Take Note!

Observe preoperatively and postoperatively for signs of brain stem herniation such as opisthotonos, nuchal rigidity, head tilt, sluggish pupils, increased blood pressure with widening pulse pressure, change in respirations, bradycardia, irregular pulse, and changes in body temperature.

BRONCHIOLITIS (RSV)

Description

- Acute inflammatory process of the bronchioles and small bronchi, nearly always caused by a viral pathogen.
- Respiratory syncytial virus (RSV) accounts for the majority of cases of bronchiolitis (adenovirus, parainfluenza, and human metapneumovirus are also important causative agents).
- The severity of disease is related inversely to the age of the child. The frequency and severity of RSV infection decrease with age.

Pathophysiology

- RSV is a highly contagious virus, contracted through direct contact with respiratory secretions or from particles on objects contaminated with the virus.
- It invades the nasopharynx, where it replicates and then spreads down to the lower airway via aspiration of upper airway secretions.

- Small airways become variably obstructed, allowing adequate inspiratory volume, but prevent full expiration leading to hyperinflation and atelectasis. Serious alterations in gas exchange occur.

Therapeutic Management

- Therapeutic management focuses on supportive treatment, including:
  - supplemental oxygen
  - nasal and/or nasopharyngeal suctioning
  - oral or IV hydration and
  - inhaled bronchodilator therapy.

Assessment Findings

Health History

- Runny nose
- Pharyngitis
- Low-grade fever
- Cough
- Wheeze
- Poor feeding.

Risk Factors

- Young age (>2 years)
- Prematurity
- Multiple births
- Birth during April to September
- History of chronic lung disease (bronchopulmonary disease)
- Cyanotic or complicated congenital heart disease (CHD)
- Immunocompromise
- Male gender
- Passive tobacco smoke exposure
- Crowded living conditions
- Daycare attendance
- School-aged siblings
- Low socioeconomic status
- Lack of breast-feeding.

Physical Examination

- Air hunger
- Cyanosis
- Tachypnea, retractions, accessory muscle use, grunting, or apnea
- Cough and audible wheeze
- Listlessness; disinterest in feeding, surroundings, or parents
- Wheezing and poor aeration on auscultation.

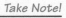 *Take Note!*

In the tachypneic infant, slowing of the respiratory rate does not necessarily indicate improvement: often, a slower respiratory rate is an indication of tiring, and carbon dioxide retention may soon be followed by apnea (American Heart Association [AHA], 2011).

Laboratory and Diagnostic Tests

- Decreased oxygen saturation per pulse oximetry.
- Hyperinflation and patchy areas of atelectasis or infiltration on chest radiographs.
- Positive identification of RSV (nasopharyngeal washings) via enzyme-linked immunosorbent assay (ELISA) or immunofluorescent antibody testing.

Nursing Interventions

- Provide supportive care: antipyretics, adequate hydration, and close observation.
- Position with the head of the bed elevated.
- Assess work of breathing, respiratory rate, breath sounds, and oxygen saturation frequently.
- Suction to maintain a patent airway.
- Maintain contact isolation to prevent spread.
- Encourage strict adherence to handwashing policies in daycare centers and when exposed to people with cold symptoms.
- To prevent RSV infection in certain high-risk children younger than 2 years, administer palivizumab (Synagis) via intramuscular injection monthly throughout the RSV season. Qualified children may include those who were born prematurely and/or have chronic lung disease (bronchopulmonary dysplasia) requiring medical intervention, certain congenital heart defects, or immunocompromise (DeNicola, Maraqua, Udeani, & Custodio, 2015).

BURNS

Description

- Children often experience burns as unintentional injury, though child abuse is a possibility in some cases.
- The majority of children younger than 4 years of age experience scald burns (Myers, 2011). Fires in the home are often related to cooking, cigarette or other smoking materials (Myers, 2011).

Pathophysiology

- Thermal injury to the skin occurs and then the tissue begins to coagulate.
- Blood vessels demonstrate increased capillary permeability, resulting in vasodilatation. This leads to increased hydrostatic pressure in the capillaries, causing water, electrolytes, and protein to leak out of the vasculature, resulting in significant edema.
- Fluid loss from burned skin occurs at an amount that is 5 to 10 times greater than that from undamaged skin, and this fluid loss continues until the damaged surface is healed or grafted.
- Initially, the severely burned child experiences a decrease in cardiac output, with a subsequent hypermetabolic response during which cardiac output increases dramatically. During this heightened metabolic state, the child is at risk for insulin resistance and increased protein catabolism.

Therapeutic Management

- Therapeutic management consists of fluid resuscitation, wound care, prevention of infection, and restoration of function.
- Burn infections are treated with antibiotics specific to the causative organism.
- If invasive burn damage occurs, surgery may be necessary.

Assessment Findings

Health History

- Mechanism of the burn injury (scald, fire, contact, etc.)
- Immunization status, especially note tetanus status.

Risk Factors

- Young or adolescent age
- Lack of adult supervision.

Physical Examination

- Erythema, blistering, weeping, or eschar.
- Superficial burns are painful, red, dry, and possibly edematous (Fig. 2.9).
- Partial-thickness and deep partial-thickness burns are very painful and edematous and have a wet appearance or blisters (Fig. 2.10).
- Full-thickness burns may be very painful or numb or pain free in some areas. They appear red, edematous, leathery, dry, or waxy and may display peeling or charred skin (Fig. 2.11).

(text continues on page 134)

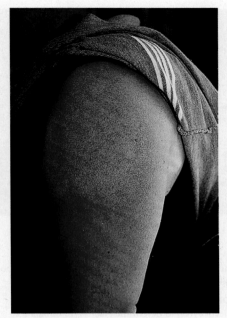

FIGURE 2.9 Superficial burn.

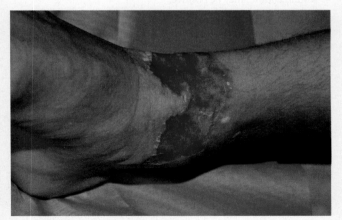

FIGURE 2.10 Partial-thickness burn.

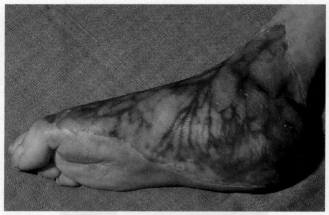

FIGURE 2.11 Full-thickness burn.

- Note whether the burn is circumferential (encircling a body part) or partially circumferential.

Laboratory and Diagnostic Tests
- Serum electrolytes: to determine electrolyte imbalance.
- CBC count: WBC elevated if infection present.
- Wound culture: may be positive.

Nursing Interventions
- Provide crystalloid IV fluid such as Ringer's lactate as ordered (warm them prior to administration).
- Strictly monitor urine output (expect at least 1 mL/kg/hour).
- Weigh the child daily.
- Monitor electrolyte levels until returned to normal.
- Maintain a neutral thermal environment; monitor the child's temperature frequently.
- Perform burn cleansing, medication application, and dressing changes as ordered.
- Provide pharmacologic and nonpharmacologic pain management.
- Administer tetanus vaccine if needed.
- Reinforce physical therapy recommendations and use of pressure garments as needed.
- Refer children and families to support networks.
- Teach families about burn care at home (see Teaching Guidelines 2.4).

Teaching Guidelines 2.4
PROVIDING BURN CARE FOR SUPERFICIAL (FIRST-DEGREE) BURNS

For Superficial (First-Degree) Burns
- Run cool water over the burned area until the pain lessens.
- Do not apply ice to the skin.
- Do not apply butter, ointment, or cream.
- Cover the burn lightly with a clean, nonadhesive bandage.
- Administer acetaminophen or ibuprofen for pain.
- Have the child seen by the physician or nurse practitioner within 24 hours.
- Ongoing care: clean in tub or shower with fragrance-free mild soap; pat or air dry.
  - Apply a thin layer of antibiotic ointment.
  - Cover with a nonadherent dressing such as Adaptic, and then cover with dry gauze.

CASTS
- Casts are used to immobilize either a bone that has been injured or a diseased joint.
- When a fracture has occurred, a cast serves to hold the bone in reduction, thus preventing deformity as the fracture heals.

Assisting with Cast Application
- Before cast or splint application:
  - Perform baseline neurovascular assessment for comparison after immobilization. Include:
    - color (note cyanosis or other discoloration)
    - movement (note inability to move fingers or toes)
    - sensation (note whether loss of sensation is present)
    - edema and
    - quality of pulses.
  - Enlist the cooperation of the child and reduce his or her fear by showing the child the cast materials and using an age-appropriate approach to describe cast application.
  - Premedicate as ordered to reduce pain when manual traction is applied to align the bone.
  - Use distraction throughout cast application and assist with application of the cast or splint.

- After the cast or splint is applied:
  - Drying time will vary on the basis of the type of material used. Splints and fiberglass casts usually take only a few minutes to dry and will cause a very warm feeling inside the cast, so warn the child that it will begin to feel very warm. Plaster requires 24 to 48 hours to dry. Take care not to cause depressions in the plaster cast while drying, as these may cause skin pressure and breakdown.
  - Instruct the child and family to keep the cast still, positioning it with pillows as needed.

Caring for the Child with a Cast

- Perform frequent neurovascular checks of the casted extremity to identify signs of compromise early. These signs include
  - increased pain
  - increased edema
  - pale or blue color
  - skin coolness
  - numbness or tingling
  - prolonged capillary refill and
  - decreased pulse strength (or absence of pulse).
- Notify the physician or nurse practitioner of changes in neurovascular status or odor or drainage from the cast.
- If the cast is plaster, petal the cast edges to prevent skin rubbing. Cut rounded-edge strips of moleskin or another soft material with an adhesive backing and apply them to the edge of cast. If a cast is lined with GORE-TEX, do not petal it.
- Position the child with the casted extremity elevated on pillows.
- Apply ice during the first 24 to 48 hours after casting, if needed.
- Teach the child with lower extremity immobilization to use crutches so that the child can maintain mobility.
- Provide home care instructions to the family about cast care (Teaching Guidelines 2.5).

Take Note!

Persistent complaints of pain may indicate compromised skin integrity under the cast.

Assisting With Cast Removal

- Children may be frightened by cast removal.
- Prepare the child using age-appropriate terminology:
  - The cast cutter will make a loud noise.

(text continues on page 138)

Teaching Guidelines 2.5
HOME CAST CARE

- For the first 48 hours, elevate the extremity above the level of the heart and apply cold therapy for 20–30 minutes, then off 1–2 hours, and repeat.
- Take your prescribed pain medication
- Assess for swelling, and have the child wiggle the fingers or toes hourly.
- For itching inside the cast:
- Never insert anything into the cast for the purposes of scratching.
- Blow cool air in from a hair dryer set on the lowest setting or tap lightly on the cast.
- Do not use lotions or powders.
- Do not pull padding out from the inside of the cast
- Protect the cast from wetness.
- Apply a plastic bag around cast and tape securely for bathing or showering. Continue to avoid placing the cast directly in water (unless it is Gore-Tex lined).
- Waterproof cast covers are available through medical supply stores (still remain cautious about submerging cast with water).
- Cover it when your child eats or drinks.
- If a cast become soiled it can be wiped clean with a slightly damp clean cloth.
- If the cast gets wet, dry it with a blow dryer on the cold setting (if warm setting is used the child could get burned). Use of a vacuum cleaner with a hose attachment to pull air through may speed drying-be careful to avoid skin.
- If the child has a large cast, change position every 2 hours during the day and while sleeping change position as often as possible.
- Check the skin for irritation.
- Press the skin back around edges of the cast.
- Use a flashlight to look for reddened or irritated areas.
- Feel for blisters or sores.
- Call the physician or nurse practitioner if:
- The casted extremity is cool to the touch, pale, blue, or very swollen.
- The child cannot move the fingers or toes.
- Severe pain occurs when the child attempts to move the fingers or toes.
- Persistent numbness or tingling occurs.
- Drainage or a foul smell comes from under the cast.
- Severe itching occurs inside the cast.
- The child runs a fever greater than 101.5°F for longer than 24 hours.
- Skin edges are red and swollen or exhibit breakdown.
- Child complains of rubbing or burning under cast.
- The cast gets wet and does not dry or is cracked, split, or softened.

Adapted from Bowden, V. R., & Greenberg, C. S. (2012). Pediatric nursing procedures (3rd ed.). Philadelphia, PA: Lippincott Williams & Wilkins; Schweich, P. (2014). Patient information: Cast and splint care (beyond the basics). UpToDate. Retrieved on October 10, 2015, from http://www.uptodate.com/contents/cast-and-splint-care-beyond-the-basics?source=see_link

Teaching Guidelines 2.6
SKIN CARE AFTER CAST REMOVAL

- Brown, flaky skin is normal and occurs as dead skin and secretions accumulate under the cast
- New skin may be tender
- Soak with warm water daily
- Wash with warm soapy water, avoiding excessive rubbing, which may traumatize the skin
- Discourage the child from scratching the dry skin
- Apply moisturizing lotion to relieve dry skin
- Encourage activity to regain strength and motion of extremity.

- The skin or extremity will not be injured (demonstrate by touching the cast cutter lightly to your palm).
- The child will feel warmth or vibration during cast removal.
- Teaching Guidelines 2.6 gives instructions related to skin care after cast removal.

CEREBRAL PALSY

Description
- Cerebral palsy is a term used to describe a range of nonspecific clinical symptoms characterized by abnormal motor pattern and postures caused by nonprogressive abnormal brain function.
- Cerebral palsy usually occurs before delivery due to abnormal development of the motor areas of the brain. However, it can also be caused by damage to the motor areas of the brain in the natal and postnatal periods. (Johnston, 2011; Zak & Chan, 2014). However, many times no specific cause can be identified.
- Cerebral palsy is the most common movement disorder of childhood; it is a lifelong condition and one of the most common causes of physical disability in children (Johnston, 2011).
- Most affected children will develop symptoms in infancy or early childhood.
- There is a large variation in symptoms and disability. For some children, it may be as mild as a slight limp; for others, it may result in severe motor and neurologic impairments.
- Primary signs include motor impairments such as spasticity, muscle weakness, and ataxia.

- Complications include mental impairments, seizures, growth problems, impaired vision or hearing, abnormal sensation or perception, and hydrocephalus. Most children can survive into adulthood but may suffer substantial impairments in function and quality of life.

Pathophysiology

- Cerebral palsy is a disorder caused by abnormal development of, or damage to, the motor areas of the brain. It results in a disruption in the brain's ability to control movement and posture.
- It is difficult to establish an exact location of the neurologic lesion, and the lesion itself does not change; thus, the disorder is considered nonprogressive because the brain injury does not progress.
- However, the clinical manifestations of the lesion change as the child grows. Some children may improve, but many either plateau in their attainment of motor skills or demonstrate worsening of motor abilities, as it is difficult to maintain the ability to move over time.

Therapeutic Management

- The overall focus of therapeutic management is to assist the child to gain optimal development and function within the limits of the disease. Treatment is symptomatic, preventive, and supportive.
- Spasticity management is a primary concern and treatment is determined by clinical findings. There is no standard treatment option for all children.

Medical Management

- Medical management is focused on promoting mobility through the use of therapeutic modalities, including physical, occupational, and speech therapy and medications.
- The earlier the treatment begins, the better chance the child has of overcoming developmental disabilities (National Institute of Neurological Disorders and Stroke, 2015).

THERAPEUTIC MODALITIES

- Physical therapists work with children to assist in the development of gross motor movements such as walking and positioning, and they help the child develop independent movement. They also assist in preventing contractures, and they instruct children and caregivers in the use of assistive devices such as walkers and wheelchairs.
- Occupational therapists may be responsible for fashioning orthotics and splints. Ankle-foot orthoses (AFOs) are the most common

orthotics used by children with cerebral palsy (Cervasio, 2011). Spinal orthotics such as braces are used in young children with cerebral palsy to combat scoliosis that develops due to spasticity. Splinting is used to maintain muscle length. Serial casting may also be used to increase muscle and tendon length. Occupational therapy also assists in the development of fine motor skills and will help the child to perform optimal self-care by working on skills such as activities of daily living.

- Speech therapy assists in the development of receptive and expressive language and addresses the use of appropriate feeding techniques in the child who has swallowing problems. Speech therapists may teach augmented communication strategies to children who are nonverbal or who have articulation problems. Many children may not communicate verbally but can use alternative means such as communication books or boards and computers with voice synthesizers to make their desires known or to participate in conversation.

PHARMACOLOGIC MANAGEMENT

- Medications are also used to treat seizure disorders in children with cerebral palsy (refer to the Epilepsy section for information related to seizure management).
- Children with athetoid cerebral palsy may be given anticholinergics to help decrease abnormal movements.
- Oral medications used to treat spasticity include baclofen, dantrolene sodium, and diazepam.
- Parenterally administered medications such as botulin toxins and baclofen are also used to manage spasticity. Botulinum toxin is injected into the spastic muscle both to balance the muscle forces across joints and to decrease spasticity. It is useful in managing focal spasticity in which the spasticity is interfering with function, producing pain, or contributing to a progressive deformity. Botulin toxin is injected by the physician or advanced practitioner and can be done in the clinic or outpatient setting.
- Intrathecal administration of baclofen has been shown to decrease tone, but it must be infused continuously because of its short half-life. Surgical placement of a baclofen pump will be considered in children with general spasticity that is limiting function, comfort, activities of daily living, and endurance. To test whether it is a suitable option, an intrathecal test dose of baclofen will be administered. If the trial is successful, a baclofen pump will be implanted. Once inserted, delivery of the drug can be individualized to meet the child's unique needs. The pump

needs to be replaced every 5 to 7 years and must be refilled with medication approximately every 3 months, depending on the type of pump. Complications with baclofen pump placement include infection, rupture, dislodgement, or blockage of the catheter.

Surgical Management

- Many children will require surgical procedures to correct deformities related to spasticity.
- Multiple corrective surgeries may be required; they usually are orthopedic or neurosurgical.
- Surgery may be used to correct contractures that are severe enough to cause movement limitations.
- Common orthopedic procedures include tendon lengthening procedures, correction of hip and adductor muscle spasticity, and fusion of unstable joints to help improve locomotion, correct bony deformities, decrease painful spasticity, and maintain, restore, or stabilize a spinal deformity.
- Neurosurgical interventions may include either placement of a shunt in children who have developed hydrocephalus or surgical interventions to decrease spasticity.
- Selective dorsal root rhizotomy is used to decrease spasticity in the lower extremities by reducing the amount of stimulation that reaches the muscles via nerves.

Assessment Findings

Health History

- The health history of the *undiagnosed child* may reveal:
  - intrauterine infections
  - prematurity with intracranial hemorrhage
  - difficult, complicated, or prolonged labor and delivery
  - multiple births
  - history of possible anoxia during prenatal life or birth
  - history of head trauma
  - delayed attainment of developmental milestones
  - muscle weakness or rigidity
  - poor feeding
  - hips and knees feel rigid and unbending when pulled to a sitting position
  - seizure activity
  - subnormal learning and
  - abnormal motor performance, scoots on back instead of crawling on abdomen, walks or stands on toes.

- The health history of the *child diagnosed with cerebral palsy* may reveal:
  - admission to the hospital for corrective surgeries or other complications of the disease, such as aspiration pneumonia and urinary tract infections (UTIs)
  - a cough, sputum production, or increased work of breathing
  - a change in muscle tone or increase in spasticity
  - presence of fever
    - feeding and weight loss and
    - other changes in physical state or medication regimen.

Physical Examination

- Delayed development, size for age, and sensory alterations such as strabismus, vision problems, and speech disorders.
- Abnormal postures may be present. While lying supine, the infant may demonstrate scissor crossing of the legs with plantar flexion. In the prone position, the infant may raise his or her head higher than normal due to arching of the back, or the opisthotonic position may be noted. The infant may also abnormally flex the arms and legs under the trunk.
- Primitive reflexes may persist beyond the point at which they disappear in a healthy infant.
- Evolution of protective reflexes may be delayed.
- Movement disorder. Infants with cerebral palsy may demonstrate abnormal use of muscle groups such as scooting on their back instead of crawling or walking.
- Hypertonicity is seen often. Increased resistance to dorsiflexion and passive hip abduction are the most common early signs. Sustained clonus may be present after forced dorsiflexion.
- Limited shoulder girdle function and tone.
- Prolonged standing on toes when supported in an upright standing position.
- Decreased hand strength.
- Limb deformity; decreased use of an extremity (as in the case of hemiparesis) may result in shortening of the extremity compared with the other one.

Laboratory and Diagnostic Tests

- Electroencephalogram is usually abnormal, but the pattern is highly variable.
- Cranial x-ray or ultrasound may show cerebral asymmetry.
- MRI or CT scan may show area of damage or abnormal development but may be normal.
- Screening for metabolic defects and genetic testing may be performed to help determine the cause of cerebral palsy.

Nursing Interventions

Provide Nursing Care Related to Therapeutic Management Modalities

- When casting, splinting, or orthotics are used:
  - Assess skin integrity frequently.
  - Pain management may also be necessary.
- Nursing management of children receiving botulin toxin focuses on assisting with the procedure and providing education and support to the child and family.
- Nursing interventions related to baclofen pump insertion include assisting with the test dose and providing preoperative and postoperative care if a pump is placed, as well as providing support and education to the child and family.
- Refer to Teaching Guideline 2.7, which gives information related to baclofen pump insertion.

Promote Nutrition

- Children with cerebral palsy may have difficulty eating and swallowing due to poor motor control of the throat, mouth, and tongue. This may lead to poor nutrition and problems with growth.
- The child may require a longer time to eat because of poor motor control.
- Special diets, such as soft or pureed, may make swallowing easier.

Teaching Guidelines 2.7
BACLOFEN PUMP: CHILD/FAMILY EDUCATION

- Check the incisions daily for redness, drainage, or swelling
- Notify the physician or nurse practitioner if the child has a temperature >101.5°F, or if the child has persistent incision pain
- Avoid tub baths for 2 weeks
- Do not allow the child to sleep on the stomach for 4 weeks after pump insertion
- Discourage twisting at the waist, reaching high overhead, stretching, or bending forward or backward for 4 weeks
- When the incisions have healed, normal activity may be resumed
- Wear loose clothing to prevent irritation at the incision site
- Carry implanted device identification and emergency information cards at all times.

- Proper positioning during feeding is essential to facilitate swallowing and reduce the risk of aspiration.
- Speech or occupational therapists can assist in working on strengthening swallowing muscles as well as assisting in developing accommodations to facilitate nutritional intake.
- Consult a dietitian to ensure adequate nutrition for children with cerebral palsy.
- In children with severe swallowing problems or malnutrition, a feeding tube such as a gastrostomy tube may be placed.

Educate and Support the Child and Family

- Cerebral palsy is a lifelong disorder that can result in severe physical and cognitive disability. In some cases, disability may require complete intensive daily care of the child. Adjusting to the demands of this multifaceted illness is difficult. Children are frequently hospitalized and need numerous corrective surgeries, which places strain on the family and its finances.
- From the time of diagnosis, the family should be involved in the child's care. Include parents in the planning of interventions and care of this child. In most cases, they are the primary caregivers and will assist the child in development of functioning and skills as well as providing daily care. They will provide essential information to the healthcare team and will be advocates for their child throughout his or her life. It is important that nurses provide ongoing education for the child and family.
- As the child grows, the needs of the family and child will change. Recognize and respect these needs.
- Providing daily intense care can be demanding and tiring. When a child with cerebral palsy is admitted to the hospital, this may serve as a time of respite for family and primary caregivers. Encourage respite care and provide support.
- Because cerebral palsy is a lifelong condition, children will need meaningful education programs that emphasize independence in the least restrictive educational environment. Refer caregivers to local resources, including education services and support groups. United Cerebral Palsy, a national organization, can be accessed at www.ucp.org. Easter Seals is an organization that helps children with disabilities and special needs and provides support to families (www.easterseals.com).
- Refer children younger than 3 years to the local early intervention service. Early intervention provides case management of developmental services for children with special needs. Each state has a coordinator for early intervention. The office of the early

intervention coordinator can then direct the healthcare professional to the local or district early intervention office.
- The website 4MyChild accessed at http://www.cerebralpalsy.org/cerebral-palsy-assistance/ provides a comprehensive list of contact information based on the state you live in.

CLEFT LIP AND PALATE

Description
- Cleft lip and palate is the most common congenital craniofacial anomaly.
- It is often associated with other anomalies such as chromosomal anomalies, heart defects, ear malformations, skeletal deformities, and genitourinary abnormality (Curtin & Boekelheide, 2010).
- Complications of cleft lip and palate include feeding difficulties, altered dentition, delayed or altered speech development, and otitis media.

Pathophysiology
- Development of the cleft occurs early in pregnancy (lip by 5 to 6 weeks' gestation; palate by 7 to 9 weeks) when either the lip or palate does not fuse.
- The cleft may be unilateral (the left side is affected more often) or bilateral and either the lip or the palate may be affected, or both.

Therapeutic Management
- Surgical repair of the lip and the palate are necessary.
- Ongoing management occurs via a specialized team that may include a plastic surgeon or craniofacial specialist, oral surgeon, dentist or orthodontist, prosthodontist, psychologist, otolaryngologist, nurse, social worker, audiologist, and speech–language pathologist.

Assessment Findings

Health History
- Maternal smoking
- Prenatal infection
- Advanced maternal age
- Use of anticonvulsants, steroids, and other medications during early pregnancy.

Physical Examination
- The characteristic physical appearance of cleft lip (Fig. 2.12)
- Visualization or palpation may identify cleft palate.

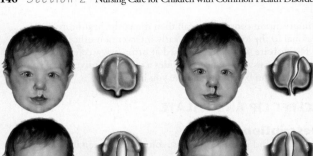

FIGURE 2.12 Cleft lip may extend all the way through the vermilion border and up to the nostril, or it may be significantly smaller. Cleft palate may be a small opening or may involve the entire palate.

Laboratory and Diagnostic Tests
- Laboratory and diagnostic tests results may include prenatal ultrasonography to identify cleft lip.

Nursing Interventions
- Encourage parent–infant bonding.
- Encourage breast-feeding in the infant with cleft lip or palate.
- If bottle-feeding, utilize specialized nipples to assist the infant to feed (Fig. 2.13). A prosthodontic device may be necessary preoperatively in some infants with cleft palate to prevent aspiration and allow nutrient ingestion.
- Provide preoperative and postoperative education, as well as family support.
  - Postoperatively, prevent injury to the suture line.
  - Place the infant in supine or side-lying positions, restraining hands as necessary.
  - Protect the repaired cleft lip with a Logan bow or butterfly adhesive.
  - Keep the suture line clean, per surgeon's preference.
  - For the repaired cleft palate, avoid putting items in the mouth that might disrupt the sutures (e.g., suction catheter, spoon, straw, pacifier, or plastic syringe).

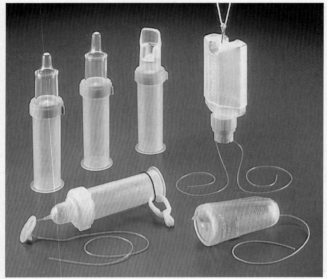

FIGURE 2.13 Feeding infants with cleft lip.

- Prevent vigorous or sustained crying in the infant by administering pain medications and providing other comfort or distraction measures, such as cuddling, rocking, and anticipation of needs.

CONGENITAL HEART DISEASE

Description
- CHD is the result of abnormal development of the heart. Abnormal openings, connections, or narrowed areas may occur.
- In some children, heart failure may occur as a result of CHD.

Pathophysiology
- CHD may result from chromosomal alterations or maternal exposure to environmental factors such as toxins, infections, chronic illnesses, and alcohol.
- Septal walls or valves may fail to develop completely, or vessels or valves may be stenotic, narrowed, or transposed. Structures that formed to allow fetal circulation may fail to close after birth, altering the pressures necessary to maintain adequate blood flow.

- Congenital heart defects are categorized on the basis of hemodynamic characteristics (blood flow patterns in the heart):
  - Disorders with decreased pulmonary blood flow: tetralogy of Fallot, tricuspid atresia
  - Disorders with increased pulmonary blood flow: patent ductus arteriosus, atrial septal defect, and ventricular septal defect
  - Obstructive disorders: coarctation of the aorta, aortic stenosis, and pulmonary stenosis
  - Mixed disorders: transposition of the great vessels, total anomalous pulmonary venous return, truncus arteriosus, and hypoplastic left heart syndrome.

Therapeutic Management

- Management depends on the severity of the child's associated symptoms. Some children lead a normal life without medical intervention. Surgical correction is required for many defects and may be a definitive treatment. However, surgical approaches may only result in palliation in some children.
- In severely cyanotic infants, prior to surgery, prostaglandin infusion will maintain patency of the ductus arteriosus, improving pulmonary blood flow.
- In children with associated heart failure, medical treatment is necessary.
- In children with failure to thrive, increased caloric intake (and/or tube feedings) is necessary.

Assessment Findings

Health History and Physical Examination

- Nursing assessment findings vary with the type and/or severity of the heart defect.
- Table 2.4 provides an illustration of each defect and common assessment findings for each defect.

Laboratory and Diagnostic Tests

- Echocardiography and cardiac catheterization reveal extent of the defect.
- Electrocardiogram may be normal or indicate abnormalities such as ventricular hypertrophy or heart failure.
- Chest radiograph demonstrates heart size and shape, as well as lung involvement if heart failure present.

Nursing Interventions

- Nursing care focuses on improving oxygenation, promoting adequate nutrition, assisting the child and family with coping,

(text continues on page 155)

TABLE 2.4	ASSESSMENT FINDINGS FOR CONGENITAL HEART DISEASES
Defect	**Assessment Findings**
Tetralogy of Fallot 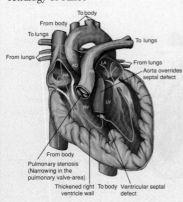	• Loud harsh murmur • Color changes associated with feeding, activity, or crying. • Hypercyanotic spells (cyanosis, hypoxemia, dyspnea, and agitation) • History of squatting or bending of the knees • History of irritability, sleepiness, or difficulty breathing • Clubbing of the digits • Tachypnea, increased work of breathing • Adventitious breath sounds (associated with heart failure)
Tricuspid Atresia 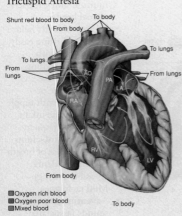	• Murmur • History of cyanosis either or a few days of age • History of rapid respirations and difficulty with feeding • Cyanosis or a pale gray color • Overactive apical impulse • Weak or poor suck • Tachypnea, increased work of breathing • Adventitious breath sounds (associated with heart failure) • Coolness or clamminess of the skin • Clubbing in the older infant or child

(continued on page 150)

ASSESSMENT FINDINGS FOR CONGENITAL HEART DISEASES *continued*

Defect	Assessment Findings
Atrial Septal Defect 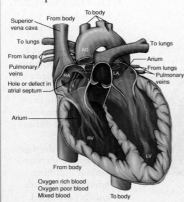	• Fixed split second heart sound and a systolic ejection murmur, best heard in the pulmonic valve area • Poor feeding as an infant • Decreased ability to keep up with peers • History of difficulty growing • Hyperdynamic precordium • Right ventricular heave along the left sternal border
Ventricular Septal Defect 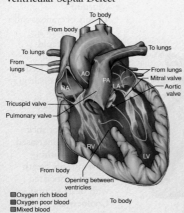	• Holosystolic harsh murmur along the left sternal border • History of heart failure • History of tiring easily, particularly with exertion or feeding • Failure to thrive • Color change or diaphoresis with nipple feeding in the infant • History of frequent pulmonary infections and shortness of breath • Extremity edema (possibly pitting) • Mild tachypnea • Adventitious breath sounds (associated with heart failure) • Palpable chest thrill

Defect	Assessment Findings
Atrioventricular Canal Defect 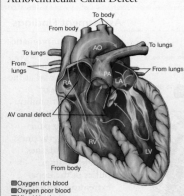	• Loud murmur • History of frequent respiratory infections, difficulty gaining weight, difficulty or increased work of breathing • Cyanosis of lips, fingernails, skin • Retractions, tachypnea, nasal flaring, and rales
Patent Ductus Arteriosus 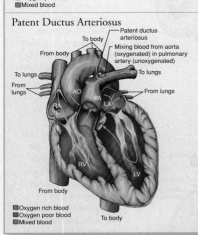	• Possibly asymptomatic • Harsh, continuous, machine-like murmur, usually loudest under the left clavicle at the first and second intercostal spaces • History of frequent respiratory infections, fatigue, poor growth, and development • Tachycardia, bounding peripheral pulses, a widened pulse pressure, tachypnea, rales

(continued on page 152)

ASSESSMENT FINDINGS FOR CONGENITAL HEART DISEASES *continued*

Defect	Assessment Findings
Coarctation of the Aorta 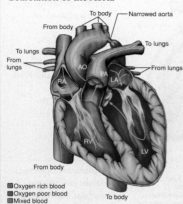	<ul><li>Possibly asymptomatic</li><li>Soft to moderately loud systolic murmur, most often heard at the base of the heart</li><li>History of irritability, frequent epistaxis, reports of leg pain with activity, dizziness, fainting, headaches</li><li>Full, bounding pulses in the upper extremities with weak or absent pulses in the lower extremities</li><li>Blood pressure in the upper extremities may be ≥20 mm Hg than that in the lower extremities</li><li>Rib notching</li></ul>
Aortic Stenosis 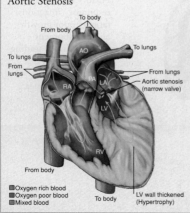	<ul><li>Typically asymptomatic</li><li>Systolic murmur best heard along the left sternal border with radiation to the right upper sternal border</li><li>History of easy fatigability, complaints of chest pain similar to anginal pain when active, dizziness with prolonged standing, difficulty with feeding</li><li>Faint pulse</li><li>Thrill at the base of the heart</li></ul>

Defect	Assessment Findings
Pulmonic Stenosis 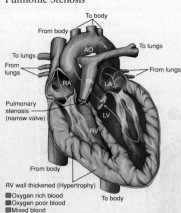	• Possibly asymptomatic • High-pitched click following the second heart sound and a systolic ejection murmur loudest at the upper left sternal border • History of mild dyspnea or cyanosis with exertion • Normal growth history
Transposition of the Great Vessels 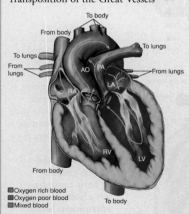	• Loud second heart sound, murmur if ductus open, or septal defect also present • Significant cyanosis without a murmur in the newborn period *or* • History of cyanosis with feeding or crying • Prominent ventricular impulse. Auscultate the heart, noting a loud second heart sound • Signs of heart failure

(continued on page 154)

ASSESSMENT FINDINGS FOR CONGENITAL HEART DISEASES *continued*

Defect	Assessment Findings
Total Anomalous Pulmonary Venous Connection 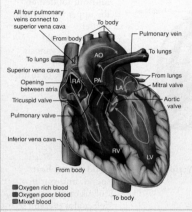	• Fixed splitting of the second heart sound and a murmur • History of cyanosis, tiring easily, difficulty feeding • Prominence of the right ventricular impulse • Retractions with tachypnea • Hepatomegaly
Truncus Arteriosus 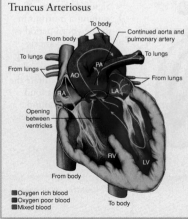	• Murmur associated with a ventricular septal defect • History of cyanosis that increases with periods of activity such as feeding, easy tiring, difficulty feeding, poor growth • Tachypnea, nasal flaring, grunting or noisy breathing, retractions, restlessness, adventitious breath sounds

Defect	Assessment Findings
Hypoplastic Left Heart Labels in diagram: To body; From body; Patent ductus arteriosus; Very small aorta; AO; To lungs; From lungs; To lungs; RA; PA; From lungs; Opening between atria; LA; Underdeveloped left ventricle; LV; RV; From body. ■ Oxygen rich blood ■ Oxygen poor blood ■ Mixed blood	• Soft systolic ejection or holosystolic murmur, gallop rhythm, or single second heart sound • Cyanosis, gradually increasing over time • History of poor feeding easy tiring • Tachycardia, tachypnea, hypothermia. • Increased work of breathing, adventitious breath sounds, extremity pallor, decreased oxygen saturation via pulse oximetry

AO, aorta; LA, left atrium; LV, left ventricle; PA, pulmonary artery; RA, right atrium; RV, right ventricle.

preventing infection, providing preoperative and postoperative nursing care, and providing child and family education.

• Frequently assess the child's cardiopulmonary status, noting alterations.
• Position the child in Fowler or semi-Fowler position; suction as needed.
• Provide humidified supplemental oxygen as ordered, warming it to prevent wide temperature fluctuations.
• For hypercyanotic spells, refer to Box 2.2, which lists interventions related to relief of hypercyanotic spells.
• Provide increased caloric intake orally or with gavage feedings. Use human milk fortifier to increase calories in the breast-fed infant. Limit nipple feeding to 20 minutes, gavaging the remainder of the feeding.

Take Note!

Breast-feeding a child before and after cardiac surgery may boost the infant's immune system, which can help fight postoperative infection. If breast-feeding is not possible, mothers can pump milk and the breast milk may be given via bottle, dropper, or gavage feeding.

BOX 2.2

RELIEVING HYPERCYANOTIC SPELLS

• Use a calm, comforting approach.
• Place the infant or child in a knee-to-chest position.
• Provide supplemental oxygen.
• Administer morphine sulfate (0.1 mg/kg IV, IM, or SQ).
• Supply IV fluids.
• Administer propranolol (0.1 mg/kg IV).

IM, intramuscularly; SQ, subcutaneously.
Adapted from Doyle, T., Kavanaugh-McHugh, A., & Fish, F. A. (2015). Management and outcome of tetralogy of Fallot. Retrieved October 10, 2015, from http://www.uptodate.com/contents/management-and-outcome-of-tetralogy-of-fallot.

• Provide support and education to the child and family. Refer to Teaching Guidelines 2.8.
• Encourage the family to participate in the child's care.
• Teach parents about prevention of infection: hand hygiene, dental care, prophylaxis for infective endocarditis as needed, and RSV prophylaxis as recommended during RSV season (children 24 months and younger; Ralston et al., 2014).
• Provide preoperative teaching based on the child's developmental level, with a tour of the intensive care unit for the older child.
• Provide postoperative care, including the following:
  • Frequently assess vital signs color of the skin and mucous membranes, capillary refill, peripheral pulses, cardiac rate and rhythm, heart sounds, breath sounds, oxygen saturation, LOC, intake and output (strict).
  • Administer supplemental oxygen as needed.
  • Monitor mechanical ventilation and suction as ordered.
  • Inspect chest tube functioning, noting amount, color, and character of drainage, maintain chest tube dressing.
  • Inspect the dressing (incision and chest tube) for drainage and intactness. Reinforce or change the dressing as ordered.
  • Assess the incision for redness, irritation, drainage, or separation.
  • Administer medications, such as digoxin or inotropic or vasopressor agents, as ordered, watching the child closely for possible adverse effects.
  • Encourage the child to turn, cough, deep breathe, use the incentive spirometer, and splint the incisional area with pillows.

- Assess the child's pain level and administer analgesics as ordered. Assist the child to get out of bed as soon as possible and as ordered.
- Assess daily weights. Administer small, frequent feedings or meals when oral intake is allowed.
- Assess the child for complications.
- Prepare the child and family for discharge (Beke, Braudis, & Lincoln, 2005).

> *Take Note!*
>
> Abrupt cessation of chest tube output accompanied by an increase in heart rate and increased filling pressure (right atrial) may indicate cardiac tamponade (Beke et al., 2005).

Teaching Guidelines 2.8
CARING FOR THE CHILD WITH A CONGENITAL HEART DISEASE

- Give medications, if ordered, exactly as prescribed.
- Weigh the child at least once a week or as ordered, at approximately the same time of the day with the same scale and wearing the same amount of clothing.
- Allow the child to engage in activity as directed. Provide time for the child to rest frequently throughout the day to prevent overexertion.
- Provide a nutritious diet, taking into account any restrictions for fluids or foods.
- Use measures to prevent infection, such as frequent handwashing, prophylactic antibiotics, and skin care.
- Adhere to schedule for follow-up diagnostic tests and procedures.
- Support the child's growth and development needs.
- Use available community support services.
- Notify the primary care provider if the child has increasing episodes of respiratory distress, cyanosis, or difficulty breathing; fever; increased edema of the hands, feet, or face; decreased urinary output; weight loss or difficulty eating or drinking; increased fatigue or irritability; decreased level of alertness; or vomiting or diarrhea.

Adapted from Cook, E. H., & Higgins, S. S. (2010). Chapter 21: Congenital heart disease. In P. J. Allen, J. A. Vessey, & N. A. Schapiro (Eds.), *Primary care of the child with a chronic condition* (5th ed., pp. 385–404). St. Louis, MO: Mosby.

CONGENITAL ADRENAL HYPERPLASIA

Description

- Congenital adrenal hyperplasia (CAH) is a group of autosomal recessive inherited disorders in which there is an insufficient supply of the enzymes required for the synthesis of cortisol and aldosterone.
- More than 90% of the cases of CAH are caused by a deficiency of 21-hydroxylase (21-OH) enzyme (Nelson-Tuttle, 2014; White, 2011). Therefore, our discussion will focus on this type.
- This condition can be life threatening and requires prompt diagnosis and treatment after birth (Nelson-Tuttle, 2014).
- Complications of CAH include hyponatremia, hyperkalemia, hypotension, shock, hypoglycemia, short adult stature, and adult testicular tumor in males.

Pathophysiology

- 21-OH enzyme deficiency results in blocking the production of adrenal mineralocorticoids and glucocorticoids. Therefore, a reduction of cortisol occurs, which leads to increased adrenocorticotropic hormone (ACTH) production by the anterior pituitary to stimulate adrenal gland production.
- Prolonged oversecretion of ACTH causes enlargement or hyperplasia of the adrenal glands and excess production of androgens leading to male characteristics appearing early or inappropriately.
- Males do not have obvious signs at birth but may enter puberty by 2 to 3 years of age. In males, the enzyme deficiency of 21-OH with excessive androgen secretion leads to a slightly enlarged penis, which may become adult-sized by school age, and a hyperpigmented scrotum.
- The female fetus develops male secondary sexual characteristics. Thus, CAH causes ambiguous genitalia in girls (Nelson-Tuttle, 2014). The clitoris is enlarged and may resemble the penis, the labia have a rugated appearance, and the labial folds are fused, but the internal reproductive organs, such as ovaries, fallopian tubes, and uterus, are normal.
- A milder form of 21-OH deficiency becomes evident later, in the toddler or preschool years, with premature adrenarche (early sexual maturation), pubic hair development, accelerated growth velocity, advanced bone age, early closure of the epiphyseal plates resulting in short stature as an adult, acne, and hirsutism (excessive body hair growth).

- Males usually have normal fertility, whereas females may have lower fertility.
- Aldosterone insufficiency also leads to fluid and electrolyte imbalances, such as hyponatremia, hyperkalemia, and hypotension due to depletion of extracellular fluid.
- Cortisol insufficiency leads to low blood glucose (hypoglycemia).

Therapeutic Management

- The goal of treatment is to stop excessive adrenal secretion of androgens while maintaining normal growth and development.
- Most children with 21-OH deficiency will take a glucocorticoid such as hydrocortisone and the mineralocorticoid fludrocortisone (Florinef) for life.
- Infants may also require sodium supplementation.
- When the medications are taken at physiologic doses, there are no adverse effects, but if the levels become elevated, hypertension, growth impairment, and acne become a problem.
- Regular follow-up care and appropriate titration maintain the dose at appropriate levels to allow normal growth and development.
- Usually when girls are born with ambiguous genitalia, standard medical treatment is to correct the external genitalia and establish adequate sexual functioning. Gender can be determined by karyotyping chromosomes. Typically, a reduction of the clitoris and opening of the labial folds is done within 2 to 6 months of life, with further surgeries at puberty (White, 2011).

Assessment Findings

Health History and Physical Examination

- History of abnormal genitalia at birth in the infant
- History of accelerated growth velocity and signs of premature adrenarche in the toddler or preschooler
- A large penis in the male infant and ambiguous genitalia in the female infant
- Pubic hair development, acne, and hirsutism in the toddler or preschooler.

Laboratory and Diagnostic Tests

- The most common type of CAH, 21-OH enzyme deficiency, is detected by newborn metabolic screening.
- If this test has not been done or the results are unavailable, random hormone levels or levels associated with ACTH stimulation may be obtained.
- Bone age is advanced and premature closure of epiphyseal plates is noted on radiographs of the long bones.

Nursing Interventions

- Nursing management of the infant or child with CAH focuses on helping the family to understand the child's response to disease and the importance of maintaining hormone supplementation.
- Provide ongoing assessment of the ill or hospitalized child with a history of CAH to recognize the development of life-threatening acute adrenal crisis.
- Signs and symptoms of acute adrenal crisis include persistent vomiting, dehydration, hyponatremia, hyperkalemia, hypotension, tachycardia, and shock.
- Monitor children with CAH closely and notify the physician or nurse practitioner if adrenal crisis is suspected.
- Teach the child and family:
  - That medication will be required throughout the child's life, as cortisone is necessary to sustain life.
  - That it is critical to maintain tight control over the levels of hydrocortisone and fludrocortisones in the bloodstream, as either underdosing or overdosing may lead to short adult stature. Low levels of the hormones may also result in adrenal crisis.
  - That these drugs are usually given orally but in some instances will need to be given via intramuscular injections.
  - How to give hydrocortisone intramuscularly if the child is vomiting and cannot keep down oral medication.
  - That if the child becomes ill, is under stress, or needs surgery, additional doses of medications may be required.
  - To obtain a medical alert identification bracelet or necklace for the child.

Take Note!

Families must keep extra steroids in an injectable form, such as SOLU-CORTEF or Decadron, at home to give during an emergency.

- Make sure the family of a newborn with ambiguous genitalia feels comfortable asking questions and exploring their feelings. There are many issues to consider, such as whether the family will reassign the child's sex or raise the child with the original assignment at birth.
- The birth certificate may pose a problem if the state requires identification of sex. Cultural attitudes, the parents' expectations, and the extent of family support influence the family's response to the child and the decision-making process related to sex assignment and surgical correction. If corrective surgery is immediately decided upon, then typical surgical concerns for newborns will need to be addressed.

- Provide families with privacy to discuss these issues, and offer emotional support.
- When referring to the infant, use terms such as "your baby" instead of the pronouns "he," "she," or "it" and describe the genitals as "sex organs" instead of "penis" or "clitoris."
- Refer families to the CARES (Congenital Adrenal Hyperplasia Research, Education, and Support) Foundation (www.caresfoundation.org, 1–866–227–3737) and the Magic Foundation (www.magicfoundation .org, 1–800–362–4423) for additional support and resources. Local parent-to-parent support groups are also helpful.

CONGENITAL HYPOTHYROIDISM

Description
- Congenital hypothyroidism is also known as cretinism.
- This disorder usually results from failure of the thyroid gland to migrate during fetal development (Lafranchi, 2011).
- This results in malformation or malfunction of the thyroid gland, which leads to insufficient production of the thyroid hormones that are required to meet the body's metabolic and growth and development needs.
- Congenital hypothyroidism leads to low concentrations of circulating thyroid hormones (T3 and T4).
- Complications include mental retardation if untreated, short stature, growth failure, and delayed physical maturation and development (Nelson-Tuttle, 2014).

Pathophysiology
- Congenital hypothyroidism is due to a defect in the development of the thyroid gland in the fetus due to a spontaneous gene mutation, an inborn error of thyroid hormone synthesis resulting from an autosomal recessive trait, pituitary dysfunction, or failure of the CNS-thyroid feedback mechanism to develop.
- Transient primary hypothyroidism may also occur. It results from transplacental transfer of maternal medications, iodine deficiency or excess, or maternal thyroid-blocking antibodies.

Therapeutic Management
- To prevent mental retardation and restore normal growth and motor development, thyroid hormone replacement with sodium L-thyroxine (Synthroid, synthetic thyroxine, or Levothroid) begins.
- There are no adverse effects with physiologic doses, but thyroid function tests are performed initially every 2 weeks to closely monitor for effects and to ensure proper dosing.

- Because thyroid hormone is vital to the infant's developing CNS, the goal is to normalize thyroid function as quickly as possible.
- This treatment will be needed lifelong to maintain normal metabolism and normal physical and mental growth and development.

Assessment Findings

Health History

- The neonatal metabolic screening test was done less than 24 to 48 hours after birth (if this is the case, a repeat test may be warranted)
- Maternal history that indicates a connection to hypothyroidism, such as maternal exposure to iodine
- Infant sensitivity to cold, constipation, feeding problems, or lethargy
- Parents remark that it is difficult to keep the baby awake (because parents like babies to sleep well, they may not complain that their baby is sleeping too much).

Physical Examination

- Most infants are asymptomatic until the first month, when they begin to develop clinical signs.
- A lethargic baby or a child with hypotonia, hypoactivity, and a dull expression.
- A combination of lethargy and irritability may exist, with an overall delayed mental responsiveness.
- Measurements of weight and height may reveal delayed growth.
- A persistent open posterior fontanel, coarse facies with short neck and limbs, periorbital puffiness, enlarged tongue, and poor sucking response may be present.
- The skin may appear pale with mottling or yellow from prolonged jaundice, or it may be cool, dry, and scaly to the touch, with sparse hair development on the older child.
- Auscultation of the chest might reveal bradycardia.
- Signs of respiratory distress and decreased pulse pressure may also be present.
- On palpation of the abdomen, there may be evidence of an umbilical hernia or a mass due to constipation.

Laboratory and Diagnostic Tests

- States mandate newborn screening for thyroid hormone levels before discharge from the hospital or 2 to 4 days after birth (American Academy of Pediatrics, 2011).
- When the test is performed within the first 24 to 48 hours along with other metabolic screenings, the result may be inaccurate because of the immediate increase in thyroid-stimulating hormone (TSH) shortly after birth (Nelson-Tuttle, 2014; American Academy of Pediatrics, 2011).

- Radioimmunoassay is used to measure levels of thyroxine (T4), which accurately reflects the child's thyroid status. If the T4 level is low, then a second confirming laboratory test is performed, as well as determining whether the TSH is elevated.
- A thyroid scan may also be used to check for the absence or ectopic placement of the gland.
- In addition to serum measurement of T4, other diagnostic tests include serum T3, radioiodine uptake, thyroid-bound globulin, and ultrasonography.

Nursing Interventions

Promoting Appropriate Growth
- Measure and record growth at regular intervals.
- Measure thyroid levels at recommended intervals, such as every 2 weeks until the target range is reached on a stabilized dose of medication, then every 1 to 3 months until the child is 1 year old, every 2 to 3 months until the child is 3 years old, and becoming less frequent as the child gets older (Lafranchi, 2014).
- A trial off the medication may be performed around the age of 3, under physician or nurse practitioner supervision, to confirm the diagnosis (Nelson-Tuttle, 2014).
- Monitor for signs of hypo- or hyperfunction, including changes in vital signs, thermoregulation, and activity level. Refer to Comparison Chart 2.1.
- Provide adequate rest periods and meet thermoregulation needs.
- If the infant's tongue is unusually large, observe feeding ability, prevent airway obstruction, and position the infant on the side.
- Fluid restrictions or a low-salt diet may be ordered.

COMPARISON CHART 2.1	HYPOTHYROIDISM VERSUS HYPERTHYROIDISM
Hyperthyroidism	**Hypothyroidism**
• Nervousness/anxiety • Diarrhea • Heat intolerance • Weight loss • Smooth, velvety skin	• Tiredness/fatigue • Constipation • Cold intolerance • Weight gain • Dry, thick skin; edema of face, eyes, and hands • Decreased growth

Take Note!

Observe for signs of thyroid hormone overdose (irritability, rapid pulse, dyspnea, sweating, fever) or ineffective treatment (fatigue, constipation, decreased appetite).

Educating and Supporting the Child and Family

- Because many infants are asymptomatic, the diagnosis may be unexpected, so reassure and convey realistic expectations to the family.
- Developmental screening may be required if the child showed any symptoms initially, or as the child gets older to ensure that drug therapy is appropriate.
- Educate the family about the disorder, the medication and method of administration, and adverse effects such as increased pulse rate (which may indicate an overdose of thyroid hormone).
- L-Thyroxine is an oral medication that is available only as a pill. It must be crushed for infants and young children. It can be mixed with a small amount of formula or breastmilk and placed in the nipple, but it should not be placed in a full bottle of formula or breastmilk because the infant will not ingest all the medication if he or she does not finish the bottle. The medication can also be mixed with a small amount of liquid and given with a dropper.
- Medication absorption is affected by soy-based formulas, fiber, and iron preparations (Lafranchi, 2014; American Academy of Pediatrics, 2011). Therefore, carefully evaluate before starting the infant on formulas such as Alsoy, Isomil, Nursoy, ProSobee, and Soyalac.
- Inform the family that this medication will be needed throughout the child's life.
- Discuss that missed doses may lead to developmental delays and poor growth.
- Tell them that frequent blood tests will be needed to evaluate thyroid function and the child's growth rate.
- Genetic counseling may be needed.
- Clinical examination, including growth and development assessment and laboratory tests, should occur frequently. More frequent monitoring may be needed if noncompliance occurs, abnormal values occur, or with any changes in medication dosage or treatment regimen. The nurse may need to help the family to find a laboratory nearby or to handle financial issues related to the therapy.
- Educate the family about infant stimulation programs if the child shows cognitive problems, retarded physical growth, or slow intellectual development.

- Some information may need to be reinforced during school-age or adolescent stages of development.
- Encourage the family to obtain a medical identification bracelet or necklace for the child.

CONSTIPATION/ENCOPRESIS

Description
- Constipation may be defined as failure to achieve complete evacuation of the lower colon. It is usually associated with difficulty in passing hard, dry, or very small stools.
- Encopresis is a term used to describe soiling of fecal contents into the underwear beyond the age of expected toilet training (4 to 5 years of age), which may occur as a result of chronic constipation and withholding of stool.
- Many psychological issues arise from chronic constipation and encopresis as the child may experience ridicule and shame (Dunn, 2013).

Pathophysiology
- Relaxation of the anal sphincter fails to occur as formed stool fills the rectum.
- Most causes of constipation are functional in nature (inorganic) as a result of withholding stool (Sood, 2015).
- As stool is withheld in the rectum, the rectal muscle can stretch over time, causing fecal impaction. Children with a stretched rectal vault may experience diarrhea, where leakage occurs around a fecal mass.

Therapeutic Management
- It may initially be managed with increased fiber and fluids.
- Behavior modification is necessary for most children.
- Laxatives are prescribed in some children.
- Mechanical disimpaction is necessary in some children.

Assessment Findings
Health History
- Altered stooling patterns (size, frequency, amount, color)
- Pain with defecation
- Withholding behaviors (postures to try to withhold the stool, such as crossing the legs, squatting or hiding in a corner, or "dancing")
- Complaints of abdominal pain and cramping

- Poor appetite
- Diarrhea leakage
- Soiling (and hiding) of undergarments.

Risk Factors
- Family history of gastrointestinal (GI) disorders
- History of rectal bleeding or anal fissures
- Report of first meconium stool after 24 hours of age
- Medication or laxative use
- History of sexual abuse.

Physical Examination
- Distended, or rounded, abdomen
- Deep pilonidal dimple with hair tuft, which is suggestive of spina bifida occulta or flat buttocks, suggestive of sacral agenesis (functional causes of chronic constipation)
- Anal fissures or soiling
- Stains or smears on underwear (indicative of soiling)
- Normal bowel sounds unless an obstruction is present (then hypoactive or absent bowel sounds)
- Dullness on percussion (fecal mass)
- Abdominal tenderness or mass.

Laboratory and Diagnostic Tests
- Stool may be positive for occult blood, which may indicate some other disease process.
- Abdominal radiographs may reveal large quantities of stool in the colon.
- Sitz marker study may detect colonic dysmotility.
- Barium enema may reveal a stricture or Hirschsprung disease.
- Rectal manometry may indicate rectal musculature dysfunction.
- Rectal suction biopsy may indicate Hirschsprung disease.

Nursing Interventions
- Teach parents how to assess for signs of constipation and withholding behaviors.
- Provide guidelines on scheduling and supervising bowel habits in reconditioning the child to use the toilet regularly.
- Teach parents to use positive reinforcement techniques.
- Encourage/provide high-fiber diet and increase fluid intake.
- Educate families about the importance of compliance with medication use, if ordered.
- Teach parents how to disimpact their children at home; this often requires an enema or stimulation therapy. See Section III, Common Laboratory and Diagnostic Tests and Nursing Procedures, for instructions on *Administering an Enema* in children.

- Provide emotional support to families (bowel retraining can be a lengthy process).

CRANIOSYNOSTOSIS

Description
- Craniosynostosis is premature closure of the cranial sutures.
- Most cases of craniosynostosis are present at birth and are evidenced by a distorted skull appearance.
- It is important that craniosynostosis be detected early if it is not evident at birth because premature closure of the suture lines will inhibit brain development.

Pathophysiology
- The cause of craniosynostosis is unknown, but in some cases, a genetic disorder is present.
- There are numerous different types of craniosynostosis depending on which cranial suture has closed.
- The prognosis is good for the majority of infants presenting with craniosynostosis, and normal brain development will occur. Exceptions to this are the infant or child who has associated genetic disorders that involve brain function and development.

Therapeutic Management
- Surgical correction may be performed. This allows for normal expansion of the brain and acceptable appearance of the head and skull.
- If one suture is fused, the surgical intervention is done mainly for cosmetic reasons.
- If more than one suture is fused, surgical intervention is essential to prevent neurologic complications.

Assessment Findings

Physical Examination
- Evident skull deformity
- A prominent bony ridge that can be palpated
- Abnormal head circumference parameters or a big change from previous measurements detected upon measurement of head circumference in children younger than 3 years.

Laboratory and Diagnostic Tests
- X-ray studies showing fusion of the sutures.

Nursing Interventions
- Observe hemoglobin and hematocrit levels due to large volumes of blood loss that can occur.

- Observe for pain, hemorrhage, fever, infection, and swelling.
- Educate the parents that due to the location of the surgery and incision line, large amounts of facial swelling may be present. This can result in an inability of the child to open his or her eyes for a few days postoperatively.
- Encourage the parents to talk to, hold, and comfort their child during this time.

CYSTIC FIBROSIS

Description
- Cystic fibrosis is an autosomal recessive disorder involving a deletion occurring on the long arm of chromosome 7 at the cystic fibrosis transmembrane regulator (CFTR).
- It is the most common debilitating disease of childhood among those of European descent. Medical advances in recent years have greatly increased the length and quality of life for affected children, with median age for survival being the late 30s (Cystic Fibrosis Foundation [CFF], n. d.).
- Complications include hemoptysis, pneumothorax, bacterial colonization, cor pulmonale, volvulus, intussusception, intestinal obstruction, rectal prolapse, gastroesophageal reflux disease (GERD), diabetes, portal hypertension, liver failure, gallstones, and decreased fertility.

Pathophysiology
- The CFTR mutation causes alterations in epithelial ion transport on mucosal surfaces, resulting in generalized dysfunction of the exocrine glands. Thickened, tenacious secretions in the sweat glands, GI tract, pancreas, respiratory tract, and other exocrine tissues occur. The increased viscosity of these secretions makes them difficult to clear.
- The sweat glands produce a larger amount of chloride, leading to a salty taste of the skin and alterations in electrolyte balance and dehydration. The pancreas, intrahepatic bile ducts, intestinal glands, gallbladder, and submaxillary glands become obstructed by viscous mucous and eosinophilic material.
- Pancreatic enzyme activity is lost and malabsorption of fats, proteins, and carbohydrates occurs, resulting in poor growth and large, malodorous stools.
- Excess mucus is produced by the tracheobronchial glands. Abnormally thick mucous plugs the small airways and then bronchiolitis and further plugging of the airways occur. Secondary bacterial

infection with *S. aureus, Pseudomonas aeruginosa,* and *Burkholderia cepacia* is common.

Therapeutic Management
- Chest physiotherapy with postural drainage is performed several times daily.
- Dornase alfa is prescribed for use with a nebulizer.
- Inhaled bronchodilators, anti-inflammatory agents, and aerosolized antibiotics are used in some children.
- Pancreatic enzymes and supplemental fat-soluble vitamins are necessary for appropriate nutrient absorption. High-calorie, high-protein diets are recommended, and sometimes supplemental high-calorie formula, either orally or via feeding tube, is needed. Some children require total parenteral nutrition to maintain or gain weight.
- Lung transplantation has been successful in some children with cystic fibrosis.

Assessment Findings

Health History
- A salty taste to the child's skin
- Meconium ileus or late, difficult passage of meconium stool in the newborn period
- Abdominal pain with or difficulty passing stool
- Bulky, greasy stools
- Poor weight gain and growth despite good appetite
- Chronic or recurrent cough and/or upper or lower respiratory infections
- Activity intolerance
- Fever
- Bone pain
- Changes in physical state or medication regimen.

Physical Examination
- Cyanosis
- Ill or fragile and thin appearance
- Nasal polyps
- Respiratory distress (tachypnea, retractions, use of accessory muscles)
- Cough, sputum production
- Barrel chest
- Digital clubbing
- Rectal prolapse
- Edema or distended neck veins

- Adventitious or diminished breath sounds, tachycardia, gallop
- Note position of comfort, frequency and severity of cough, and quality and quantity of sputum produced.

Laboratory and Diagnostic Tests
- Sweat chloride test: suspicious if the level of chloride in collected sweat is above 50 mEq/L and diagnostic if the level is above 60 mEq/L
- Decreased oxygen saturation: via pulse oximetry
- Chest radiographs: may reveal hyperinflation, bronchial wall thickening, atelectasis, or infiltration
- Pulmonary function tests: may indicate a decrease in forced vital capacity and forced expiratory volume, with increases in residual volume.

Nursing Interventions
- Perform chest physiotherapy, involving percussion, vibration, and postural drainage, several times a day to assist with mobilization of secretions. See Section III, Common Laboratory and Diagnostic Tests and Nursing Procedures, for instructions on the chest physiotherapy technique. For older children and adolescents, the flutter-valve device, positive expiratory pressure therapy, or a high-frequency chest compression vest may also be used. The vest airway clearance system provides high-frequency chest wall oscillation to increase airflow velocity to create repetitive cough-like shear forces and to decrease the viscosity of secretions.
- Encourage breathing exercises as well as physical exercise.
- Administer dornase alfa as ordered, as well as inhaled bronchodilators and anti-inflammatory agents if prescribed.
- Administer pancreatic enzymes with all meals and snacks (and additional enzyme capsules when high-fat foods are being eaten). In the infant or young child, the enzyme capsule can be opened and sprinkled on cereal or applesauce.
- A well-balanced, high-calorie, high-protein diet is necessary to ensure adequate growth. Some children require up to 1.5 times the recommended daily allowance of calories for children their age.
- Provide supplementation with vitamins A, D, E, and K. Administer gavage feedings or total parenteral nutrition as prescribed to provide for adequate growth.
- Provide emotional support and education to the child and family.

- Refer parents to a local support group for families of children with cystic fibrosis. The CFF has chapters throughout the United States (www.cff.org).
- Assist with anticipatory grieving and decision making related to end-of-life care. Parents of children with a terminal illness might face the death of their child at an earlier age than expected.

DEHYDRATION

Description

- Dehydration occurs when fluid loss exceeds intake, resulting in decreased body fluid volume.
- It may be isotonic (electrolytes within normal limits), hypotonic (electrolyte levels decreased), or hypertonic (electrolyte levels increased).
- Dehydration occurs more readily in infants and young children than it does in adults because they have an increased extracellular fluid percentage and a relative increase in body water compared with adults.
- Dehydration left unchecked leads to shock, so early recognition and treatment of dehydration are critical to prevent progression to hypovolemic shock.
- The goals of therapeutic management of dehydration are to restore appropriate fluid balance and to prevent complications.

Pathophysiology

- Increased basal metabolic rate, increased BSA, immature renal function, and increased insensible fluid loss through temperature elevation also contribute to dehydration.
- Dehydration may occur when fluid is lost via diarrhea, vomiting, or drainage tube, or when fluid intake is inadequate.

Therapeutic Management

- Oral rehydration solution may be used in children who are not vomiting.
- In the severely dehydrated child, or in the child with persistent vomiting, isotonic IV fluids may be necessary.

Assessment Findings

Health History
- Diarrhea
- Vomiting

- Decreased oral intake
- Sustained high fever
- Diabetic ketoacidosis (DKA)
- Extensive burns.

Physical Examination
- Tachycardia
- Normal blood pressure
- Weight loss
- Depressed fontanel or sunken eyes
- Sticky or dry oral mucosa
- Cool, pale extremities
- As dehydration progresses, LOC changes and decreased urine output and poor skin turgor may be noted.

Laboratory and Diagnostic Tests
- Increased, decreased, or normal electrolyte levels.

Nursing Interventions
- Provide oral rehydration to children with mild to moderate states of dehydration (see Teaching Guidelines 2.9).
- Administer IV fluids to children with severe dehydration. Initially, administer 20 mL/kg of normal saline or lactated Ringer's and then reassess the hydration status.
- Once initial fluid balance is restored, administer IV fluids at the prescribed rate (maintenance rate or as much as 1.5 times maintenance). Refer to Box 2.3 for calculation of fluid maintenance.

 Teaching Guidelines 2.9
ORAL REHYDRATION THERAPY

- ORS should contain 75 mmol/L sodium chloride and 13.5 g/L glucose (standard ORS solutions include Pedialyte, Infalyte, and Ricelyte).
- Tap water, milk, undiluted fruit juice, soup, and broth are *not* appropriate for oral rehydration.
- Children with mild to moderate dehydration require 50–100 mL/kg of ORS over 4 hours.
- After reevaluation, oral rehydration may need to be continued if the child is still dehydrated.

ORS, oral rehydration solution.

BOX 2.3

FORMULA FOR FLUID MAINTENANCE

- 100 mL/kg for first 10 kg
- 50 mL/kg for next 10 kg
- 20 mL/kg for remaining kg
- Add together for total mL needed per 24-hour period.
- Divide by 24 for mL/hour fluid requirement.
- Thus, for a 23-kg child:
  - $100 \times 10 = 1,000$
  - $50 \times 10 = 500$
  - $20 \times 3 = 60$
  - $1,000 + 500 + 60 = 1,560$
  - $1,560/24 = 65$ mL/hour

Adapted from Engorn, B., & Flerlage, J. (2015). *The Harriet Lane handbook* (20th ed.). Philadelphia, PA: Saunders.

Take Note!

The same anatomic and physiologic differences that make infants and young children susceptible to dehydration also make them susceptible to overhydration. Thus, continuously evaluate hydration status and be aware of the appropriateness of IV fluid orders.

DEVELOPMENTAL DYSPLASIA OF THE HIP

Description

- Developmental dysplasia of the hip (DDH) refers to abnormalities of the developing hip that include dislocation, subluxation, and dysplasia of the hip joint. It may affect just one or both hips.
- In DDH, the femoral head has an abnormal relationship to the acetabulum. Frank dislocation of the hip may occur, in which there is no contact between the femoral head and acetabulum. Subluxation is a partial dislocation, meaning that the acetabulum is not fully seated within the hip joint. Dysplasia refers to an acetabulum that is shallow or sloping instead of cup-shaped.
- Complications of DDH include avascular necrosis of the femoral head, loss of range of motion, recurrently unstable hip, femoral nerve palsy, leg-length discrepancy, and early osteoarthritis.

Pathophysiology

- Although dislocation may occur during a growth period in utero, the laxity of the newborn's hip allows dislocation and relocation of the hip to occur.
- The hip can develop normally only if the femoral head is appropriately and deeply seated within the acetabulum. If subluxation and periodic or continued dislocation occur, then structural changes in the hip's anatomy occur.
- Continued dysplasia of the hip leads to limited abduction of the hip and contracture of muscles.

Therapeutic Management

- The goal of therapeutic management is to maintain the hip joint in reduction so that the femoral head and acetabulum can develop properly. Treatment varies on the basis of the child's age and the severity of DDH. Follow-up continues until the age of skeletal maturity.
- Infants younger than 6 months may be treated with a Pavlik harness, which reduces and stabilizes the hip by preventing hip extension and adduction and maintaining the hip in flexion and abduction (Sankar, Horn, Wells, & Dormans, 2011; Grossman, 2014). The Pavlik harness is successful in the treatment of DDH in the majority of infants younger than 6 months if it is used on a full-time basis and applied properly (Sankar et al., 2011).
- Children between 4 months and 2 years of age often require closed reduction (Sankar et al., 2011). Skin or skeletal traction may be used first to gradually stretch the associated soft tissue structures. Closed reduction occurs under general anesthesia, with the hip being gently maneuvered back into the acetabulum. A spica cast worn for 12 weeks maintains reduction of the hip. After the cast is removed, the child must wear an abduction brace full time (except for baths) for 2 months (Sankar et al., 2011). The brace is then worn at night and during naps until development of the acetabulum is normal.
- Children older than 2 years or those who have failed to respond to prior treatment require an open surgical reduction, followed by a period of casting (Sankar et al., 2011).

Assessment Findings

Health History

- Hip pain in previously undiagnosed children.

Risk Factors

- Family history of DDH
- Female gender
- Oligohydramnios or breech birth

- Native American or Eastern European descent
- Associated lower limb deformity, metatarsus adductus, hip asymmetry, torticollis, or other congenital musculoskeletal deformity.

Physical Examination

- Ongoing screening assessments are required throughout for at least the first several months of the infant's life.
- The physical examination may reveal the following:
  - Asymmetry of thigh or gluteal folds with the infant in a prone position
  - Shortening of affected femur observed as a limb-length discrepancy
  - Trendelenburg gait in older children
  - Limited hip abduction (<75 degrees) and adduction (<30 degrees) when passive range of motion is performed
  - A "clunk" felt or heard as the femoral head dislocates (positive Barlow sign) or reduces (positive Ortolani sign) back into the acetabulum.

Laboratory and Diagnostic Tests

- Ultrasonography of the hip allows for visualization of the femoral head and the outer edge of the acetabulum.
- Plain hip radiographs may be used in the infant or child older than 6 months.

Nursing Interventions

- Practice excellent assessment skills and report any abnormal findings.
- Encourage breast-feeding throughout the harness treatment period but provide advice on creative positioning of the infant.
- Perform postoperative nursing care in the case of surgery, including pain management and monitoring for bleeding.
- Teach parents the use of the harness and assessment of the baby's skin. If started early, harness use usually continues for about 3 months (Teaching Guidelines 2.10).
- Teach families how to care for the cast at home (refer to section on cast care).

Teaching Guidelines 2.10
CARING FOR A CHILD IN A PAVLIK HARNESS

- Do not adjust the straps without checking with the physician or nurse practitioner first.

- Until your physician or nurse practitioner instructs you to take the harness off for a period of time each day, it must be used continuously (for the first week or sometimes longer).
- Change your baby's diaper while in the harness.
- Place your baby to sleep on his or her back.
- Check skin folds, especially behind the knees and diaper area, for redness, irritation, or breakdown. Keep these areas clean and dry.
- Once the baby is permitted to be out of the harness for a short period, you may bathe your baby while the harness is off.
- Long knee socks and an undershirt are recommended to prevent rubbing of the skin against the brace.
- Note location of the markings on the straps for appropriate placement of the harness.
- Wash the harness with mild detergent by hand and air dry. If using the dryer, use *only* the air fluffing setting (no heat).
- Call the physician or nurse practitioner, if
  - your baby's feet are swollen or bluish
  - the harness appears to small
  - skin is raw or a rash develops and
  - your baby is unable to actively kick his or her legs.

DIABETES INSIPIDUS (DI)

Description
- Diabetes insipidus (DI) can be classified into two types: central DI and nephrogenic DI.
- Nephrogenic DI can be transmitted genetically (e.g., sex-linked, autosomal dominant, or autosomal recessive forms) or be acquired because of chronic renal disease, hypercalcemia, hypokalemia, or use of certain drugs such as lithium, amphotericin, methicillin, and rifampin (Breault & Majzoub, 2011). This variant of DI is not associated with the pituitary gland and is related to decreased renal sensitivity to antidiuretic hormone (ADH).
- Central DI is a disorder of the posterior pituitary gland and is the most common form of DI (Children's Hospital of Boston, 2012).
- It is characterized by excessive thirst (polydipsia) and excessive urination (polyuria), which is not affected by decreasing fluid intake.
- Typically, this disorder occurs in children as a result of complications from head trauma or cranial surgery to remove hypothalamic–pituitary tumors such as craniopharyngioma.
- Other causes include genetic mutations, granulomatous disease, infections such as meningitis or encephalitis, vascular anomalies, congenital malformations, infiltrative disease such as leukemia, or

administration of certain drugs that are associated with inhibition of vasopressin release, such as phenytoin (Breault & Majzoub, 2011).

- However, 10% of DI cases in children are idiopathic (Breault & Majzoub, 2011). Some cases of central DI can be hereditary.
- DI is usually permanent and requires treatment throughout life.

Pathophysiology

- Central DI results from a deficiency in the secretion of ADH.
- This hormone, also known as vasopressin, is produced in the hypothalamus and stored in the pituitary gland.
- ADH is involved in concentrating the urine from the kidneys by stimulating reabsorption of water in the renal collecting tubules through increased membrane permeability. This conserves water and maintains normal osmolality.
- In ADH deficiency, the kidney loses massive amounts of water and retains sodium in the serum.

Therapeutic Management

- Unless a tumor is present (in which case it is removed by surgery), the usual treatment of central DI involves a low solute diet (low sodium and low protein), daily replacement of ADH, and/or use of a thiazide diuretic (Bichet, 2013a).
- The drug of choice for home treatment is DDAVP, a long-acting vasopressin analog (Breault & Majzoub, 2011; Nelson-Tuttle, 2014). In children, it is typically given intranasally. However, it can also be administered subcutaneously or orally. The drug is given every 8 to 12 hours. The dose depends on the child's age, urine output, and urine specific gravity.

Take Note!

A metered nasal spray form of DDAVP is available, but the prescribed dose must be greater than 10 µg/0.1 mL in order for the child to use the spray (Bichet, 2013a).

- Treatment of DI and the use of DDAVP in infants and small children is challenging and complicated due to their inability to access fluids and articulate thirst (Bichet, 2013a). In neonates and young infants, the treatment is often solely fluid therapy due to their large volume requirements of nutritive fluid (i.e., the drive behind an infant's fluid intake is hunger rather than thirst) (Breault & Majzoub, 2011). However, research has shown that subcutaneously administered DDAVP may be more effective than oral or intranasal therapy in infants and small children related to variable

absorption and the challenge of administering accurate doses via these routes (Bichet, 2013a).
- In the hospital, the child may receive aqueous vasopressin, 8-arginine vasopressin (Pitressin), intravenously (Breault & Majzoub, 2011). This is a short-acting drug, so the dosage can be adjusted quickly.
- For nephrogenic DI, the treatment involves diuretics, high fluid intake, and restricted sodium intake as well as a high-protein diet.

Take Note!

Monitor blood pressure closely when initiating vasopressin.

Assessment Findings

Health History
- History of any conditions that led to the development of the disorder, including information about the neonatal period, as well as a current history of infections such as meningitis, diseases such as leukemia, or familial patterns
- Abrupt onset of symptoms, most commonly polyuria and polydipsia (Breault & Majzoub, 2011; Bichet, 2013b)
- Complaints representing the early signs of dehydration
- Except for unconscious children, the child typically maintains adequate perfusion by drinking water.
- Report of frequent trips to the bathroom, nocturia, or enuresis
- When the child cannot compensate for the excessive loss of water by increasing fluid intake, other symptoms will be reported, such as weight loss or signs of dehydration. For example, irritability may be due to the early signs of dehydration or the frustration the child feels at being unable to quench his or her thirst.
- Other signs may include intermittent fever, vomiting, and constipation.

Physical Examination
- Weight loss or failure to thrive in the young infant
- Signs of dehydration, such as dry mucous membranes or decreased tears
- Urine excretion greater than 3 L/m^2/day
- Tachycardia or increased respiratory rate may be signs of compensation for the decrease in fluid volume
- Slightly depressed fontanels or decreased skin turgor

Laboratory and Diagnostic Tests
- Radiographic studies such as CT scan, MRI, or ultrasonography of the skull and kidneys to determine whether a lesion or tumor is present
- Urinalysis: Urine is dilute, osmolarity is less than 3,000 mOsm/L, specific gravity is less than 1.005, and sodium level is decreased

- Serum osmolarity is greater than 300 mOsm/L
- Serum sodium level is elevated
- Fluid deprivation test measures vasopressin release from the pituitary in response to water deprivation. Normal results will show decreased urine output, increased urine specific gravity, and no change in serum sodium.

Take Note!

During a fluid deprivation test, the child may be irritable and frustrated because fluid is being withheld. Don't drink in front of the child.

Nursing Interventions

Promoting Hydration

- The goal of treatment is to achieve hourly urine output of 1 to 2 mL/kg and urine specific gravity of at least 1.010.
- Maintain fluid intake regimens as ordered.
- Monitor fluid status by measuring vital signs, fluid intake and output, and daily weights (using the same scale at the same time of day).
- Feed infants more frequently, because they excrete more dilute urine, consume larger volumes of free water, and secrete lower amounts of vasopressin than older children.
- Monitor for signs and symptoms of dehydration during the fluid deprivation test as well as when starting the treatment regimen.
- If the child is unconscious or has brain injury, maintain hydration and nutrition with nasogastric or gastrostomy feedings.

Take Note!

Notify the physician or nurse practitioner if the urine output is >1,000 mL/hour for two consecutive voids.

Promoting Activity

- Establish appropriate activity for the child and allow time for him or her to regain strength and the desire to increase level of activity.
- Assess the child's abilities daily, schedule frequent bathroom breaks, keep fluids the child likes available at all times, and fit the treatment plan to the child's activity.

Educating and Supporting the Child and Family

- Involve the family in development of the fluid intake regimens.
- A journal or daily log is essential in maintaining the regimen and identifying problems.

- Children with intact thirst centers can self-regulate their need for fluids, but if this is not the situation, help the family develop a plan for 24-hour fluid replacement. This may require instruction on nasogastric or gastrostomy feedings.
- Infants will need fluid intake at night.
- Educate the family about the symptoms of water intoxication (drowsiness, listlessness, headache, confusion, sudden weight gain, and anuria) and dehydration.
- Help the family develop a plan to inform the school and other individuals in the child's life about the need for liberal bathroom privileges and extra fluids to prevent accidents or dehydration. Recommend that the family obtain a medical alert bracelet or necklace for the child.
- Encourage compliance with follow-up appointments, which will probably be every 6 months.
- Educate the family about the medication regimen. See Teaching Guidelines 2.11.

Teaching Guidelines 2.11
DDAVP INTRANASAL ADMINISTRATION

Keep DDAVP in the refrigerator at all times (if directed, some products no longer require refrigeration, refer to product insert).
- Clear the nostrils (the medication may be poorly absorbed if the child has nasal congestion).
- Insert the measuring tube into the bottle.
- Fill to proper dosage and hold the top of the tube closed while inserting the medication-filled end into the nostril.
- Blow the liquid out of the tubing into the nostril.
- When using metered nasal spray, spray must be primed before first use
- If the child sneezes, repeat the dosage.
- Measure urine specific gravity to monitor effectiveness of the drug.
- Monitor for signs and symptoms of overdosage such as confusion, headache, drowsiness, and rapid weight gain due to fluid retention.

DIABETES MELLITUS (DM)

Description
- DM is a common chronic disease seen in children and adolescents.
- In DM, carbohydrate, protein, and lipid metabolism is impaired.
- Its cardinal feature is hyperglycemia.

- If DM goes unrecognized, DKA or fat catabolism develops, resulting in anorexia, nausea and vomiting, presence of ketones in urine, sweet-smelling breath, Kussmaul respirations, air hunger, and, if left untreated, coma and death. DKA is a medical emergency.
- Long-term complications of DM include failure to grow, poor wound healing, recurrent infections, retinopathy, neuropathy, vascular complications, nephropathy, microaneurysms, and cardiovascular disease.
- The major forms of diabetes are classified as type 1, which is caused by a deficiency of insulin secretion due to pancreatic beta cell damage, and type 2, which is a consequence of insulin resistance that occurs at the level of skeletal muscle, liver, and adipose tissue with different degrees of beta cell impairment (Alemzadeh & Ali, 2011). However, clinical presentation and disease progression of DM can vary considerably. Therefore, in some cases, children cannot be clearly defined as having DM type 1 or type 2 (American Diabetes Association, 2014).

Pathophysiology

Diabetes Mellitus Type 1

- DM type 1 is an autoimmune disorder that occurs in genetically susceptible individuals who may also be exposed to one of several environmental or acquired factors, such as chemicals, viruses, or other toxic agents implicated in the development process.
- As the genetically susceptible individual is exposed to environmental factors, the immune system begins a T-lymphocyte–mediated process that damages and destroys the beta cells of the pancreas, resulting in inadequate insulin secretion.
- Insulin cannot alter peripheral cells to transport glucose across the cell membrane.
- The end result is hyperglycemia, glucose accumulation in the blood, and the body's inability to use its main source of fuel efficiently.
- The kidneys try to lower blood glucose, resulting in glycosuria and polyuria, and protein and fat are broken down for energy.
- The metabolism of fat leads to a buildup of ketones and acidosis.

Diabetes Mellitus Type 2

- In DM type 2, the pancreas usually produces insulin but the body is resistant to the insulin or there is an inadequate compensatory insulin secretion response (the body can produce insulin but not enough to meet its needs).
- Eventually, insulin production decreases (resulting from the pancreas working overtime to produce insulin), with a result similar to DM type 1.

- Historically, DM type 2 occurred mostly in adults; however, the incidence has been increasing in children.
- Many children with type 2 diabetes have a relative with DM type 2 and/or are overweight.
- The rate of type 2 DM is higher in certain minority ethnic groups, such as among Hispanic and African-American children (Dabelea et al., 2014).

Other Types of Diabetes Mellitus

- Other types of DM, or exacerbation of insulin deficiency and resistance forms, develop as a result of the following conditions:
  - Diseases of the exocrine glands (e.g., cystic fibrosis)
  - Endocrine pathologies (e.g., Cushing syndrome)
  - Drug or chemical-induced problems (e.g., corticosteroid overuse)
  - Genetic defects of insulin action (e.g., congenital lipodystrophy)
  - Genetic syndromes associated with diabetes (e.g., Down syndrome, Klinefelter syndrome, Turner syndrome, Prader–Willi syndrome)
  - Infection (e.g., congenital rubella CMV)
  - Gestational diabetes (Alemzadeh & Ali, 2011).

Therapeutic Management

- Treatment involves a multidisciplinary healthcare team, with the child and family as a central part of that team.
- The general goals for therapeutic management include:
  - achieving normal growth and development
  - promoting optimal serum glucose regulation, including fluid and electrolyte levels and near-normal glycosylated hemoglobin (which is hemoglobin that glucose is bound to; it monitors long-term control of blood sugars and diabetes) levels
  - preventing complications; and
  - promoting positive adjustment to the disease, with ability to self-manage in the home.
- Established glucose control is essential in reducing the risk of long-term complications associated with DM.
- The key to success is to educate the child and family so that they can self-manage this chronic condition.
- Treatment involves blood glucose monitoring; daily injections of insulin, and/or oral hypoglycemic medications, a realistic diet; an exercise program; and self-management and decision-making skills.

Monitoring Glycemic Control

- Consistent glycemic control leads to less long-term diabetes-related complications.

- Two important methods for monitoring glycemic control include blood glucose monitoring and monitoring hemoglobin $A1_c$ (HbA1c) levels.

BLOOD GLUCOSE MONITORING
- Blood glucose monitoring evaluates short-term glycemic control and allows for tighter glucose control because supplemental insulin can be used to correct or prevent hyperglycemia.
- Blood glucose monitoring enables children and healthcare providers to provide better management.
- Children who are in the hospital for management of their DM require blood glucose monitoring before meals and at bedtime if not more frequently.
- Additional glucose checks may be necessary if glycemic control has not occurred, during times of illness, during episodes of hypoglycemic or hyperglycemic symptoms, or changes in therapy.

MONITORING HEMOGLOBIN $A1_c$ LEVELS
- Evaluates long-term control of glucose levels.
- Glycemic control goals need to be individualized and need to take into account the risks of severe hypoglycemia, but the American Association of Diabetes (2014) has developed standards related to HbA1c goals in children with type I diabetes. These include:
  - infants and young children 0 to 6 years of age: HbA1c less than 8.5% and less than 8.0% if this can be achieved without excessive hypoglycemia
  - children 6 to 12 years of age: HbA1c less than 8%; and
  - children and adolescents 13 to 19 years of age: HbA1c less than 7.5%.

Insulin Replacement Therapy
- Insulin replacement therapy is the cornerstone of management of DM type 1.
- Insulin is administered daily by subcutaneous injections into adipose tissue over large muscle masses with a traditional insulin syringe or a subcutaneous injector.
- U-100 insulin may also be administered with a portable insulin pump.
- The frequency, dose, and type of insulin are based on how much the child needs to achieve a normal, average blood glucose concentration and to prevent hypoglycemia.
- Typically, two or four daily injections are commonly used, with dosage depending on the needs of the child.
- The dose may need to be increased during the pubertal growth spurt as well as during illness or stress.

- Types of insulin include rapid-acting, short-acting, intermediate-acting, and long-acting types (Table 2.5). Each type works at a different pace, and most children will use more than one type.
- In some cases, premixed combinations of intermediate and short or rapid acting, such as 70% NPH and 30% regular, may be used. Again this depends on the needs of the child.
- Insulin can be kept at room temperature (insulin that is administered cold may increase discomfort with injection) but should be discarded 1 month after opening, even if refrigerated.
- Any extra, unopened vials should be stored in the refrigerator.
- An *insulin pump* is a device that administers a continuous infusion of rapid-acting insulin.
  - It comprises a computer, a reservoir of rapid-acting insulin, thin tubing through which the insulin is delivered, and a small needle inserted into the abdomen.
  - Insulin pumps attempt to mimic the physiologic insulin release by delivering small continuous infusion of insulin with additional bolus units administered at meal times, for planned carbohydrate intake, and if glucose testing results show it is needed.
  - Advantages of insulin pump therapy include the following:
    - Fewer injections and less trauma.
    - Children's food intake can be unpredictable, so insulin delivery can occur after a meal and adjusted on the basis of actual intake.
    - Children can be sensitive to insulin and require only minute doses, which the pump can deliver with precision.
    - The pumps can store different basal rates for different times during the day and days of the week (i.e., a higher basal rate may be needed in the morning when the child is sitting at his or her desk, and a lower rate may be necessary during the afternoon when the child is more active with recess and physical education classes). Also, rates can be programmed differently for school days versus weekend days when the child may sleep later and have differing activity levels.

Take Note!

Insulin glargine (Lantus) is usually given in a single dose at bedtime. Lantus may not be mixed with other insulins.

Oral Diabetic Medications

- In DM type 2, oral diabetic medications, also referred to as hypoglycemic, antidiabetic, or antihyperglycemic medications, are used if glycemic control cannot be achieved by diet and exercise.

(text continues on page 186)

TABLE 2.5 INSULIN TYPE, ACTION, AND DURATION

Type	Generic (Brand) Name	Onset	Peak	Duration
Rapid acting	Aspart/(NovoLog) Lispro/ (Humalog) Glulisine/ (Apidra)	Within 15 minutes	30–90 minutes	3–5 hours
Short acting	Regular (Humulin R, Novolin R)	30–60 minutes	2–4 hours	5–8 hours
Intermediate acting	NPH (Humulin N, Novolin N)	1–3 hours	4–10 hours	10–16 hours
Long acting	Glargine (Lantus) Detemir (Levemir)	1–2 hours	No clear peak, offer continuously steady coverage	6–24 hours

Adapted from National Diabetes Information Clearinghouse (NDIC), (2013). What I need to know about diabetes medicines: Types of Insulin. Retrieved October 10, 2015 from http://www.niddk.nih.gov/health-information/health-topics/Diabetes/diabetes-medicines/Pages/insert_C.aspx

- Oral diabetic medications work in a variety of ways.
  - Sulfonylureas (such as glipizide [Glucotrol] and glyburide [Diabeta]) and meglitinides (such as repaglinide [Prandin] and nateglinide [Starlix]) stimulate insulin secretion by increasing the response of beta cells to glucose.
  - Another group, the biguanides, reduces glucose production from the liver. Metformin is an example and is an effective initial therapy unless significant liver or kidney impairment is present.
  - Insulin sensitizers help decrease insulin resistance and improve the body's ability to use insulin in the liver and skeletal tissues.
  - Alpha-glucosidase inhibitors slow digestion of starch in the small intestines so that glucose from the starch enters the bloodstream more slowly and can be matched more effectively with the impaired insulin response of the body.
  - Combination agents are also available.
  - Common adverse effects of these oral agents include headache, dizziness, flatulence, and GI distress, edema, and liver enzyme elevation. If the oral hypoglycemics fail to maintain a normal glucose level, then insulin injections will be required.

Other Therapies

- Other therapies involve diet and exercise protocols and management of complications.
- The American Dietetic Association in conjunction with the American Diabetes Association recommends goals that do not exclude any foods and reflect the growth needs of the child.
  - The recommendations suggest that approximately 55% of calories come from carbohydrates, such as grains, breads, fruit, milk, and vegetables; 15% from protein, such as meat, beans, eggs, cheese, and legumes; and 30% from fats, such as butter, oil, or mayonnaise (Alemzadeh & Wyatt, 2007).
- Exercise has an important influence on the hypoglycemic effects of insulin, so the child should maintain or increase his or her activity levels.
  - If the child is taking insulin, the family should know how to change the dosage or add food to maintain blood glucose control.
  - Children with DM type 2 are often overweight, so the exercise plan is very important in helping the child to lose weight as well as assisting with the hypoglycemic effects of the medications.

Assessment Findings

- The first phase of assessment involves identifying the child who may have DM.
- The second phase involves identifying problems that might develop in the child with DM.

Health History
- During the *initial diagnosis* of DM, the history may reveal
  - problems at home or in school related to some of the mental and behavior changes that may occur in a hyperglycemic state (e.g., weakness, fatigue, mood changes)
  - blurred vision, headaches, or bedwetting and
  - a history of poor growth.
- In the *child who is known to have DM,* the health history includes:
  - any problems with hyperglycemia or hypoglycemia
  - diet
  - activity and exercise patterns; and
  - medications (insulin, oral diabetic medications), including dose and times of administration, ability to administer insulin, and monitor blood glucose levels.

Risk Factors
- The American Diabetes Association (2014) recommends screening for type 2 diabetes if a child is *overweight or obese* and also has *any two* of the following risk factors:
  - Family history; a parent or relative with DM type 2
  - Ethnic background of Native American, African American, Latino American, Asian American, or Pacific Islander
  - Older than 10 years or if onset of puberty occurs before age 10 (American Diabetes Association, 2014).

Physical Examination
Comparison Chart 2.2 gives information about common history and physical examination findings in children with DM type 1 versus type 2.
- Type I diabetes typically presents with acute symptoms and hyperglycemia, whereas type 2 diabetes can frequently go undiagnosed until complications appear (American Diabetes Association, 2011).

Laboratory and Diagnostic Tests
- A HbA1c greater than 6.5%, a random glucose level greater than 200 mg/dL (accompanied by typical symptoms of diabetes), a fasting glucose level of 126 mg/dL or greater, and a 2-hour plasma glucose level of 200 mg/dL or greater during an oral glucose tolerance test are laboratory criteria for the diagnosis of DM (American Diabetes Association, 2014). With each of these tests, if hyperglycemia is not explicit, the results should be confirmed with a repeat test on a different day (American Diabetes Association, 2014).
- Other laboratory and diagnostic tests include serum measurements of islet cell antibodies.
- Serum levels of urea nitrogen, creatinine, calcium, magnesium, phosphate, and electrolytes such as potassium and sodium may be drawn.

COMPARISON CHART 2.2 TYPE 1 VERSUS TYPE 2 DIABETES MELLITUS

History and Physical Findings Usually Present at Diagnosis	Type 1	Type 2
Family history	Less tendency than type 2	Yes
Prone ethnic groups	All	Native American, African American, Hispanic/Latino, Asian/Pacific Island descent
Polydipsia, polyuria, polyphagia	Yes	Yes, may be mild or absent
Weight	Possibly weight loss	Usually obese
Age of onset	Usually younger children	Usually pubertal children
Incidental finding on screening urinalysis	Rare	Common
Antecedent influenza-like illness/symptoms	Common	Possible
Autoimmune antibodies	Yes	No
Diabetic ketoacidosis	Common	Possible
Hypertension	No	Common
Acanthosis nigricans	No	Common
Dyslipidemia	No	Common

Adapted from Alemzadeh, R., & Ali, O. (2011). Section 6: Diabetes mellitus in children. In R. M. Kleigman, B. F. Stanton, J. W. St. Geme III, N.F. Schor, & R.E. Behrman (Eds.), *Nelson textbook of pediatrics* (19th ed., pp. 1968–1997). Philadelphia, PA: Saunders.

- Additional tests include a CBC count, urinalysis, and immunoassay to measure levels of C-peptides after a glucose challenge to verify endogenous insulin secretion.

Nursing Interventions

Regulating Glucose Control

- Consistent and established glucose control can reduce the risk of long-term complications associated with diabetes. Therefore, regulating glucose is a very important nursing function.
- In children with type 1 diabetes and sometimes in cases of type 2 diabetes, glucose is regulated by subcutaneous injections of insulin.
  - Many times the regimen consists of three injections of intermediate-acting insulin, with the addition of rapid-acting insulin before breakfast and dinner or three injections of a short-acting insulin with a long-acting injection at bedtime.
  - Insulin doses are typically ordered on a sliding scale related to the serum glucose level and how the insulin works.
  - Insulin doses and frequency are based on the needs of the child.
  - In children due to continual growth, onset of puberty, varying activity levels with unpredictable schedules, unpredictable eating habits, and the inability to always verbalize the way they are feeling, regulating glucose can be more challenging. Close monitoring of changing glucose levels and insulin needs is essential.
  - Adjustment of insulin dosing based on carbohydrate intake is essential to manage blood sugar levels. The use of carbohydrate counting can help children enjoy more freedom to choose their type or amount of food and can allow them to vary their meal and snack times. Parents will need extensive education and continual follow-up in order to ensure successful use of this method.

Take Note!

Blood sugar level should never be the only factor considered when calculating insulin dosing. Food intake and recent or expected activity/exercise must be factored.

- Figure 2.14 shows appropriate sites for subcutaneous injection of insulin.
- Sites should be rotated to avoid adipose hypertrophy (fatty lumps that absorb insulin poorly).
- If using an insulin pump, additional education will be needed.

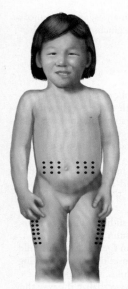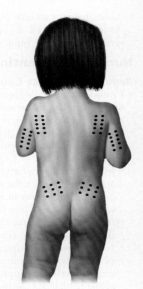

FIGURE 2.14 Sites for subcutaneous injection of insulin.

Take Note!

When giving a combination of short- and long-acting insulin, draw up the clear (short-acting) insulin first to prevent contamination with the long-acting insulin.

Monitoring for Complications

- While the child is in the hospital, monitor for signs of complications such as acidosis, coma, hyperkalemia or hypokalemia, hypocalcemia, cerebral edema, or hyponatremia and assess for the development of hypoglycemia or hyperglycemia every 2 hours (see Comparison Chart 2.3).
- Monitor the child's status closely during peak times of insulin action.
- Perform blood glucose testing as ordered or as needed if the child develops symptoms.
- In the case of a child *presenting with DKA:*
  - Monitor the glucose level hourly to prevent it from falling more than 100 mg/dL/hour. A too rapid decline in blood glucose predisposes the child to cerebral edema.

COMPARISON CHART 2.3	HYPOGLYCEMIA VERSUS HYPERGLYCEMIA
Hypoglycemia	**Hyperglycemia**
Behavioral changes (tearfulness, irritability, naughtiness), confusion, slurred speech, belligerence	Mental status changes, fatigue, weakness
Diaphoresis	Dry, flushed skin
Tremors	Blurred vision
Palpitations, tachycardia	Abdominal cramping, nausea, vomiting, fruity breath odor

- Fluid therapy is given to treat dehydration, correct electrolyte imbalances (sodium and potassium due to osmotic diuresis), and improve peripheral perfusion.
- Administration of regular insulin per physician or nurse practitioner order, given intravenously, is preferred during DKA (only regular insulin may be given intravenously).
- Usually the child with DKA is treated in the pediatric intensive care unit.
- When the child is having a hypoglycemic reaction:
  - Administer glucagon (a hormone produced by the pancreas and stored in the liver) either subcutaneously or intramuscularly. Children under 20 kg receive 0.5 mg; children over 20 kg receive 1 mg (Alemzadeh & Ali, 2011).
  - Dextrose (50%) may be given intravenously if needed.
  - If the child is coherent, glucose paste or tablets may be used.
  - Offer 10 to 15 g of a simple carbohydrate such as orange juice if the child feels some symptoms and glucose monitoring indicates a drop in blood glucose level. Follow this with a more complex carbohydrate such as peanut butter and crackers to maintain the glucose level.
- When the child is having a hyperglycemic reaction:
  - Administer insulin. The dosage is usually based on a sliding scale or determined after consultation with the physician or nurse practitioner.

Take Note!

Double-check all insulin doses against the order sheet and with another nurse to ensure accuracy.

Educating and Supporting the Child and Family

- Education is the priority intervention because it will enable the child and family to self-manage this chronic condition. The nurse should always be alert for opportunities to provide education that will expand the understanding and skills of the child and family.
- Daily management of the child with diabetes is complex and dynamic. It will require frequent monitoring, medications, including oral diabetic medications and insulin injections, and individual meal plans while the child is at school.
- The school nurse will be a principal contact person for both staff and family. With appropriate management, involvement of the community, and confidence and compliance by the family, the child can maintain a happy, productive life.
- Challenges related to educating children with diabetes include the following:
  - Children lack the maturity to understand the long-term consequences of this serious chronic illness.
  - Children do not want to be different from their peers and having to make lifestyle changes may result in anger or depression.
  - Poor families may not be able to afford appropriate food, medication, transportation, and telephone service.
  - Families may demonstrate unhealthy behaviors, making it difficult for the child to initiate change because of the lack of supervision or role modeling.
  - Family dynamics are affected because management of diabetes must occur all day, every day.
- The initial goal of education is for the family to develop basic management and decision-making skills.
- Assess the family's ability to learn the basic concepts and offer psychological support.
- Teach about specific topics in sessions lasting 15 to 20 minutes for the children and 45 to 60 minutes for the caregivers.
- Teaching must be geared toward the child's level of development and understanding.
- Among the topics to include when teaching children and their families about diabetes management are
  - Fingerstick method and blood glucose measurement. Teaching Guidelines 2.12 presents information to cover when teaching the family about blood glucose monitoring.
  - Urine ketone testing
  - Medication use:
    - Oral diabetic agents
    - Subcutaneous insulin injection or insulin pump use

Teaching Guidelines 2.12
BLOOD GLUCOSE MONITORING

Obtain glucose levels before meals and bedtime snacks.

- Perform monitoring more often during prolonged exercise, if you are ill, if you have eaten more food than usual, or if you suspect nighttime hypoglycemia.
- Use the manufacturer's recommendations and perform quality control measures as directed.
- Look for patterns. For example, 3–4 days of a consistent pattern of glucose values above 200 mg/dL before dinner indicates a need to adjust the insulin dose.
- Blood glucose measurements are the best way to determine daily insulin dosages.
- Normal levels are as follows: nondiabetics: 70–110 mg/dL; toddlers and children with type 1 DM younger than 6 years old: before meals 100–180 mg/dL, at bedtime 110–200 mg/dL; children with type 1 DM ages 6–12: before meals 90–180 mg/dL, at bedtime 100–180 mg/dL; adolescents 13–19 years of age, before meals 90–130 mg/dL, at bedtime 90–150 mg/dL (American Diabetes Association, 2014).

- Subcutaneous site selection and rotation
- When to alter insulin dosages
- Use of glucagon
- Signs and symptoms of hypoglycemia and hyperglycemia (refer to Comparison Chart 2.3 Hypoglycemia Versus Hyperglycemia)
- Treatment for hypoglycemia and hyperglycemia at home or other setting such as school
- Complications
- Laboratory testing and follow-up care
- Teach families how to give insulin, how to use the insulin pump, and how to rotate injection sites (see earlier).
- Sick-day instructions may include the following:
  - Contact the physician.
  - Perform blood glucose monitoring more often.
  - Use a sliding scale to calculate the insulin dosage.
- Review basic nutritional information with the child and family and provide sample meals.
- Incorporate the family's cultural preferences when planning meals.
- Encourage the child and family to keep a food diary.

- For the child who needs to lose weight, suggest low-carbohydrate snacks, and encourage appropriate daily physical activity (See Teaching Guidelines 2.13).
- Referral to a dietitian may be appropriate; they can help the family with detailed meal planning and dietary guidelines.
- The diagnosis of a chronic illness that will require self-management can be difficult and the child and family will need support.
- The child and family first need time to adjust to the diagnosis.
- Children with diabetes and their families may have difficulty coping if they lack confidence in their self-management skills.
- Assess the ability of the child and family to handle situations.
- Role-play specific situations related to symptoms or complications to help them see different ways to solve problems.
- Work with the child and family to enhance their conflict resolution skills.
- Provide opportunities for them to express their feelings.
- Observe for signs of depression, especially in adolescents.
- To enhance the child's confidence and promote feelings of mastery and inclusion, refer him or her to special camps for children with diabetes and refer families to local support groups, parent-to-parent networks, or one of many national support resources and foundations.

Teaching Guidelines 2.13
DIET AND EXERCISE FOR CHILDREN WITH DIABETES MELLITUS

- Provide sufficient calories and good nutrition for normal growth and development. The diet should be low in saturated fats and concentrated carbohydrates.
- Learn to identify carbohydrate, protein, and fat foods.
- Make adjustments during periods of rapid growth and for issues such as travel, school parties, and holidays.
- Consult a dietitian with expertise in diabetes education as needed.
- Provide three meals per day and midafternoon and bedtime snacks. Consistency of intake can help prevent complications and maintain near-normal blood glucose levels.
- Encourage the child to exercise routinely to help the body use insulin efficiently, thus reducing the insulin requirement.
- Encourage the child to participate in age-appropriate sports.
- When exercising, monitor insulin dose and nutritional and fluid intake, and observe for hypoglycemic reactions. Add an extra snack containing 15–30 g carbohydrate for each 45–60 minutes of exercise. Avoid exercising excessively when insulin is peaking.

DIARRHEA

Description
- Diarrhea is either an increase in the frequency or a decrease in the consistency of stool. It can either be acute or chronic.

Pathophysiology
- Acute diarrhea in children is most commonly caused by viruses, but it may also be related to bacterial or parasitic enteropathogens.
- Viruses injure the absorptive surface of mature villous cells, resulting in decreased fluid absorption and disaccharidase deficiency.
- Bacteria produce intestinal injury by directly invading the mucosa, damaging the villous surface, or releasing toxins.

Therapeutic Management
- Therapeutic management of diarrhea is usually supportive (maintaining fluid balance and nutrition).
- Probiotic supplementation may decrease the length and extent of diarrhea (Hoffenberg et al., 2014).
- Bacterial and parasitic causes of diarrhea may be treated with antibiotics and antiparasitic medications, respectively.

Assessment Findings

Health History
- Increased number, frequency, and/or volume of stools
- Abdominal pain
- Cramping
- Nausea
- Vomiting
- Fever
- Presence of blood or mucus in the stool.

Risk Factors
- Family history of similar symptoms
- Recent ingestion of undercooked meats
- Exposure to farm animals
- Foreign travel
- Daycare attendance
- Well water use.

Physical Examination
- Altered hydration status
- Abdominal distention or concavity
- Decreased urine output
- Anal redness or rash

• Hypoactive or hyperactive bowel sounds
• Abdominal tenderness to palpation.

Laboratory and Diagnostic Tests

• Stool culture: may indicate presence of bacteria
• Stool for ova and parasites (O&P): may indicate the presence of parasites
• Stool viral panel or culture: to determine the presence of rotavirus or other viruses
• Stool for occult blood: may be positive if inflammation or ulceration is present in the GI tract
• Stool for leukocytes: may be positive in cases of inflammation or infection
• Stool pH/reducing substances: to see if the diarrhea is caused by carbohydrate intolerance
• Electrolyte panel: may indicate dehydration
• Abdominal x-rays (KUB and upright): the presence of stool in colon may indicate constipation or fecal impaction (hardened immobile bulk of stool); air–fluid levels may indicate intestinal obstruction.

Nursing Interventions

• Teach the parents the importance of oral rehydration therapy (see Teaching Guidelines 2.9).
• Continue the child's regular diet if the child is not dehydrated.
• Administer probiotic supplementation or antimicrobials if ordered.

> *Take Note!*
> Avoid prolonged use of clear liquids in the child with diarrhea because "starvation stools" may result. Also, avoid fluids high in glucose, such as fruit juice, gelatin, and soda, which may worsen diarrhea (Fleisher, 2014).

ENURESIS

Description

• Enuresis is continued incontinence of urine past the age of toilet training.
• Nocturnal enuresis generally subsides by 6 years of age; if it does not, further investigation and treatment may be warranted (Dunn, 2013).
• Occasional daytime wetting or dribbling of urine is usually not a cause for concern, but frequent daytime wetting concerns both the child and the parents.

Pathophysiology

- The most frequent cause of daytime enuresis is dysfunctional voiding or holding of urine, though giggle incontinence and stress incontinence also occur.
- Nocturnal enuresis may be related to a high fluid intake in the evening, obstructive sleep apnea, sexual abuse, a family history of enuresis, or inappropriate family expectations.
- In some children, enuresis may occur secondary to a physical disorder such as DM or DI, sickle cell anemia, ectopic ureter, or urethral obstruction, urine-concentrating defect, UTI, constipation, and emotional distress (sometimes serious).

Therapeutic Management

- Behavioral or motivation therapies may be used. Enuresis alarms are successful in some children.
- Occasionally, medications such as oxybutynin, imipramine, or desmopressin are warranted.

Assessment Findings

Health History

- History of achievement of successful daytime and nighttime dryness
- Urine-holding behaviors such as squatting, dancing, or staring as well as rushing to the bathroom (diurnal enuresis)
- Large fluid intake in the evening.

Risk Factors

- Family disruption or other stressors
- Chronic constipation
- Excessive family demands related to toileting patterns
- History of being difficult to arouse from sleep
- Family history of enuresis.

Physical Examination

- Physical examination is usually normal.
- Short stature or elevated blood pressure may be present if the child has a renal abnormality.

Laboratory and Diagnostic Tests

- Normal urinalysis.

Nursing Interventions

- For the child with diurnal enuresis, encourage him or her to increase the amount of fluid consumed during the day in order to increase the frequency of the urge to void.
- Set a fixed schedule for the child to attempt to void throughout the day.

- For nocturnal enuresis, teach the family that the child is not lazy, nor does he or she wet the bed intentionally.
- Encourage the parents to limit intake of bladder irritants such as chocolate and caffeine.
- Teach parents to limit fluid intake after dinner and ensure that the child voids just before going to bed. Waking the child to void at 11 PM may also be helpful.
- Provide child and family support and encouragement. A reward system for dry nights may be helpful.
- Teach the family how to use the enuresis alarm system if recommended, or how to administer medications if prescribed.

Take Note!

Enuresis is a source of shame and embarrassment for children and adolescents. It affects the child's life emotionally, behaviorally, and socially. The family's life is also significantly affected. Enuresis is associated with childhood and adolescent low self-esteem (Dunn, 2013).

EPILEPSY

Description

- Epilepsy is a condition in which seizures are triggered recurrently from within the brain.
- The International League Against Epilepsy (ILAE) recently altered the practical definition of epilepsy and it is now defined by the presence of any of the following conditions:
  - Two or more unprovoked (or reflex) seizures, which occur more than 24 hours apart,
  - One unprovoked (or reflex) seizure and a chance of further seizures the same as the general recurrence risk (at least 60%) after two unprovoked seizures, happening over the next 10 years
  - Diagnosis of an epilepsy syndrome (Fisher et al., 2014)
- Epilepsy may be acquired and related to brain injury, or it may be a familial tendency, but in most cases the cause is unknown (Centers for Disease Control and Prevention, 2015).

Pathophysiology

- Recurrent or unprovoked seizures are the clinical manifestation of epilepsy and result from a disruption of electrical communication among the neurons of the brain (Table 2.6 for most common seizure types).

(text continues on page 204)

TABLE 2.6   COMMON TYPES OF SEIZURES

Type	Description	Characteristics
Epileptic spasm such as infantile spasms	Mode of seizure onset unknown whether focal or generalized Type of epileptic spasm seen in infancy Usually seen between 3 and 12 months of age, peak incidence 3–7 months and rarely seen after the age of 18 months	Occurs in series or clusters, Presents as flexing or extending, in variant clinical patterns, of the neck, arms, legs, and trunk, symmetric and at the same time May see: • Extension of neck, trunk, arms, and legs • Flexion of neck, trunk, and extremities with contracting of abdominal muscles (may cause body to bend forward often referred to as "jackknife seizures") • Cry may precede or follow Majority of infants have some brain disorder before seizures begin. The infant seems to stop developing and may lose skills that he or she has already attained after the onset of infantile spasms. Hormonal therapy (mainly corticotropin) and anticonvulsants (most commonly vigabatrin) are common forms of treatment.

(continued on page 200)

COMMON TYPES OF SEIZURES continued

Type	Description	Characteristics
Absence (formerly petit mal)	Type of generalized seizure; Uncommon before age 5	Abrupt onset and offset Sudden cessation of motor activity or speech with a blank facial expression or rhythmic twitching of the mouth, eyebrows, chin, eyelids, or other parts of the face Child may experience countless seizures in a day. Not associated with a postictal (after seizure) state May go unrecognized or mistaken for inattentiveness because of subtle change in child's behavior Myoclonic absence seizure consists of jerks of the shoulder and arms may result in lifting of the arms. Eyelid myoclonia brief (6 seconds) jerking of the eyelids with eyeballs rolling back; multiple seizures occur daily
Clonic	Type of generalized seizure that presents with repeated jerking movements	Muscles will spasm, jerk then relax Spasm/jerking cannot be stopped by restraining or repositioning Clonic seizures alone are rare; may precede a tonic–clonic seizure
Tonic	Type of generalized seizures that presents with stiffening of the muscles, typically the back, legs, arms	Consciousness usually preserved; Tightening of chest muscles may lead to cyanosis; seen Lennox–Gastaut syndrome

Type	Description	Characteristics
Tonic–clonic (formerly grand mal)	Extremely common generalized seizures. Most dramatic seizure type	Associated with an aura Loss of consciousness occurs and may be preceded by a piercing cry. Presents with entire body experiencing tonic contractions followed by rhythmic clonic contractions alternating with relaxation of all muscle groups Cyanosis may be noted due to apnea. Saliva may collect in the mouth due to inability to swallow. Child may bite tongue. Loss of sphincter control, especially the bladder, is common. Postictal phase: child will be semicomatose or in a deep sleep for approximately 30 minutes to 2 hours; usually responds only to painful stimuli Child will have no memory of the seizure; may complain of headache and feeling fatigue Safety of the child is a primary concern.
Myoclonic	Type of generalized seizure that involves the motor cortex of the brain. May occur along with other seizure forms	Sudden, brief, massive muscle jerks that may involve the whole body or one body part Child may or may not lose consciousness.
Atonic	Type of generalized seizure often referred to as "drop attacks." Seen in children with Lennox–Gastaut syndrome	Sudden loss of muscle tone. In children, may only be a sudden drop of the head. Child will regain consciousness within a few seconds to a minute. Can result in injury related to violent fall

(continued on page 202)

COMMON TYPES OF SEIZURES *continued*

Type	Description	Characteristics
Focal seizure without impairment of consciousness (previously referred to as simple partial seizure)	Type of partial seizure that occurs in one part of the brain. The symptoms seen will depend on which area of the brain is affected.	Motor activity characterized by clonic or tonic movements involving the face, neck, and extremities Can include sensory signs such as numbness, tingling, paresthesia, changes in vision and hearing, possible hallucinations, or pain Can include autonomic symptoms such as changes in blood pressure, heart rhythm, bowel function Can include psychic symptoms such as triggering emotions of fear, anxiety, joy sadness Child remains conscious and may verbalize during the seizure No postictal state
Focal seizure with impaired consciousness (dyscognitive) previously known as complex partial	Common type of partial seizure May begin with a simple partial seizure then progress	May or may not have a preceding aura Consciousness will be impaired Automatisms and complex purposeful movements are common features in infants and children. Infants will present with behaviors such as lip smacking, chewing, swallowing, and excessive salivation; can be difficult to distinguish from normal infant behavior In older children, will see picking or pulling at bed sheets or clothing, rubbing objects, or running or walking in a nondirective and repetitive fashion These seizures can be difficult to control.

Type	Description	Characteristics
Status epilepticus	Common neurologic emergency in children. Can occur with any seizure activity. Febrile seizures are the most common type. In children with epilepsy, it commonly occurs early in the course of epilepsy. Can be life threatening	Prolonged or clustered seizures where consciousness does not return between seizures The age of the child, cause of the seizures, and duration of status epilepticus influence prognosis Prompt medical intervention is essential to reduce morbidity and mortality Treatment: • Basic life support—ABCs (airway, breathing, circulation) • Administration of anticonvulsants to cease seizures is crucial. Common medications include benzodiazepines such as lorazepam and diazepam, and fosphenytoin. • Blood glucose levels and electrolytes along with evaluation of the underlying cause should be initiated.

Adapted from Mikati, M. A. (2011). Chapter 586. Seizures in Childhood. In R. M. Kliegman, B. F. Stanton, J. W. St. Geme III, N. F. Schor & R. E. Behrman (Eds.), *Nelson textbook of pediatrics* (19th ed., pp. 2013–2039). Philadelphia, PA: Saunders; Zak, M., & Chan, V. W. (2014). Chapter 46: Pediatric neurologic disorders. In S. M. Nettina (Ed.), *Lippincott manual of nursing practice* (10th ed., pp. 1545–1575). Philadelphia, PA: Wolters/Kluwer Health: Lippincott Williams & Wilkins.

- This disruption results from an imbalance between the excitatory and inhibitory mechanisms in the brain, causing the neurons to either fire when they are not supposed to or not fire when they should.

Therapeutic Management

- Focuses on controlling seizures or reducing their frequency.
- Anticonvulsant medications are the primary mode of treatment.
- If seizures remain uncontrolled, another option for managing them is surgery. Depending on the area of the brain that is affected, it may be possible to remove the area that is responsible for the seizure activity or to interrupt the impulses from spreading and therefore stop or reduce the seizures. The adverse effects range from mild to severe, depending on the area of the brain that is affected.
- Other nonpharmacologic treatments that may be considered in children with intractable seizures include a ketogenic diet or placement of a vagal nerve stimulator.

Assessment Findings

Health History of the Undiagnosed Child

- Occurrence of a seizure while sleeping, eating, playing, or just after waking
- Description of child's behavior during the event—What types of movements were observed, how did the movements progress, how long did the seizure last, were there any changes in respiratory status, or presence of apnea?
- Particular actions by the child after the event, including LOC, nausea or vomiting, complaints of headache, and ability to speak and interact.
- Recurring seizure episodes. If so, ask how frequent.
- Precipitating factors such as a fever, fall, activity, anxiety, infection, or exposure to strong stimuli such as flashing lights or loud noises before the occurrence of the seizure.

Risk Factors

- Family history of seizures or epilepsy
- Any complications during the prenatal, perinatal, or postnatal periods
- Changes in developmental status or delays in developmental milestones
- Any recent illness, fever, trauma, or toxin exposure

Health History of Children Diagnosed with Epilepsy

- Children known to have epilepsy are often admitted to the hospital for other health-related issues or complications and treatment of their seizure disorder. The health history should include questions related to the following:

- Age of onset of seizures.
- Seizure control—What medications is the child taking and has he or she been able to take them; when was his or her last seizure?
- Description and classification of seizures—Does the child lose consciousness; does the child become apneic?
- Precipitating factors that may contribute to onset of seizures.
- Adverse effects related to anticonvulsant medications.
- Compliance with medication regimen.

Physical Examination

- Perform a complete neurologic examination.
- Careful assessment of the child's mental status, language, learning, behavior, and motor abilities can help provide information about any neurologic deficits.
- If you observe seizure activity directly, provide a thorough and accurate description of the event. This description needs to include the following:
  - Time of onset and length of seizure activity.
  - Alterations in behavior such as a cry or changes in facial expression, motor abilities, or sensory alterations prior to the seizure that may indicate an aura.
  - Precipitating factors such as fever, anxiety, just waking, or eating.
  - Types of movements and progression of movements.
  - Increased respiratory effort or apnea.
  - Changes in color (pallor or cyanosis).
  - Altered position of mouth, injury to mouth or tongue, inability to swallow, or excessive salivation.
  - Loss of bladder or bowel control.
  - State of consciousness during seizure and postictal (after seizure) state—During the seizure, the nurse may ask the child to remember a word; after the seizure, assess if child is able to recall it, to help accurately establish current mental state.
  - Assess orientation to person, place, and time; motor abilities; speech; behavior; alterations in sensation postictally.
  - Duration of postictal state.

Laboratory and Diagnostic Tests

- Serum glucose, electrolytes, and calcium: to rule out metabolic causes such as hypoglycemia and hypocalcemia.
- Lumbar puncture: to analyze CSF to rule out meningitis or encephalitis.
- Skull x-ray examinations: to evaluate for the presence of fracture or trauma.

- CT and MRI studies to identify abnormalities, intracranial bleeds, and rule out tumors.
- Electroencephalographs (EEGs): EEG findings may be noted with certain seizure types, but a normal EEG does not rule out epilepsy because seizure activity rarely occurs during the actual testing time. EEGs are useful in evaluating seizure type and assisting in medication selection. They can be useful in differentiating seizures from nonepileptic activity.
- Video EEGs: provide the opportunity to see the child's actual behavior on video, accompanied with EEG changes; can improve the chance of catching a seizure because the monitoring is done over a period of time.

Nursing Interventions

- Focus on preventing injury during seizures.
- Administer appropriate medication and treatments to prevent or reduce seizures.
- Administer antibiotics if ordered.
- Institute seizure precautions:
  - Pad side rails and other hard objects.
  - Raise side rails on the bed at all times when child is in the bed.
  - Keep oxygen and suction at bedside.
  - Provide supervision, especially during bathing, ambulation, or other potentially hazardous activities.
  - Encourage the use of a protective helmet during activity.
  - Make sure that the child wears a medical alert bracelet.
- Educate the child and family:
  - Instruct parents and family members, along with those in the community who may care for the child, on how to respond in case of a seizure. Instruct parents and caregivers to do the following:
    - Remain calm.
    - Time seizure episode.
    - If the child is standing or sitting, ease the child to the ground if possible.
    - Loosened tight clothing and jewelry around the neck if possible.
    - Place the child on one side and open airway if possible.
    - Do not restrain the child.
    - Remove hazards in the area.
    - Do not forcibly open jaw with a tongue blade or fingers.
    - Document length of seizure and movements noted, as well as cyanosis or loss of bladder or bowel control and any other characteristics.
    - Remain with child until fully conscious.

- Call emergency medical services if
  - the child stops breathing
  - any injury has occurred
  - seizure lasts for >5 minutes
  - this is the child's first seizure or
  - the child is unresponsive to painful stimuli after seizure.
- Provide the child and family teaching and instruction regarding the administration of anticonvulsant therapy and its importance. Included in this discussion should be common adverse effects, the need to continue the medication unless instructed otherwise by the physician, and the need to call the physician if the child is ill and vomiting and unable to take his or her medication.
- Educate not only the child and family but also the community, including the child's teachers and caregivers, on the reality and facts of the disorder.
- Encourage parents to be involved in the management of their child's seizures but to allow the child to learn about the disorder and its management as soon as he or she is old enough.
- Encourage parents to treat the child with epilepsy just as they would a child without this disorder.
- Educate parents and children on any restrictions and encourage parents to place only the necessary restrictions on the child. Any activity restrictions, such as limiting swimming or participation in sports, will be based on the type, frequency, and severity of the seizures the child has.
- Referral to support groups is appropriate. The Epilepsy Foundation can be accessed at www.epilepsyfoundation.org. Additional resources can be found at www.paceusa.org and www.epilepsyinstitute.org.

EXTERNAL FIXATION

Description
- External fixation may be used for complicated fractures, especially open fractures with soft tissue damage.
- A series of pins or wires is inserted into the bone and then attached to an external frame.

Caring for the Child With an External Fixator
- Provide care of an external fixator, including:
  - maintaining skin integrity
  - preventing infection and
  - preventing injury.

- Provide routine neurovascular and skin assessment, including:
  - routine pin care
  - elevation of the extremity to help prevent swelling
  - move the fixator by grasping the frame, as the fixator can tolerate ordinary movement and
  - encourage weight bearing as prescribed.
- Provide appropriate education to the child and family, including:
  - encourage the child to look at the apparatus
  - teach the child not to pick or manipulate the pins and
  - encourage the child to wear baggy or loose clothing over the device. Velcro sewn into the seams can be helpful and allows clothes to slip over the device.

FEVER MANAGEMENT

- Fever is one of the most common reasons parents seek medical attention.
- Many parents have great concerns about fever. They fear febrile seizures, neurologic complications, and a potential serious underlying disease.
- Healthcare providers need to educate parents that fever is a protective mechanism the body uses to fight infection.
- Fever is typically managed at home, so it is important for nurses to give guidance and instruction on how to manage fever (Teaching Guidelines 2.14).

Teaching Guidelines 2.14
FEVER MANAGEMENT

Fever is a sign of illness and not a disease; it is the body's weapon to fight infection.

- Diurnal variation may allow temperature changes as much as 1°C (1.8°F) over a 24-hour period, peaking in the evening.
- Antipyretics are used if the child demonstrates discomfort. Always check correct doses before administration. Never give aspirin or aspirin-containing products to a child <19 years of age with a fever.
- In some children, fever can be associated with a seizure or dehydration, but this will not lead to brain damage or death. Discuss the facts about febrile seizures.
- Watch for the signs and symptoms of dehydration; it is important to provide oral rehydration by increasing fluid intake.
- Dress the child lightly and avoid warm, binding clothing or blankets.

- The use of sponging with tepid water is controversial; if used, encourage the parent to give an antipyretic before sponging. Ensure the sponging does not produce shivering (which causes the body to produce heat and maintain the elevated set point), and reinforce the importance of using tepid water and not cold water or alcohol. Instruct the parent to stop if the child experiences discomfort.
- Call the physician for
  - any child <3 months of age who has a rectal temperature above 38°C (100.4°F)
  - any child who is lethargic or listless, regardless of temperature
  - fever lasting >3–5 days; and
  - fever >40.6°C (105°F).
- Any child who is immunocompromised by illness, such as cancer or HIV, will need further evaluation and treatment.

FOREIGN BODY ASPIRATION

Description
- Foreign body aspiration occurs when any solid or liquid substance is inhaled into the respiratory tract.
- It is common in infants and young children and can present in a life-threatening manner (Federico et al., 2014).

Pathophysiology
- The object may lodge in the upper or lower airway, causing varying degrees of respiratory difficulty.
- Small, smooth objects such as peanuts are the most frequently aspirated, but any small toy, article, or piece of food smaller than the diameter of the young child's airway can be aspirated.

Therapeutic Management
- If the object is lodged in small or large airway, bronchoscopy may be used to remove it.

> **Take Note!**
>
> Items smaller than 1.25 inches (3.2 cm) can be aspirated easily. A simple way for parents to estimate the safe size of a small item or toy piece is to gauge its size against a standard toilet paper roll, which is generally about 1.5 inches in diameter (Safe Kids, 2015).

Nursing Assessment

Health History
- Sudden onset of cough, wheeze, or stridor (though sometimes it may be a gradual onset).

Risk Factors
• Young age.

Physical Examination
• Respiratory distress
• Audible stridor
• Wheezing, rhonchi, or decreased aeration.

Laboratory and Diagnostic Tests
• A chest radiograph will demonstrate the foreign body only if it is radiopaque.

Nursing Interventions
• The most important nursing intervention related to foreign body aspiration is prevention.
• Anticipatory guidance for families with 6 month olds should include a discussion of aspiration avoidance. This information should be repeated at each subsequent well-child visit through age 5.
• Teach parents the following points about preventing aspiration:
  • Do not let young children (particularly those younger than 3 years) play with toys with small parts.
  • Keep coins and other small objects out of the reach of young children.
  • Do not feed peanuts and popcorn to children until they are at least 3 years old.
  • Chop all foods (especially carrots, grapes, and hot dogs) so that they are small enough to pass down the trachea should children neglect to chew them up thoroughly.

FRACTURE

Description
• Fractures occur frequently in children and adolescents, especially in the forearm and the wrist (Haut, 2014).
• Greenstick and buckle fractures are common pediatric fractures.

Pathophysiology
• Fractures in children result most frequently from accidental trauma (Haut, 2014).
• Nonaccidental trauma (child abuse) and other disease processes are other causes of fractures.
• In children younger than 2, most fractures that occur are the result of another person causing the injury (Haut, 2014).
• Fractures in children heal more rapidly and result in less disability and deformity than in adults.

- The younger the child, the more quickly the bone heals. Spiral, pelvic, and hip fractures are rare in children. Table 2.7 explains common types of fractures in children.
- Midclavicular, humerus, or femur fractures can occur as a result of birth trauma. They typically heal well but may require limiting mobility or splinting.

Take Note!

Any type of fracture can be the result of child abuse, but spiral femur fractures, rib fractures, and humerus fractures, particularly in the child younger than 2 years, should always be thoroughly investigated to rule out the possibility of abuse (Wells, Sehgal, & Dormans, 2011).

Therapeutic Management

- The vast majority of childhood fractures would heal well with splinting only, but casting of these fractures is performed to provide further comfort to the child and to allow for increased activity while the fracture is healing.
- Displaced fractures require manual traction to align the bones, followed by casting.
- More severe fractures may require traction for a period of time, usually followed by casting.
- Severe or complicated fractures may alternatively require open reduction and internal fixation for healing to occur.
- Complex fractures are often treated with external fixation.

Take Note!

Significant swelling may occur initially after immobilization with a splint. Splinting and then delaying casting for a few days provide time for some of the swelling to subside, allowing for successful casting a few days after the injury.

Assessment Findings

Health History

- Recent injury, trauma, or fall
- Complaint of pain
- Difficulty bearing weight
- Limp
- Refusal to use an extremity
- Young children often demonstrate sudden onset of irritability and refusal to bear weight.
- Inconsistencies between the history and the clinical picture or mechanism of injury (inconsistency may be an indicator of child abuse)

TABLE 2.7	COMMON TYPES OF FRACTURES	
Fracture Type	**Description**	**Illustration**
Plastic or bowing deformity	Significant bending without breaking of the bone	A
Buckle fracture	Compression injury; the bone buckles rather than breaks.	B
Greenstick fracture	Incomplete fracture of the bone	C
Complete fracture	Bone breaks into two pieces.	D

Risk Factors
- Rickets
- Renal osteodystrophy
- Osteogenesis imperfecta
- Participation in sports, particularly contact sports
- Failure to use protective equipment as recommended for various physical activities and sports (e.g., wrist guards while rollerblading).

Physical Examination
- Perform the physical examination of the child with a potential fracture carefully, so as not to cause further pain or trauma.
- The physical examination may reveal
  - bruising, erythema, or swelling of the skin
  - deformity of an extremity
  - neglect of an extremity or inability to bear weight
  - a limp, if ambulating
  - point tenderness upon palpation, which is a reliable indicator of fracture in children; or
  - altered neurovascular status, including distal extremity temperature, spontaneous movement, sensation, numbness, capillary refill time, and quality of pulses.

Laboratory and Diagnostic Tests
- Plain x-ray films will reveal most simple fractures.
- CT scan or MRI may diagnose complicated fractures that require surgical intervention.

Nursing Interventions
- Immediately after the injury, immobilize the limb above and below the site of injury in the most comfortable position with a splint.
- Use cold therapy to reduce swelling in the first 48 hours after injury.
- Elevate the injured extremity above the level of the heart.
- Perform frequent neurovascular checks.
- Assess pain level and administer pain medications as needed.
- Utilize nonpharmacologic methods of pain relief as needed.
- Administer tetanus vaccine in the child with an open fracture if he or she has not received a tetanus booster within the past 5 years.

Take Note!

Assess the injured, splinted, or casted extremity frequently for the "5 P's," which may indicate compartment syndrome: pain (increased out of proportion), pulselessness, pallor, paresthesia, and paralysis. Report these findings immediately.

- Unless bed rest is prescribed, explain that children with upper extremity casts and "walking" leg casts can resume increased levels of activity as the pain subsides.
- Explain that children who require crutches while in a cast may return to school, but those in spica casts will be at home for several weeks.
- Provide distraction and find ways to keep up with schoolwork.
- Teach the child and families how to care for the cast (refer to the section on cast care).
- Provide education on ways to prevent fractures, including the following:
  - Discourage risky behavior such as climbing trees and performing tricks on bicycles.
  - Provide appropriate supervision, particularly with outdoor activity.
  - Encourage appropriate use of protective equipment, such as wrist guards with rollerblading and shin guards with soccer.
  - Ensure that playground equipment is in good working order and intact; there should not be protruding screws or unbalanced portions of equipment, which may increase the risk for falling.

FUNGAL SKIN INFECTIONS

Description
- Fungi may cause infections on children's skin. Tinea is a fungal disease of the skin occurring on any part of the body. Candidiasis may occur in the diaper area of infants and young children.

Pathophysiology
- The three organisms most often responsible for tinea are *Epidermophyton, Microsporum,* and *Trichophyton.*
- *Candida albicans* also causes skin infections, particularly in a warm, moist area such as the diaper area.

Therapeutic Management
- Treatment includes appropriate hygiene and administration of an antifungal agent.
- Topical antifungal cream (for tinea corporis, diaper candidiasis) and oral antifungal agent (for tinea pedis).

Assessment Findings

Health History
- Exposure to another person with a fungal infection
- Exposure to a pet
- Wearing diapers.

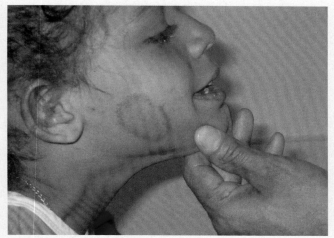

FIGURE 2.15 **Tinea corporis.**

Risk Factors
- Immunosuppression
- Young age
- Recent barber visit (tinea capitis).

Physical Examination
- Annular lesion with raised peripheral scaling and central clearing (tinea corporis; Fig. 2.15)
- Patches of scaling in the scalp with central hair loss or kerion (tinea capitis; Fig. 2.16)
- Fiery red lesions, scaling in the skin folds, and satellite lesions located further out from the main rash (diaper candidiasis; Fig. 2.17).

Laboratory and Diagnostic Tests
- Scraping and KOH preparation: branching hyphae
- Wood's lamp examination: fluoresces yellow-green if tinea capitis caused by *Microsporum*
- Fungal culture of a plucked hair: most reliable for diagnosis of tinea capitis.

Nursing Interventions
- Maintain appropriate hygiene and administer antifungal agents as prescribed.
- Child may return to daycare or school once treatment has begun. Identify and treat family members or other contacts.

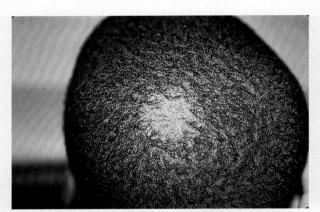

FIGURE 2.16   **Tinea capitis.**

- Counsel the child with tinea capitis and parents that hair will usually regrow in 3 to 12 months. Wash sheets and clothes in hot water to decrease the risk of the infection spreading to other family members.
- For management of diaper candidiasis, follow the suggestions listed in Teaching Guidelines 2.15 on diaper dermatitis.

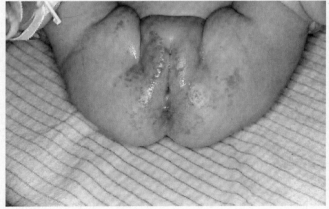

FIGURE 2.17   **Diaper candidiasis.**

Teaching Guidelines 2.15
DIAPER DERMATITIS

* Change diapers frequently. Stool-soiled diapers should be changed as soon as possible.
* Gently wash the diaper area with a soft cloth, avoiding harsh soaps.
* Baby wipes may be used in most children, but avoid wipes that contain fragrance or preservatives.
* Once the rash has occurred, allow the infant or child to go diaper-less for a period of time each day to allow the rash to heal.
* Blow-dry the diaper area with the dryer set on the warm (not hot) setting for 3–5 minutes.
* Avoid rubber pants.

GASTROESOPHAGEAL REFLUX DISEASE

Description
* Passage of gastric contents into the esophagus, resulting in vomiting and/or respiratory complications

Pathophysiology
* Transient relaxation of the lower esophageal sphincter occurs during swallowing, crying, or other Valsalva maneuvers that increase intra-abdominal pressure, resulting in the reflux of highly acidic gastric contents into the esophagus.

Therapeutic Management
* Conservative medical management: elevating the head of the bed and keeping the infant or child upright for 30 minutes after feeding smaller, more frequent feedings
* Antacids and prokinetic agents
* Surgical intervention with a Nissen fundoplication (gastric fundus is wrapped around the lower 2 to 3 cm of the esophagus; Fig. 2.18)

Assessment Findings
Health History
* Recurrent vomiting or regurgitation
* Weight loss or poor weight gain
* Infant irritability
* Respiratory symptoms such as chronic cough, wheezing, stridor, asthma, or apnea
* Hoarseness/sore throat
* Halitosis

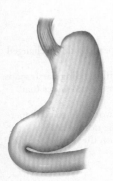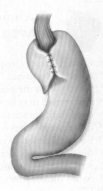

FIGURE 2.18 Nissen fundoplication.

- Heartburn
- Chest pains
- Abdominal pain
- Abnormal neck posturing (Sandifer syndrome)
- Hematemesis
- Dysphagia or feeding refusal
- Chronic sinusitis
- Otitis media
- Poor dentition.

Risk Factors
- Prematurity
- Certain dietary habits (e.g., chocolate, coffee, spicy or fatty foods, caffeine, formula-fed or breast-fed, overeating, or overfeeding)
- Smoking/alcohol use (older children)
- Food allergies
- Other GI disorders (gastric outlet dysfunction/hiatal hernia)
- Congenital abnormalities
- Certain feeding or sleeping positions and patterns (especially important in infants).

Physical Examination
- Small for age, or undernourished appearance
- Irritability
- Wheezing or other adventitious breath sounds
- Normal abdominal examination
- Cyanosis, altered mental status, and alterations in tone may be present if an acute life-threatening event (ALTE) has occurred (Hoffenberg et al., 2014).

Take Note!

Not all infants with GERD actually vomit. Some may only demonstrate irritability associated with feeding or posturing (arching back during or after feeding [Sandifer syndrome]) and grimacing. Episodes of GERD often cause bradycardia, so if these signs occur, they should be reported to the physician or nurse practitioner, even if the baby is not vomiting (Winter, 2015a).

Laboratory and Diagnostic Tests
- Upper GI series: may show some reflux
- Esophageal pH probe study: quantifies gastroesophageal reflux episodes as they correlate to symptoms
- Esophagogastroduodenoscopy (EGD): shows esophageal and gastric tissue damage from GERD
- CBC count: may demonstrate anemia
- Hemoccult: may be positive if chronic esophagitis is present.

Nursing Interventions
- Give infants smaller, more frequent feedings, using a nipple that controls flow well.
- Frequently burp the infant during feedings.
- Thicken the formula with products such as rice or oatmeal cereal.
- Keep infants upright for 30 to 45 minutes after feeding. For infants, elevate the head of the crib 30 degrees. Placing infants in infant seats or swings is not recommended, as this increases intra-abdominal pressure (Winter, 2015b). For older children, elevate the head of the bed as much as possible and restrict meals for several hours before bedtime.
- Maximize reflux precautions to keep the risk of airway involvement to a minimum.
- Teach parents cardiopulmonary resuscitation.
- In rare instances, GERD causes apnea or an ALTE. In these cases, use an apnea/bradycardia monitor to monitor for such episodes. (Hoffenberg et al., 2014).
- Administer medications if prescribed.
- Provide postoperative Nissen fundoplication care, including the following:
  - Assess for pain, abdominal distention, and return of bowel sounds.
  - Keep gastrostomy tube open to straight drain as ordered.
  - When bowel sounds have returned and the infant or child is stable, introduce feedings slowly (typically via the gastrostomy tube).
  - Assess for tolerance of feedings (absence of abdominal distention or pain, minimal residual, and passage of stool).
  - If the abdomen becomes distended or the child has discomfort, open the gastrostomy tube to air to decompress the stomach.

- Assess the insertion site of the gastrostomy tube for redness, edema, or drainage. Keep the site clean and dry per surgeon or hospital protocol.
- Teach the parents how to care for the gastrostomy tube and the insertion site and how to use the tube for feeding.

GROWTH HORMONE DEFICIENCY

Description

- Growth hormone (GH) deficiency is also known as hypopituitarism or dwarfism. It is characterized by poor growth and short stature.
- GH deficiency is often first identified when the physician or nurse practitioner assesses growth patterns.
- Children may start with a normal birth weight and length, but within a few years, the child is less than the third percentile on the growth chart.
- Possible complications related to GH deficiency and its treatment include altered carbohydrate, protein, and fat metabolism, hypoglycemia, glucose intolerance/diabetes, slipped capital femoral epiphysis, pseudotumor cerebri, leukemia, recurrence of CNS tumors, infection at the injection site, edema, and sodium retention.

Pathophysiology

- GH deficiency is generally a result of the failure of the anterior pituitary or hypothalamic stimulation on the pituitary to produce sufficient GH.
- GH is vital for postnatal growth. It is released throughout the day, with most secreted during sleep. GH stimulates linear growth, bone mineral density, and growth in all body tissues.
- The lack of GH impairs the body's ability to metabolize protein, fat, and carbohydrates.
- Primary causes of GH deficiency include an injury or destruction of the anterior pituitary gland or hypothalamus because of a tumor such as craniopharyngioma, infection, infarction, CNS irradiation, abnormal formation of these organs in utero, or result from damage or trauma during *birth* or after.
- GH deficiency may also be part of genetic syndromes, such as Prader–Willi syndrome or Turner syndrome, or the result of a genetic mutation or deletion.
- In some cases, the cause may be idiopathic, nutritional deprivation, or psychosocial issues and reversible.

Therapeutic Management

- Treatment of primary GH deficiency involves the use of supplemental GH.

- Secondary GH deficiency requires removal of any tumors that might be the underlying problem, followed by GH therapy.
- Biosynthetic GH, derived from recombinant DNA, is given by subcutaneous injection. The weekly dosage is 0.2 to 0.3 mg/kg, divided into equal doses given daily for best growth (Nelson-Tuttle, 2014). Treatment stops when the epiphyseal growth plates fuse and the final height is achieved.

Assessment Findings

Health History

- It may reveal a familial pattern of short stature or a prenatal history of maternal disorders such as malnutrition.
- The history may be significant for birth history of intrauterine growth retardation or history of severe head trauma or a brain tumor such as craniopharyngioma.
- Evaluate previous and current growth patterns.
- Note history of chronic illness such as cardiac, kidney, or intestinal disorders that may contribute to a decreased growth pattern.
- Assess the child's feelings about being short.

Physical Examination

- Linear height being at or below the third percentile on standard growth charts
- Higher weight-to-height ratio
- Prominent subcutaneous deposits of abdominal fat
- A childlike face with a large prominent forehead
- A high-pitched voice
- Delayed sexual maturation (e.g., micropenis and undescended testes in boys)
- Delayed dentition
- Delayed skeletal maturation
- Decreased muscle mass.

> **Take Note!**
>
> Infants with congenital defects of the pituitary gland or hypothalamus may present as a neonatal emergency. The symptoms include apnea, cyanosis, severe hypoglycemia with possible seizures, and prolonged jaundice (Parks & Felner, 2011).

Laboratory and Diagnostic Tests

- Bone age (as shown by x-ray) will be two or more standard deviations below normal.
- CT scan or MRI rules out tumors or structural abnormalities.

- Pituitary function testing confirms the diagnosis. This test consists of providing a GH stimulant such as glucagon, clonidine, insulin, arginine, or L-DOPA to stimulate the pituitary to release a burst of GH. Peak GH levels below 7 to 10 ng/mL in at least two tests confirm the diagnosis.

Nursing Interventions

Promoting Growth
- The goal of growth promotion is for the child to demonstrate an improved growth rate, as evidenced by at least 3 to 5 inches in linear growth in the first year of treatment without complications.
- At the beginning of treatment, monitor for height increase and possible side effects related to the medications. Measure the child's height at least every 3 to 6 months and plot growth over time on standardized growth charts.
- Provide information to the child and family about normal development and growth rates, bone age, and growth potential.
- Explore with the child and family the expectations and their understanding of what is normal so that they will have realistic expectations of treatment.
- Consult a dietitian whether the child and family need assistance in providing adequate nutrition for growth and development.

Take Note!
Growth measurements are often inaccurate and unreliable in children. Improved accuracy, especially in performing linear measurements, could yield earlier detection and diagnosis of growth disorders (Foote et al., 2011). Evidence-based clinical practice guidelines on linear growth measurement of children have been developed and have been endorsed by the Pediatric Endocrinology Nursing Society (PENS, 2014). These guidelines can be found at http://pens.org/PENS%20Documents/Clinical%20Practice%20Guideline%20on%20Linear%20Growth%20Measurement.pdf

Enhancing the Child's Self-Esteem
- Encourage the child to express positive feelings about his or her self-image, as shown by comments during healthcare visits as well as involvement with peers.
- Encourage the child to voice concerns.
- Emphasize the child's strengths and assets.
- Provide information about community support groups or websites related to GH deficiency.
- Evaluate for long-term learning problems that may develop if the child had a tumor and surgery or irradiation to remove it.

• Treat and communicate with the child in an age-appropriate manner, even though he or she may appear younger.

Educating and Supporting the Child and Family

• Explain how to prepare GH and give the correct dosage.
• Encourage rotation of sites in the subcutaneous tissue to prevent skin irritation.
• Have the family provide a return demonstration to make sure they understand correct dilution and administration of GH.
• Continue to provide periodic evaluation and ongoing support.
• Instruct the family to report headaches, rapid weight gain, increased thirst or urination, or painful hip or knee joints as possible adverse reactions.
• Inform the child and family that the child should visit the pediatric endocrinologist every 3 to 6 months to monitor for growth, for potential adverse effects, and for compliance with therapy.
• Stress the importance of complying with the GH replacement therapy and frequent supervision by a pediatric endocrinologist.
• Educate the family about the financial costs of therapy, which may be high; the family may need help in obtaining assistance and require referral to social services.
• Guide the child and family in setting realistic goals and expectations based on age, personal abilities and strengths, and the effectiveness of the GH replacement therapy. For example, the family may want to encourage the child to choose sports that are not dependent on height.
• Encourage the family to dress the child according to age and not size. Refer the child and family to counseling if indicated.
• Inform families about support groups such as the Short Stature Foundation (1–800–243–9273), the Human Growth Foundation (www.hgfound.org/, 1–800–451–6434), or the Magic Foundation (http://www.magicfoundation.org/www, 800–362–4423).

HEAD TRAUMA

Description

• Head injury is the most common cause of injury-related death and disability in childhood (ChildTrends, 2014).
• Common causes of head trauma in children include falls, motor vehicle accidents, pedestrian and bicycle accidents, and child abuse.

Pathophysiology

• See Table 2.8 for descriptions of common head injuries seen in children.

(text continues on page 227)

TABLE 2.8 COMMON HEAD INJURIES SEEN IN CHILDREN

Types	Description	Characteristics
Skull fractures	A break in the bone surrounding the brain	In infants and children younger than 2 years old, a great deal of force is needed to produce a skull fracture. Because of the flexibility of the immature skull, it can withstand a great degree of deformation before a fracture will occur. Can result in little or no brain damage but may have serious consequences if the underlying brain tissue is injured
Linear skull fracture	A simple break in the skull that follows a relatively straight line	Most common skull fracture. Can result from minor head injuries such as being struck by a rock, stick, or other object; falls; or motor vehicle accidents. Not usually serious unless there is additional injury to the brain
Depressed skull fractures	The bone is locally broken and pushed inward, causing pressure on the brain	Can result from forceful impact from a blunt object, such as a hammer or another heavy but fairly small object Surgery is often required to elevate the bony pieces. Inspect the brain for evidence of injury
Diastatic skull fracture	A fracture through the skull sutures	Most commonly occurs in the lambdoid sutures Usually treatment is not required but observation will be necessary.
Compound skull fracture	A laceration of the skin and splintering of the bone	The fracture can be linear or depressed. Generally, it is the result of blunt force. Usually requires medical intervention and surgery may be necessary

Types	Description	Characteristics
Basilar skull fracture	A fracture of the bones that form the base of the skull	Can result from severe blunt head trauma with significant force. Because of the proximity to the brainstem, this is a serious head injury. Findings include CSF rhinorrhea and otorrhea, bleeding from the ear, and orbital or postauricular ecchymosis (bruising behind ear is referred to as Battle sign), and these children are at increased risk for infection because the fracture may allow a portal of entry into the CNS
Concussion	A type of traumatic brain injury that is caused by a bump, blow, jolt, jarring, or shaking and results in disruption or malfunction of the electrical activities of the brain	Most common head injury. Results from a blow or jolt to the head caused by sports injuries, motor vehicle accidents, and falls. Confusion and amnesia after the head injury are seen. Loss of consciousness may or may not occur. Noted symptoms may include increased distractibility and difficulty with concentration. Treatment includes rest and monitoring for neurologic changes that could indicate a more severe injury, such as increased sleepiness, worsening headache, increased vomiting, worsening confusion, difficulty walking or talking, changes in LOC, and seizures
Contusion	Bruising of cerebral tissue	Results from a blow to the head from incidents such as a motor vehicle accident, falls, or abuse such as SBS. May cause focal disturbances in vision, strength, and sensation. The signs and symptoms will vary on the basis of the extent of vascular injury and can range from mild weakness to prolonged unconsciousness and paralysis. Treatment includes close monitoring for neurologic changes. Surgery is usually not necessary.

(continued on page 226)

COMMON HEAD INJURIES SEEN IN CHILDREN *continued*

Types	Description	Characteristics
Subdural hematoma	Collection of blood between the dura and cerebrum	Low incidence of fracture. Most common in children younger than 2 years, especially infants. Results from birth trauma, falls, bicycle injuries, and abuse such as SBS. Usually consists of venous bleeding. Symptoms may occur within 3 days of trauma or as late as 20 days. Symptoms include vomiting, failure to thrive, changes in LOC, seizures, and retinal hemorrhage. Treatment depends on clinical symptoms, size of clot, and area of the brain involved. In some cases, the bleeding may be closely monitored for resolution. In other cases, treatment may include subdural taps in infants and surgical evacuation in older children. Close monitoring of neurologic status and for signs of increased intracranial pressure is indicated.
Epidural hematoma	Collection of blood located outside the dura but within the skull	Relatively uncommon. Often results from skull fracture. Seen when head trauma is severe. Usually arterial bleeding, therefore brain compression occurs rapidly and can result in impairment of the brainstem and respiratory or cardiovascular function. Symptoms include vomiting, headache, and lethargy. Treatment depends on clinical symptoms, the size of the clot, and the area of the brain involved. Treatment includes prompt surgical evacuation and cauterization of the artery. The earlier the bleed is recognized and treated, the more favorable the outcome. Close monitoring of neurologic status is indicated.

LOC, level of consciousness; SBS, shaken baby syndrome.

Therapeutic Management

- Management of the child with head trauma depends on the seriousness of the injury. Initial management will focus on airway, breathing, and circulation (ABCs). Refer to the section entitled Managing Emergencies starting on page 73.

Take Note!

It is vital to keep the child's spine stabilized after a head injury until spinal cord injury is ruled out.

Assessment Findings

Health History

- Loss of consciousness or change in consciousness
- Irritability
- Lethargy
- Abnormal behavior
- Vomiting
- Seizure activity
- Complaints of headache
- Visual changes
- Neck pain.

Physical Examination

- The physical examination may reveal altered neurologic function such as altered LOC, abnormal pupillary response, and seizure activity.

Take Note!

Fixed and dilated pupils, fixed and constricted pupils, or sluggish pupillary reaction to light will warrant prompt intervention.

Laboratory and Diagnostic Tests

- X-rays of the head and neck, CT scans, and MRI provide a more definitive diagnosis of the severity and type of head trauma.

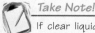

Take Note!

If clear liquid fluid is noted draining from the ears or nose, notify the physician or advanced practitioner. If the fluid tests positive for glucose, this is indicative of leaking CSF.

Nursing Interventions

- Most children with mild to moderate closed head injury, which refers to brain injury without any penetrating injury to the brain, who suffered no loss of consciousness, no other injury to their head or body, are acting normally after the injury, and were healthy before the injury can be cared for and observed at home. Provide parents and caregivers with clear instructions regarding the care of their child at home. Explain that they must seek medical attention if the child's condition worsens at any time during the first several days after injury. See Teaching Guidelines 2.16.

- Children with more severe head injury may require intensive care initially until stabilized. Focus will be on
  - maintaining the child's airway
  - monitoring breathing, circulation, and neurologic status closely
  - preventing and ceasing any seizure activity; and
  - treating any other injuries that may have occurred as a result of the trauma.

- Individualize care to the specific needs of the child. Interventions include the following:
  - Maintain a quiet environment to help reduce restlessness and irritability.
  - Manage pain and administer sedation as ordered. Observe the level of sedation closely to ensure that LOC will not become altered, which would hinder the ability to assess adequately for neurologic changes.
  - Monitor for the development of complications, which include hemorrhage, infection, cerebral edema, and herniation.

Teaching Guidelines 2.16
MONITORING THE CHILD WITH CLOSED HEAD INJURY AT HOME

Instruct parents and caregivers:
- Stay with the child for the first 24 hours and be ready to take the child to the hospital if necessary.
- Wake the child every 2 hours to ensure that he or she moves normally, wakes enough to recognize the caregiver, and responds to the caregiver appropriately.
- Closely observe the child for a few days
- Call the medical provider or bring child to the emergency room if the child exhibits any of the following:
  - Constant headache that gets worse
  - Slurred speech
  - Dizziness that does not go away or happens repeatedly
  - Extreme irritability or other abnormal behavior
  - Vomiting more than two times
  - Clumsiness or difficulty walking

- Oozing blood or watery fluid from ears or nose
- Difficulty waking up
- Unequal-sized pupils
- Unusual paleness that lasts longer than 1 hour
- Seizures
- Review signs and symptoms of increased intracranial pressure and provide parents with a number they can call if they have questions or concerns.

Take Note!

Parents are extremely helpful resources in evaluating a child's behavior for changes or abnormalities. They can provide insight into whether a behavior seen is normal or abnormal for this child. Examples include the ease at which a child is normally aroused, how much the child normally sleeps during the day, and what is the child's normal visual and hearing acuity.

- Educate the child and family. Include the following:
  - Encourage involvement in the child's care.
  - The extent of residual neurologic damage and recovery may be unclear for the child with a head injury. This can be frustrating and stressful for parents and family. Encourage verbalization of their feelings and concerns.
- Encourage involvement in the rehabilitation process. Rehabilitation should begin as soon as possible in the hospital setting and may continue for months to years. This can place a strain on the family and its finances.
- Ensure the parents and family are involved with the interdisciplinary team.
- Educate on ways to prevent head injuries such as
  - helmet use with certain sports
  - bicycle and motorcycle safety
  - car seat and seat belt use; and
  - providing adequate supervision of children to help prevent injuries and accidents—and resultant head trauma—from occurring.

HEAD TRAUMA, NONACCIDENTAL

Description
- In the United States, inflicted or nonaccidental head trauma is the leading cause of traumatic death and morbidity during infancy (Christian & Endom, 2014).

- Causes include violent shaking, referred to as shaken baby syndrome (SBS), blows to the head, and intentional cranial impacts against the wall, furniture, or floor.

Pathophysiology

- The infant's large head size and weak neck muscles place him or her at an increased risk for head trauma due to violent shaking or cranial impacts from adults.
- As a result of inflicted head injuries, the majority of children will suffer some impairment of motor and cognitive abilities, language, vision, and behavior. These inflicted injuries may also contribute to later problems with education and social attainment.

Therapeutic Management

- Treatment will be similar to that for the child with accidental head trauma (see the earlier section, Head Trauma).

Assessment Findings

Health History

- Discrepancies between the physical injuries and the history of injury given by the parent. For example, if the stories are conflicting or if the caregivers are unable to give an explanation for the injury.
- Previous intracranial or skeletal injuries that cannot be explained

Physical Examination

- External bruising of the head and face
- In less severe cases:
  - Poor feeding or sucking
  - Vomiting
  - Lethargy or irritability
  - Failure to thrive
  - Increased sleeping
  - Difficulty arousing.
- In more severe cases:
  - Seizure activity
  - Apnea
  - Bradycardia
  - Decreased LOC
  - Bulging fontanel.

Take Note!

No evidence of external trauma, but the presence of intracranial or intraocular hemorrhages, is the classic presentation of SBS. Retinal hemorrhages are seen in the majority of cases, which is a rare finding in accidental or nontraumatic events.

BOX 2.4

RISK FACTORS ASSOCIATED WITH SHAKEN BABY SYNDROME

- Single parent
- Young parent
- Substance abuse by a parent
- Any external factors present such as financial, social, or physical burdens that place stress on the parent
- Premature or sick infant
- Infant with colic.

Laboratory and Diagnostic Tests

- CT scan and MRI provide a more definitive diagnosis of the severity and type of head trauma.
- Ophthalmologic examination may indicate retinal hemorrhages.
- Skeletal survey radiographs may reveal other injuries and help determine the extent and type of injury.

Nursing Interventions

- Prevention of nonaccidental head trauma, including SBS, is a major concern for all healthcare professionals.
- Be aware of risk factors related to the potential for SBS to occur. Recognizing these risk factors will allow appropriate intervention and protection of the child to take place. See Box 2.4 for risk factors related to SBS.
- Teach parents and caregivers on appropriate ways to handle stress and ways to cope with a crying infant can help to prevent nonaccidental head trauma (see Teaching Guidelines 2.17).
- Teach parents and caregivers that shaking a baby, even for only a few seconds, can cause serious brain damage and death.

Teaching Guidelines 2.17
TIPS TO CALM A CRYING BABY

Instruct parents and caregivers:
- Try to Figure out what is upsetting the baby.
  - Is the baby hungry?
  - Is the baby's diaper dry?
  - Is the baby cold or hot?
  - Is the baby overtired or overstimulated?

- Is the baby in pain?
- Is the baby sick or running a fever?
- Try to help the baby relax.
  - Turn down the lights.
  - Swaddle the baby.
  - Walk the baby.
  - Rock the baby.
  - Give the baby a breast, bottle, or pacifier.
  - Shhh, talk to, or sing to the baby.
  - Talk the baby for a stroller or car ride.
- Sometimes the baby may continue to cry after all your efforts. If you feel overwhelmed, frustrated, or angry, focus on keeping the baby safe.
  - Stop what you are doing, take a deep breath, and count to 10.
  - Place the baby in a safe place, such as the crib or playpen.
  - Leave the room and shut the door, and find a quiet place for yourself.
  - Check on the baby every 5–15 minutes.
  - Do not be afraid to call for help; call a friend, relative, or neighbor.

HEART FAILURE

Description

- Heart failure refers to a set of clinical signs and symptoms that reflect the heart's inability to pump effectively to provide adequate blood, oxygen, and nutrients to the body organs and tissues (Francis, Wilson Tang, & Walsh, 2011; Darst, Collins, & Miyamoto, 2014).
- Heart failure occurs most often in children with CHD and also occurs secondary to other conditions such as cardiomyopathy, myocarditis, fluid volume overload, hypertension, anemia, or sepsis or as a toxic effect of certain chemotherapeutic agents used in the treatment of cancer.

Pathophysiology

- In the event of reduced cardiac output, multiple compensatory mechanisms are activated. When the ventricular contraction is impaired (systolic dysfunction), reduced ejection of blood occurs and therefore cardiac output is reduced (Francis et al., 2011; Darst et al., 2014).
- Diminished ability to receive venous return (diastolic dysfunction) occurs when high venous pressures are required to support ventricular function.

- As a result of decreased cardiac output, the renin–angiotensin–aldosterone system is activated as a compensatory mechanism. Fluid and sodium retention as well as improved contractility and vasoconstriction then occur.

Therapeutic Management

- Management of heart failure is supportive, with promotion of oxygenation and ventilation being of utmost importance.
- Digitalis, diuretics, inotropic agents, vasodilators, antiarrhythmics, and antithrombotics may be used. Intensive care may also be necessary.
- Augmenting nutrition and ensuring adequate rest are also critical.

Assessment Findings

Health History

- Failure to gain weight or rapid weight gain
- Failure to thrive, difficulty feeding, sucking, and then tiring quickly
- Fatigue, exercise intolerance, dizziness, syncope, or irritability
- Shortness of breath
- Decreased number of wet diapers.

Take Note!

Subtle signs may occur in infants with heart failure. Be alert to parental statements such as "the baby drinks a small amount of breast milk (or formula) and stops, but then wants to eat again very soon afterward"; "the baby seems to perspire a lot during feedings"; or "the baby seems to be more comfortable when he's sitting up or on my shoulder than when he's lying flat."

Physical Examination

- Recent rapid weight gain or lack of weight gain
- Tachycardia, tachypnea, decreased blood pressure
- Pallor, cyanosis, diaphoresis (profuse sweating)
- Facial or extremity edema
- Increased work of breathing, nasal flaring, retractions, cough (possibly with bloody sputum), adventitious breath sounds
- Gallop rhythm or an accentuated third heart sound
- Weak or thready peripheral pulses, or clammy, cool skin
- Ascites, hepatomegaly, or splenomegaly.

Laboratory and Diagnostic Tests

- Chest x-ray, revealing an enlarged heart and/or pulmonary edema
- Electrocardiogram, indicating ventricular hypertrophy
- Echocardiogram, revealing the underlying cause of heart failure, such as a congenital heart defect.

Nursing Interventions

- Nursing care focuses on improving oxygenation, supporting cardiac function, promoting adequate nutrition, and promoting rest.
- Position the infant or child in a semi-upright position.
- Suction as needed and/or provide chest physiotherapy and postural drainage.
- Administer supplemental oxygen as ordered and monitor oxygen saturation via pulse oximetry.

Take Note!

In a child with a large left-to-right shunt, oxygen will decrease pulmonary vascular resistance while increasing the systemic vascular resistance, which leads to increased left-to-right shunting. Monitor the child carefully and use oxygen only as prescribed.

- Administer digitalis, angiotensin-converting enzyme (ACE) inhibitors and diuretics as prescribed.
- During digitalization (24-hour period), monitor the electrocardiogram for a prolonged PR interval and decreased ventricular rate.
- Monitor the child for signs of digoxin toxicity. Measure blood pressure before and after the administration of ACE inhibitors, holding the dose and notifying the physician if the blood pressure falls by more than 15 mm Hg. Observe for signs of hypotension such as lightheadedness, dizziness, or fainting.
- Weigh the child daily and maintain accurate records of intake and output, restricting fluid intake as ordered.
- Carefully monitor potassium levels, administering potassium supplements if prescribed.
- Provide increased caloric intake (continuous or intermittent gavage feeding may be necessary).
- Ensure adequate time for sleep and group nursing interventions to provide for uninterrupted rest.
- Provide age-appropriate activities that can be performed quietly or in bed.

HEMOLYTIC UREMIC SYNDROME

Description

- Hemolytic uremic syndrome (HUS) is defined by three features—hemolytic anemia, thrombocytopenia, and acute renal failure.
- Typical HUS features an antecedent diarrheal illness. Watery diarrhea progresses to hemorrhagic colitis and then to the triad of HUS.

Pathophysiology

- The features of HUS, as well as effects on other organs, are caused primarily by microthrombi and ischemic changes within the organs. The thrombotic events in the small blood vessels of the glomerulus lead to occlusion of the glomerular capillary loops and glomerulosclerosis, resulting in renal failure.
- A verotoxin-producing strain of *Escherichia coli* O157:H7, causes the majority of cases, though *Streptococcus pneumoniae, Shigella dysenteriae,* and other bacteria may also be the cause (Tan & Silverberg, 2015). Undercooked ground beef, animal feces, unpasteurized dairy products and fruit products, and human feces via public swimming pools account for transmission of *E. coli* O157:H7.
- HUS may progress to acute or chronic renal failure.

Therapeutic Management

- Maintenance of fluid balance, correction of hypertension, acidosis, and electrolyte abnormalities, blood transfusion, and provision of dialysis are the treatment options for HUS.

Assessment Findings

Health History

- Watery diarrhea, which after several days becomes bloody and eventually improves
- Abdominal cramping
- Vomiting.

Risk Factors

- Ingestion of ground beef
- Visits to a water park or to a petting zoo before the onset of the diarrheal illness
- Use of antidiarrheal medications or antibiotics.

Physical Examination

- Pallor, toxic appearance
- Edema
- Oliguria or anuria
- Elevated blood pressure
- Abdominal tenderness
- Neurologic involvement: altered LOC, seizures, posturing, or coma.

Laboratory and Diagnostic Tests

- Urinalysis: positive for blood, protein, pus, and/or casts
- BUN and creatinine: elevated
- CBC count: decreased hemoglobin, hematocrit; platelet count: elevated reticulocyte count, WBC count (with shift to left)

- Bilirubin and lactic dehydrogenase (LDH) levels: increased
- Electrolytes: decreased sodium, increased potassium, and phosphate.

Nursing Interventions

- Institute and maintain contact precautions to prevent spread of *E. coli* O157:H7 to other children (bacteria are shed for up to 17 days after resolution of the diarrhea).
- Maintain strict intake and output monitoring.
- Carefully monitor IV infusions and blood chemistries.
- Administer diuretics as ordered.
- Assess blood pressure frequently and report elevations to the physician.
- Administer antihypertensives as ordered and monitor their effectiveness.
- Encourage adequate nutritional intake within the constraints of prescribed dietary restrictions.
- Monitor for bleeding, fatigue, and pallor.
- Preventing HUS:
  - Teach children to wash their hands after using the bathroom, before eating, and after petting farm animals.
  - Encourage the use of "swim diapers," which contain feces, for children who are not toilet trained.
  - Teach parents to thoroughly cook all meats to a core temperature of 155°F or until the meat is gray or brown throughout and the juices from the meat are clear rather than pink.
  - Wash all fruits and vegetables thoroughly.
  - Ensure that drinking water and the water used for recreation are appropriately treated.
  - Avoid unpasteurized dairy products and fruit juices (including cider).

HEMOPHILIA A

Description

- Hemophilia A is an X-linked recessive disorder that results in deficiency of the coagulation factor, factor VIII.
- The coagulation factors in the blood are essential for clot formation either spontaneously or from an injury. When these factors are absent, bleeding will be difficult to stop.

Pathophysiology

- X-linked recessive disorders are transmitted by carrier mothers to their sons. Therefore, usually only males are affected by hemophilia A.

- Factor VIII is essential in the activation of factor X, which is required for the conversion of prothrombin into thrombin.
- When factor VIII is deficient, then the platelets are unable to participate in clot formation, because the clotting factor cascade has been disrupted.
- Hemophilia is classified according to the severity of the disease, ranging from mild to severe. The more severe the disease, the more likely it is that there will be bleeding episodes.

Therapeutic Management
- The primary goal of managing hemophilia is to prevent bleeding.
- Factor administration is provided prophylactically on a scheduled basis in severely affected children, with injury or bleeding episodes, or prior to any surgeries, procedures, or other traumas that can lead to bleeding, such as intramuscular injections and dental care.

Assessment Findings
Health History
- Factors leading to the bleeding episode or bruise
- History of hemorrhagic episodes in other systems, such as the GI tract (e.g., black tarry stools, hematemesis)
- Injury resulting in joint hemorrhage, or hematuria
- Inquire about length of bleeding and amount of blood loss.

Physical Examination
- Spontaneous bleeding
- Joint swelling
- Bruising
- Epistaxis
- Chest or abdominal pain (indicating internal bleeding)
- Late findings of poor pulse quality and tachycardia (associated with hypovolemia).

Laboratory and Diagnostic Tests
- Factor levels may be quantified with blood testing.
- Decreased hemoglobin and hematocrit may occur if bleeding is prolonged or severe.

Nursing Interventions
- Administer factor VIII replacement by slow IV push as prescribed. Document the product name, number of units, lot number, and expiration date.
- Educate families about the lack of hepatitis and HIV transmission via pooled-donor factor since dry heat treatment began in 1986 (National Hemophilia Foundation, 2009). Factor replacement has also been produced using recombinant DNA technology.

- If external bleeding occurs, apply pressure to the area until bleeding stops.
- If joint bleeding occurs, apply ice or cold compresses to the area and elevate any injured extremities, except when contraindicated by further injury.
- Inform the family that the child should wear a health alert bracelet.
- Instruct all school personnel to call the parent immediately if the child sustains a head, abdominal, or orbit injury at school.
- Teach parents and caregivers how to administer the IV infusion of factor VIII.
- Involve children as developmentally appropriate in the infusion process.
- Educate and support the parents and child. Refer families to the National Hemophilia Foundation (116 West 32nd Street, 11th Floor, New York, NY 10001; 1–800–42-HANDI or 1–212–328–3700; www.hemophilia.org/).
- Instruct the child to avoid activities with a high potential for injury (e.g., football, riding motorcycles, skateboarding) and encourage the child to participate in activities with the least amount of contact (e.g., swimming, running, tennis).

HIV INFECTION

Description
- Worldwide, 3.2 million children younger than 18 years old are living with HIV infection and about 650 become infected with HIV each day (UNAIDS, 2014).
- Infants primarily become infected through their mothers, whereas adolescents primarily contract HIV infection through sexual activity or IV drug use (McFarland, 2014).

Pathophysiology
- HIV affects immune function via alterations mainly in T-cell function, but it also affects other cells. HIV infects the CD4 (T-helper) cells and replicates within them, rendering the cell dysfunctional.
- Immunodeficiency results as the number of normal, functioning CD4 cells drops.
- Eventually, CD8 counts also fall. Helper T-cell function decreases, T cells lose response to recall antigens, and B-cell defects occur leading to an increased risk of serious bacterial infection. Natural killer cell function decreases, as does the ability to fight other viral infections.
- HIV rapidly invades the CNS in infants and children and is responsible for progressive HIV encephalopathy, acquired

microcephaly, motor deficits, or loss of previously achieved developmental milestones.

Therapeutic Management

Currently, there is no cure for HIV infection, though survival has improved since the advent of highly active antiretroviral therapy (HAART).

Medication therapy ranges from single-drug therapy in the asymptomatic HIV-exposed newborn to HAART, consisting of a combination of antiretroviral drugs. Medications are prescribed on the basis of the severity of the child's illness.

In addition to improved survival, improved growth, neurodevelopment, and immune function occur with HAART (Fahrner & Romano, 2010; McFarland, 2014).

Assessment Findings

Health History

- Failure to thrive
- Recurrent bacterial infections
- Opportunistic infections
- Chronic or recurrent diarrhea
- Recurrent or persistent fever
- Developmental delay
- Prolonged candidiasis
- Adolescent or childhood sexual abuse
- Substance use or abuse (including IV drug use)
- Participation in vaginal or anal sex without the use of a condom.

Risk Factors

- Parent with HIV infection
- Unprotected sex
- IV drug use.

Physical Examination

- Fever
- Delayed growth
- Developmental delay
- Candidiasis
- Lymphadenopathy
- Hepatosplenomegaly
- Increased work of breathing or adventitious breath sounds (with pneumonitis or pneumonia); altered LOC (with HIV encephalopathy).

Laboratory and Diagnostic Tests

- Positive polymerase chain reaction test and/or positive ELISA test (less accurate in children younger than 2 years due to the presence of maternal antibodies)

- Low CD4 count
- High platelet count (severe HIV infection).

Nursing Interventions

- Administer a 6-week course of zidovudine therapy to all infants born to HIV-positive mothers (Fahrner & Romano, 2010).
- Discourage breast-feeding in the HIV-infected mother and instruct her about safe alternatives to breast-feeding.
- Educate sexually active adolescents about HIV transmission and urge them to use condoms. Urge teens to limit the number of sexual partners.
- Discourage substance use. Warn teens of the risk of contracting HIV infection via shared needles (as with IV drug use or via unclean needles used in tattooing).
- Administer antiretroviral therapy as ordered.
- Educate the family about the importance of complying with the medication regimen.
- Administer prophylactic antibiotics as prescribed in any HIV-exposed infant in whom HIV infection has not yet been excluded.
- Provide tuberculosis screening and childhood immunization in accordance with national guidelines.
- For the infant, provide high-calorie formula as tolerated. For the child, provide high-calorie, high-protein meals and snacks.
- Document growth through weekly measurements of weight and height/length.
- Educate caregivers about the medication regimen, the ongoing follow-up that is needed, and when to call the infectious disease provider.
- Provide emotional support and refer families and caretakers to appropriate local resources and support groups.
- Respect the family's desire about disclosure of the diagnosis to the child. When disclosure occurs, discuss with the child in an age-appropriate manner.

Take Note!

Do not administer live vaccines to the immunocompromised child without the express consent of the infectious disease or immunology specialist. Immunosuppression is a contraindication to vaccination with live vaccines (Atkinson, Wolfe, & Hamborsky, 2012).

HYDROCEPHALUS

Description

- Hydrocephalus is not a specific disease, but it results from underlying brain disorders.

- It results from an imbalance in the production and absorption of CSF.
- CSF accumulates within the ventricular system and causes the ventricles to enlarge and increases in ICP to occur.
- Common disorders or illnesses that are associated with hydrocephalus include neural tube defects such as myelomeningocele; intraventricular hemorrhage in premature infants; meningitis; intrauterine viral infections; lesions or malformations of the brain such as posterior fossa brain tumors; Chiari malformations; and nonaccidental injury.
- Prognosis for the child with hydrocephalus depends mainly on the cause and whether or not brain damage has occurred prior to recognition and treatment. These children are at increased risk for developmental disabilities, visual problems, abnormalities in memory, and reduced intelligence. Long-term follow-up and multidisciplinary care are necessary.

Pathophysiology

- CSF is formed primarily in the ventricular system by the choroids plexus. It flows as a result of the pressure gradient that exists between the ventricular system and the venous channels.
- CSF is absorbed primarily by the arachnoid villi.
- Hydrocephalus results when there is an obstruction in the ventricular system or obliteration or malfunction of the arachnoid villi. This results in impaired absorption or circulation of the CSF.

Therapeutic Management

- Treatment needs to be initiated in order to prevent brain tissue damage that can result from the increased ICP that hydrocephalus creates.
- Specific treatment will depend on the cause.
- The goals of treatment include relieving hydrocephalus and managing complications associated with the disorder, such as growth and developmental delay.
- With few exceptions, most cases of hydrocephalus are treated with the surgical placement of an extracranial shunt. (Most often a ventriculoperitoneal shunt [VP shunt] is placed.)
- Endoscopic third ventriculostomy is an alternative to shunt placement to treat hydrocephalus in select patients.
- The shunt will need to be replaced as the child grows. Therefore, the child will undergo shunt revision surgery at various times during his or her life.
- Infections of shunts are treated with IV antibiotics. Intrathecal administration of antibiotics may be performed by the physician or nurse practitioner.

- If the infection is persistent, the shunt will be removed and an external ventricular drainage (EVD) system will be put into place until the CSF is sterile and then a new shunt will be placed after the infection has cleared.
- Intrathecal administration of antibiotics may be performed by the physician or nurse practitioner to treat infection.

Assessment Findings

Pregnancy History and Past Medical History
- Intrauterine infections
- Prematurity with intracranial hemorrhage
- Meningitis
- Mumps encephalitis.

Health History of the Undiagnosed Child
- Irritability
- Lethargy
- Poor feeding
- Vomiting
- Complaints of headache in older children
- Altered, diminished, or changes in LOC.

Health History of the Diagnosed Child
- Children known to have hydrocephalus are often admitted to the hospital for shunt malfunctions or other complications of the disease
- The health history should include questions related to the following:
  - Neurologic status—Have there been changes or decreases in LOC, changes in personality, deterioration in school performance?
  - Complaints of headache
  - Vomiting
  - Visual disturbances
  - Any other changes in physical or cognitive state.

Physical Examination
- A rapid increase in head circumference and wide-open, bulging fontanels in the infant
- Loss of development and changes in personality in the older child
- Positive Macewen sign (This is when a "cracked pot" sound is heard during percussion and can indicate separation of the sutures. Advance practitioners perform percussion.)
- Signs and symptoms associated with increased ICP may be seen (see Comparison Chart 2.4).

| COMPARISON CHART 2.4 | EARLY VERSUS LATE SIGNS OF INCREASED INTRACRANIAL PRESSURE |

Early Signs	Late Signs

• Headache
• Vomiting, possibly projectile
• Blurred vision, double vision (diplopia)
• Dizziness
• Decreased pulse and respirations
• Increased blood pressure or pulse pressure
• Pupil reaction time decreased and unequal
• Sunset eyes
• Changes in level of consciousness, irritability
• Seizure activity
• In infant, the following will also be seen:
  • Bulging, tense fontanel
  • Wide sutures and increased head circumference
  • Dilated scalp veins
  • High-pitched cry
	• Lowered level of consciousness
	• Decreased motor and sensory responses
	• Bradycardia
	• Irregular respirations
	• Cheyne–Stokes respirations
	• Decerebrate or decorticate posturing
	• Fixed and dilated pupils

Laboratory and Diagnostic Tests
• Skull x-ray studies may reveal separation of sutures.
• CT and MRI will reveal the presence of hydrocephalus and can also aid in identifying the cause of hydrocephalus.

Nursing Interventions
• Focus nursing management of the child with hydrocephalus on
  • maintaining cerebral perfusion
  • minimizing neurologic complications
  • maintaining adequate nutrition
  • promoting growth and development
  • supporting and educating the child and family; and
  • administering proper antibiotics.
• Prevent and recognize shunt infection and malfunction: It is important for healthcare professionals and parents to be able to recognize when a shunt needs replacing or when complications are occurring, to decrease the possibility of death or disability that may occur due to increased ICP.

- Signs and symptoms of a *shunt infection* include elevated vital signs, poor feeding, vomiting, decreased responsiveness, seizure activity, and signs of local inflammation along the shunt tract.
- Signs and symptoms of *shunt malfunction* include vomiting, drowsiness, and headache. Signs and symptoms of increased ICP as listed earlier can also be indicative of shunt complications.
- Perform proper management of an EVD device, if present:
  - Ensure all connections are secure and label catheter as EVD.
  - Regularly check that drip chamber of manometer is set at the height prescribed in relation to the client (i.e., zero at clavicle).
  - Clamp the drain in the event of client movement or movement anticipated with care. Rezero and open clamps when done.
  - Accurately document volume and color of CSF every hour (CSF is normally clear and colorless; cloudiness indicates infection). Notify the physician or charge nurse of any significant increase in the amount of drainage (if exceeds 10 mL more than previous volumes).
  - If minimal or no drainage, check tubing for kinks, blockage, or closed clamps. Check to see if CSF is oscillating in tubing. If blockage is suspected, notify neurosurgery department immediately.
  - Dress the entry site into the skull with a sterile occlusive dressing; change it if it is soiled or nonocclusive.
  - Send routine CSF samples for culture and analysis.
  - Administer prophylactic antibiotics if ordered (may be ordered because of increased risk of infection from the drain).

Take Note!

Rapid drainage of CSF, which may occur if the child sits up without the EVD system being clamped, will decrease ICP and can lead to extreme headache, collapse of the ventricles, formation of subdural hematomas, and neurologic deterioration.

- Educate the child and family.
- Teach the child and families about signs and symptoms of shunt infection and malfunction. Early recognition of complications is essential to prevent neurologic damage.
- Support the family and assist them in establishing realistic goals and helping the child to achieve his or her developmental and educational potential.
- Involve the family in the child's care from the time of diagnosis.

- Provide parents with accurate information regarding the procedure and be available both to listen to parents' concerns and to answer questions that arise.
- Provide ongoing education about the illness and its treatment, including signs and symptoms of shunt complications.
- Refer the child and family to support groups, which can be helpful for both the family and the child. The National Hydrocephalus Foundation can be accessed at www.nhfonline.org. Additional resources can be found at www.hydroassoc.org and www.hydro-cephalus.org.

HYPERTROPHIC PYLORIC STENOSIS

Description
- Frequent and forceful (often projectile) nonbilious vomiting developing at 2 to 4 weeks of life

Pathophysiology
- The circular muscle of the pylorus becomes hypertrophied, causing thickness in the luminal side of the pyloric canal and subsequent gastric outlet obstruction.

Therapeutic Management
- Requires surgical intervention: A pyloromyotomy is performed to cut the muscle of the pylorus and relieve the gastric outlet obstruction.

Assessment Findings
Health History
- Forceful, nonbilious vomiting unrelated to feeding position
- Hunger soon after vomiting episode
- Weight loss due to vomiting
- Lethargy.

Physical Examination
- Alteration in hydration status
- Palpable mass in right upper quadrant (a hard, moveable "olive").

Laboratory and Diagnostic Tests
- Pyloric ultrasonography may identify a thickened hypoechoic ring in the region of the pylorus.
- Serum electrolyte panel may reveal metabolic alkalosis.

Nursing Interventions
- Preoperatively, administer IV fluids and correct abnormal electrolyte values.

- Provide family emotional support and education.
- After surgery, follow physician's orders for slow resumption of oral feedings usually over 1 to 2 days.

HYPOSPADIAS/EPISPADIAS

Description
- Hypospadias is a urethral defect in which the opening is on the ventral surface of the penis rather than at the end of the penis (Fig. 2.19).
- Epispadias is a urethral defect in which the opening is on the dorsal surface of the penis.
- In either case, the opening may be near the glans of the penis, midway along the penis, or near the base.

Pathophysiology
- The defect occurs during embryonal development, sometime between 8 and 20 weeks' gestation.

Therapeutic Management
- Surgical correction usually occurs sometime after about 1 year of age to provide for an appropriately placed meatus that allows for normal voiding and ejaculation (Pfeil & Lindsay, 2010).
- The meatus is moved to the glans penis and the urethra is reconstructed as needed.

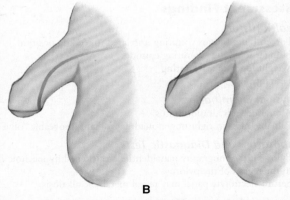

A   B

FIGURE 2.19 **A**: Hypospadias: the urethral opening is located on the ventral side of the penis. **B**: Epispadias: the urethral opening is located on the dorsal side of the penis.

Assessment Findings

Health History
- Reports of an unusual urine stream.

Physical Examination
- Off-center placement of urethral meatus or the presence of the meatus somewhere along the shaft of the penis
- Chordee (fibrous band causing the penis to curve downward)
- Associated anomalies include cryptorchidism, hydrocele, and inguinal hernia

Nursing Interventions
- Teach the newborn's parents that circumcision should be delayed until after surgical repair of the urethral meatus.
- Postoperatively, assess urinary drainage from the urethral stent or drainage tube.
- Ensure that the urinary drainage tube remains carefully taped with the penis in an upright position to prevent stress on the urethral incision.
- Administer antibiotics if prescribed.
- Assess for pain, which is usually not extensive, and administer analgesics or antispasmodics (oral oxybutynin or B & O suppository) as needed for bladder spasms.
- Double diapering is a method used to protect the urethra and stent or catheter after surgery; it also helps keep the area clean and free from infection. The inner diaper contains stool and the outer diaper contains urine, allowing separation between the bowel and bladder output (see Section III, Common Laboratory and Diagnostic Tests and Nursing Procedures, for technique on how to double diaper the child). Change the outside (larger) diaper when the child is wet; change both diapers when the child has a bowel movement.
- If the child is to be discharged with the urinary catheter in place (which is common), teach the parents how to care for the catheter and drainage system.
- Tub baths are generally prohibited until it is time to remove the penile dressing.
- Roughhousing, ride-on toys, or any activity involving straddling is not allowed for 2 to 3 weeks.

INTELLECTUAL DISABILITY

Description
- Intellectual disability refers to a functional state in which significant limitations in intellectual status and adaptive behavior (functioning in daily life) develop before the age of 18 years.

- Though intellectual disability includes the definition of intellectual quotient (IQ) less than 70 to 75, the range of impairments associated with the low IQ is variable. Impairments in the adaptive domains of conceptual, social, or practical assist with determining the severity of ID (from mild to profound) (Pivalizza & Lalani, 2014).

Pathophysiology

- The exact cause may remain unknown.
- May occur as a result of a prenatal error in CNS development or from an insult to the brain in the prenatal, perinatal, or postnatal period from a variety of causes. Prenatal exposure to alcohol or other drugs may impact cognitive development as well.
- Intellectual disability may be categorized according to severity (summarized in Table 2.9).

Therapeutic Management

- The primary goal of therapeutic management of children with intellectual disability is to provide appropriate educational experiences that allow the child to achieve a level of functioning and self-sufficiency needed for existence in the home, community, work, and leisure settings.
- The majority of people with intellectual disability require only minimal support in the school or home setting. These people are able to achieve some level of self-sufficiency.

Assessment Findings

Health History
- Family history of intellectual disability
- Problems with pregnancy and birth
- Delayed attainment of developmental milestones
- History of motor, visual, or language difficulties
- Concomitant seizure disorder
- Orthopedic problems, speech problems, or vision or hearing deficit
- Determine the child's ability to toilet, dress, and feed himself or herself
- Ask the parents about involvement with school and community services and support.

Risk Factors
- Preterm or postterm birth
- Low birth weight
- Birth injury
- Prenatal or neonatal infection
- Prenatal alcohol or drug exposure
- Genetic syndrome
- Chromosomal alteration

(text continues on page 250)

TABLE 2.9 SEVERITY OF INTELLECTUAL DISABILITY

Classification	IQ (generally)	Conceptual	Social	Practical
Mild	between 50–55 and 70	Requires academic supports	Immature social skills and personal judgment	Usually independent in activities of daily living
Moderate	between 35–40 and 50–55	Complex tasks require substantial support	Social cues, judgment and life decisions need regular support	Independent self-care with moderate supports
Severe	between 20–25 and 35–40	Little understanding of written language; require extensive supports	Benefit from healthy supportive interactions	Require significant and ongoing supervision for activities of daily living
Profound	less than 20–25	May use objects in a goal-directed fashion	May understand gestures and emotional cues; use nonverbal expression	Dependent upon support for all activities of daily living

- Metabolic disease
- Exposure to toxins (e.g., lead)
- Head injury or other trauma
- Nutritional deficiency
- Cerebral malformation
- Other brain disease or mental health disorder.

Physical Examination

- Altered language, sensory, or psychomotor functioning
- Dysmorphic features consistent with certain syndromes
- Assess language, sensory, and psychomotor functioning.

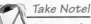 *Take Note!*

Because of the extent of cognition required to understand and produce speech, the most sensitive early indicator of intellectual disability is delayed language development.

Laboratory and Diagnostic Tests

- Newborn metabolic screening test may reveal an inborn error of metabolism, resulting in developmental delay and intellectual disability.
- Thyroid function tests may be ordered to rule out thyroid problems leading to developmental delay.
- Chromosome studies may show Down syndrome or other chromosome defect associated with intellectual disability.
- CT scan or MRI may determine damage to the brain.
- IQ tests demonstrate IQ of less than 70 to 75.

Nursing Interventions

- Continue the child's home routine while hospitalized.
- Follow through with feeding and motor supports that the child uses.
- Ensure that the child is closely supervised and remains free from harm.
- Allow parents time to verbalize frustrations or fears. Arrange for respite care as available.
- Support the child's strengths, and assist the child and family to follow through with therapy or treatment designed to enhance the child's functioning.
- Assist with the development of the child's IEP as appropriate.

IRON DEFICIENCY ANEMIA

Description

- Iron deficiency anemia occurs when the body does not have enough iron to produce hemoglobin.
- In the United States, iron deficiency anemia has a peak prevalence in children between 6 and 24 months of age, and again at the age of puberty (Ambruso, Nuss, & Wang, 2014).

- Delayed growth may occur if iron deficiency anemia persists; cognitive delays and behavioral changes may be noted.

Take Note!

For appropriate growth to occur in adolescence, increased amounts of iron must be consumed and absorbed.

Pathophysiology

- The heme portion of hemoglobin consists of iron surrounded by protoporphyrin. When not enough iron is available to the bone marrow, hemoglobin production is reduced.
- As hemoglobin levels decrease, the oxygen-carrying capacity of the blood is decreased, resulting in weakness and fatigue.
- Adequate dietary intake of iron is required for the body to make enough hemoglobin.
- Cow's milk consumption contributes to iron deficiency anemia in older infants and young children due to its poor iron availability (Bryant, 2010).

Therapeutic Management

- Iron supplementation is needed in most cases of iron deficiency anemia. Supplements are usually provided in the form of ferrous sulfate or ferrous fumarate and are available over the counter.
- In more severe cases, transfusion of packed red blood cells (PRBCs) may be needed (Bryant, 2010).

Assessment Findings

Health History

- Irritability
- Headache
- Dizziness
- Weakness
- Shortness of breath
- Pallor
- Fatigue
- Difficulty feeding
- Pica
- Muscle weakness
- Unsteady gait.

Risk Factors

- Maternal anemia during pregnancy
- Poorly controlled diabetes during pregnancy
- Prematurity, low birth weight, or multiple birth

- Cow's milk consumption before 12 months of age or excessive cow's milk consumption (more than 24 ounces a day)
- Infant consumption of low iron formula
- Lack of iron supplementation after 6 months of age in breast-fed infants
- Excessive weight gain
- Chronic infection or inflammation
- Chronic or acute blood loss
- Restricted diets
- Use of medication interfering with iron absorption, such as antacids
- Low socioeconomic status
- Recent immigration from a developing country (Ambruso et al., 2014; Bryant, 2010).

Physical Examination
- Fatigue
- Lethargy
- Pallor of the skin, conjunctivae, oral mucosa, palms, and soles
- Nail spooning (concave shape)
- Low oxygen saturation via pulse oximetry
- Tachycardia
- Splenomegaly.

Laboratory and Diagnostic Tests
- Decreased hemoglobin and hematocrit
- Decreased reticulocyte count
- Microcytosis
- Hypochromia
- Decreased serum iron and ferritin levels
- Increased free erythrocyte protoporphyrin level.

Nursing Interventions
- Provide close observation of the anemic child. Assist the older child with ambulation. Educate the parents on how to protect the child from injury due to an unsteady gait or dizziness.
- Ensure breast-fed infants begin iron supplementation around the 4 or 5 months of age.
- For children older than 1 year, limit cow's milk intake to 24 ounces/day.
- Limit fast-food consumption and encourage intake of iron-rich foods such as red meats (iron from red meat is the easiest for the body to absorb), tuna, salmon, eggs, tofu, enriched grains, dried beans and peas, dried fruits, leafy green vegetables, and iron-fortified breakfast cereals.
- Teach the parents about dietary intake of iron (see Box 2.5).
- Refer families who meet the financial limits and who have children 5 years and younger to the Women, Infants, and Children (WIC)

BOX 2.5

RECOMMENDED DIETARY DAILY INTAKE FOR IRON IN CHILDREN

- 0–6 months: 0.27 mg
- 6–12 months: 3 mg
- 1–3 years: 7 mg
- 4–8 years: 11 mg
- 9–13 years: 8 mg
- Boys 14–18 years: 11 mg
- Girls 14–18 years: 15 mg

Adapted from Haemer, M., Primark, L. E., & Krebs, N. R. (2012). Normal childhood nutrition and its disorders. In W. W. Hay, M. J. Levin, R. R. Deterding, & M. J. Abzug, (Eds.), *Current pediatric diagnosis and treatment* (22nd ed.). New York, NY: McGraw-Hill.

---

program, which provides for supplementation of infant's and children's diets.

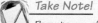

Take Note!

Parents are often concerned that a diagnosis of iron deficiency anemia or referral to the WIC program may lead to interventions from children's services. Assure the family that as long as appropriate measures are taken to address the anemia, referrals of this nature are not generally made.

- Teach parents proper administration of iron supplements. Liquid should be placed behind the teeth to avoid tooth staining.
- Encourage parents to increase fiber and fluid in the child's diet to decrease the occurrence of constipation due to iron supplementation.

JUVENILE IDIOPATHIC ARTHRITIS

Description

- Juvenile idiopathic arthritis is a chronic disease in which the child may experience healthy periods alternating with flare-ups of joint pain.
- In some children, the disease resolves as they approach adolescence or adulthood, whereas others will have more severe disease that continues throughout the adult years (Jones & Higgins, 2010).
- Table 2.10 explains the three most common types.

TABLE 2.10 TYPES OF JUVENILE IDIOPATHIC ARTHRITIS

Type	Definition	Nonjoint Manifestations	Complications
Pauciarticular	Involvement of four or fewer joints; quite often the knee is involved. Most common type	Eye inflammation, malaise, poor appetite, poor weight gain	Iritis, uveitis, uneven leg bone growth
Polyarticular	Involvement of five or more joints; frequently involves small joints and often affects the body symmetrically	Malaise, lymphadenopathy, organomegaly, poor growth	Often a severe form of arthritis; rapidly progressing joint damage, rheumatoid nodules
Systemic	In addition to joint involvement, fever and rash may be present at diagnosis	Enlarged spleen, liver, and lymph nodes; myalgia; severe anemia	Pericarditis, pericardial effusion, pleuritis, pulmonary fibrosis

Adapted from Jones, K. B., & Higgins, G. C. (2010). Juvenile rheumatoid arthritis. In P. J. Allen, J. A. Vessey, & N. A. Schapiro (Eds.), *Primary care of the child with a chronic condition* (5th ed., pp. 587–606). St. Louis, MO: Mosby.

Pathophysiology

- Juvenile idiopathic arthritis is an autoimmune disorder in which the autoantibodies mainly target the joints.
- Inflammatory changes in the joints cause pain, redness, warmth, stiffness, and swelling.
- Stiffness usually occurs after inactivity (as in the morning, after sleep).
- Some forms also affect the eyes or other organs.

Therapeutic Management

- Therapeutic management focuses on inflammation control, pain relief, promotion of remission, and maintenance of mobility.
- NSAIDs, corticosteroids, and antirheumatic drugs such as methotrexate and etanercept are prescribed, depending on the type and severity of the disease.
- NSAIDs are helpful with pain relief, but disease-modifying (antirheumatic) drugs are necessary to prevent disease progression.

Assessment Findings

Health History

- Irritability or fussiness (especially in the infant or very young child)
- Complaints of pain
- History of withdrawal from play
- Difficulty getting the child out of bed in the morning (joint stiffness after inactivity)
- Fever (above 39.5°C for 2 weeks or more in systemic disease).

Physical Examination

- Fever (present with systemic disease)
- Evanescent, pale red, nonpruritic macular rash (may be present at diagnosis of systemic disease)
- Limp
- Guarding of a joint or extremity
- Delayed growth
- Joint edema, redness, warmth, or tenderness
- Flexed positioning of joints.

Laboratory and Diagnostic Tests

- CBC count: may reveal mild to moderate anemia
- Elevated ESR
- Positive antinuclear antibody in young children with the pauciarticular form or a positive rheumatoid factor in adolescents with polyarticular disease.

Nursing Interventions

- Refer the child to a pediatric rheumatologist to ensure that he or she receives the most up-to-date treatment.

- Encourage regular eye examinations and vision screening both to allow for early treatment of visual changes and to prevent blindness.
- Administer medications as prescribed to control inflammation and prevent disease progression.
- Maintain joint range of motion and muscle strength via exercise (physical or occupational therapy).
- Teach families appropriate use of splints prescribed to prevent joint contractures. Monitor for pressure areas or skin breakdown with splint or orthotic use.
- Encourage adequate sleep to allow the child to cope better with symptoms and to function better in school. Warm baths at bedtime may promote sleep.
- Sleep may be promoted by a warm bath at bedtime and warm compresses to affected joints or massage.
- Encourage the child to attend school and ensure that teachers, the school nurse, and classmates are educated about the child's disease and any limitations on activity.
- Encourage children and families to become involved with local support groups, so they can see that they are not alone.

KAWASAKI DISEASE

Description
- Kawasaki disease is an acute systemic vasculitis occurring mostly in children 6 months to 5 years of age
- It is a self-limited syndrome but can cause cardiovascular complications such as coronary artery aneurysm, and cardiomyopathy among others (Sundel, 2015).

Pathophysiology
- Kawasaki disease appears to be an autoimmune response mediated by cytokine-induced endothelial cell surface antigens that leads to vasculitis.
- Neutrophils, followed by mononuclear cells, T lymphocytes, and IgA-producing plasma cells, infiltrate the vessels and then inflammation occurs.
- Coronary dilatation (ectasia) or aneurysm may occur (either acutely or as a long-term sequela).

Therapeutic Management
- In the acute phase, high-dose aspirin in four divided doses daily and a single administration of intravenous immunoglobulin (IVIG) are used.

• Children whose fever persists longer than 48 hours after initiation of aspirin therapy may receive a second dose of IVIG.

Assessment Findings

Health History
• Fever, chills
• Headache, malaise, extreme irritability
• Vomiting, diarrhea, abdominal pain
• Joint pain.

Take Note!

Of particular note is a history of high fever (39.9°C) of at least 5-day duration that is unresponsive to antibiotics.

Physical Examination
• Significant bilateral conjunctivitis without exudate
• Dry, fissured lips, strawberry (cracked and reddened) tongue, and pharyngeal and oral mucosa erythema
• Hyperdynamic precordium
• Diffuse, erythematous, polymorphous rash
• Edema of the hands and feet, erythema, and painful induration of the palms and soles
• Desquamation (peeling) of the perineal region, fingers, and toes, extending to the palms and soles
• Possible jaundice
• Cervical lymphadenopathy (usually unilateral)
• Hepatomegaly
• Joint tenderness to palpation
• Tachycardia, gallop, or murmur.

Laboratory and Diagnostic Tests
• CBC count: mild to moderate anemia, an elevated WBC count during the acute phase, and significant thrombocytosis (elevated platelet count [500,000 to 1 million]) in the later phase
• ESR and the C-reactive protein (CRP) level are elevated.
• Echocardiogram is obtained as soon as possible to provide a base-line of a healthy heart or to evaluate for coronary artery involvement. Repeat echocardiograms may be obtained during the illness and as part of long-term follow-up.

Nursing Interventions
• Administer aspirin and immunoglobulin as ordered.
• Administer IV and oral fluids as ordered, evaluating intake and output carefully.

- Assess frequently for signs of developing heart failure such as tachycardia, gallop, decreased urine output, or respiratory distress.
- Evaluate quality and strength of pulses and provide cardiac monitoring as ordered, reporting arrhythmias.
- Prepare the child for echocardiography.
- Provide acetaminophen for fever management and apply cool cloths as tolerated.
- Keep the environment quiet and cluster nursing care activities to decrease stimulation and hence irritability; provide comfortable positioning, particularly if the child has joint pain or arthritis.
- Apply petrolatum jelly or another lubricating ointment to the lips; encourage the older child to suck on ice chips, whereas the younger child may suck on a cool, moist washcloth; popsicles are also soothing.
- Provide ongoing support and education to the child and family.
- Ensure the family understands the importance of cardiology follow-up after discharge.

LATEX ALLERGY

Description
- Latex allergy occurs in particular subsets of children, but potentially any child could become allergic to latex.

Pathophysiology
- Latex allergy is an IgE-mediated response to exposure to latex, a natural rubber product used in many common items (especially gloves in the healthcare setting).
- An immediate allergic reaction of itching, redness, and hives may occur if a latex-allergic child comes in to contact with latex.
- Anaphylaxis may also occur, resulting in respiratory distress and arrest.

Therapeutic Management
- Avoidance of exposure to latex products is recommended for those who are allergic to it.

Assessment Findings
Health History
- Known allergic response to latex
- Hives after rubber glove exposure
- Coughing/wheezing/shortness of breath after glove exposure
- Swelling or mouth itching after a dental examination.

Risk Factors

- Previous exposure and known allergy to pear, peach, passion fruit, plum, pineapple, kiwi, fig, grape, cherry, melon, nectarine, papaya, apple, apricot, banana, chestnut, carrot, celery, avocado, tomato, or potato.

Physical Examination

- Hives
- Wheeze
- Cough
- Shortness of breath
- Nasal congestion and rhinorrhea
- Sneezing
- Nose, palate, or eye pruritus
- Hypotension.

Nursing Interventions

- Prevent exposure to latex products.
- Document latex allergy on the chart, child's identification band, the medication administration record, and the physician's order sheet.
- Instruct children and their families to avoid foods with a known cross-reactivity to latex such as those listed earlier.
- If the child is exposed to latex, remove the irritating substance and cleanse the area with soap and water. Assess for the need for resuscitation and perform it if needed.
- Become familiar with the institution's latex allergy policy. Know which products contain latex and which do not.
- Refer families to resources for people with latex allergy.

MEDICAL CHILD ABUSE

Description

- Medical child abuse has historically been termed Münchausen syndrome by proxy (MSBP). It is a type of child abuse in which the parent creates physical and/or psychological symptoms of illness or impairment.

Pathophysiology

- The adult parent meets his or her own psychological needs by having an ill child. Medical child abuse is difficult to detect and may remain hidden for years. In most cases, the biologic mother is the perpetrator (Endom, 2015).

Therapeutic Management

- Ensure the safety and well-being of the child.

- Because of the psychological issues of the perpetrator, management of medical child abuse is complex. The perpetrator must receive psychotherapy.

Assessment Findings
- Detailed documentation of the history and physical examination is the basis for determining that medical child abuse is present.

Health History
- Child with one or more illnesses that do not respond to treatment or that follow a puzzling course
- A similar history in siblings
- Symptoms that do not make sense or that disappear when the perpetrator is removed or not present. The symptoms are witnessed only by the caregiver (e.g., cyanosis, apnea, seizure).
- Physical and laboratory findings that do not fit with the reported history
- Repeated hospitalizations failing to produce a medical diagnosis, transfers to other hospitals, discharges against medical advice
- Parent who refuses to accept that the diagnosis is not medical (Endom, 2015).

Physical Examination
- Observe the mother's behavior with the child, spouse or partner, and staff.
- Use of covert video surveillance may reveal maternal actions causing illness in the child.

Nursing Interventions
- When an actual abusive activity is identified, notify the social services and risk management departments of the hospital.
- Ensure that the local child protection team and the caregiver's family or support system is present when the caregiver is confronted.
- Inform the caregiver of the plan of care for the child and of the availability of psychiatric assistance for the caregiver.

MYELOMENINGOCELE

Description
- Myelomeningocele is a type of spina bifida cystica, and clinically the term "spina bifida" is often used to refer to myelomeningocele.
- In myelomeningocele, the spinal cord often ends at the point of the defect, resulting in absent motor and sensory functions beyond that point.
- Long-term complications include paralysis, orthopedic deformities, and bladder and bowel incontinence.

- The presence of neurogenic bladder and frequent catheterization puts the child at an increased risk for UTIs, pyelonephritis, and hydronephrosis, which may result in long-term renal damage if managed inappropriately.
- Accompanying hydrocephalus is common due to the improper development and the downward displacement of the brain into the cervical spine resulting in CSF flow being blocked. The lower the deformity is on the spine, the lower the risk of developing hydrocephalus (Kinsman & Johnston, 2011).
- These children usually require multiple surgical procedures and due to frequent catheterizations are at an increased risk of developing a latex allergy (Kinsman & Johnston, 2011; Zak & Chan, 2014).
- Learning problems and seizures are common in these children, but the majority of those surviving with myelomeningocele have average intelligence (Kinsman & Johnston, 2011).
- Ambulation is possible for some children, depending on the level of the lesion.

Pathophysiology

- The cause is unknown, but risk factors are consistent with other neural tube defects, such as maternal drug use, malnutrition, and a genetic predisposition (Kinsman & Johnston, 2011).
- The neural tube fails to close at the end of the fourth week of gestation. As a result, an external sac-like protrusion that encases the meninges, spinal fluid, and, in some cases, nerves is present on the spine.
- The degree of neurologic deficit will depend on the location and size of the lesion (Kinsman & Johnston, 2011). An increase in neurologic deficit is seen with higher lesions as more nerves are affected.

Therapeutic Management

- Surgical closure will be performed as soon as possible after birth, especially if a CSF leak is present or if there is a danger of the sac rupturing. The goal of early surgical intervention is to prevent infection and to minimize further loss of function, which can result from the stretching of nerve roots as the meningeal sac expands after birth.
- A new option is becoming available but remains experimental. In utero fetal surgery to repair the myelomeningocele has been performed in the United States, with the first randomized trial showing improved outcomes for the fetuses but is not without risks to the mother and fetus (Robinson, 2011; Committee on Obstetric Practice, 2013)
- Ongoing management of this disorder remains complex and *necessitates* lifelong follow-up; a multidisciplinary approach is needed, involving specialists in neurology, neurosurgery, urology, orthopedics, therapy, and rehabilitation along with intense nursing care.

Assessment Findings

Health History of Undiagnosed Child
• High-risk deliveries.

Risk Factors
• Lack of prenatal care
• Lack of preconception and/or prenatal folic acid supplementation
• Previous child born with neural tube defect or family history of neural tube defects
• Maternal consumption of certain drugs that antagonize folic acid, such as anticonvulsants (carbamazepine and phenobarbital).

Health History of a Diagnosed Child
• Current mobility status and any changes in motor abilities
• Current genitourinary function and regimen and any changes
• Current bowel function and regimen and any changes
• Signs or symptoms of urinary infections
• History of hydrocephalus with the presence of a shunt
• Signs or symptoms of shunt infection or malfunction (refer to the section on hydrocephalus)
• Latex sensitivity
• Changes in nutritional status, including changes in weight
• Changes in physical or cognitive state.

Physical Examination
• At birth, physical examination may reveal
  • a visible external sac protruding from the spinal area (with or without an intact sac cover)
  • neurologic anomalies; or
  • flaccid paralysis, absence of deep tendon reflexes, lack of response to touch and pain stimuli, skeletal abnormalities such as club feet, constant dribbling of urine, and a relaxed anal sphincter.
• In the older infant or child, physical examination may reveal
  • decreased functional performance
  • specific level of paralysis or paresthesia
  • skin breakdown; or
  • decreased motor capabilities.

Laboratory and Diagnostic Tests
• Ultrasonography may detect myelomeningocele prenatally around 16 to 18 weeks' gestation.
• Blood test may detect increases in AFP prenatally.
• Analysis of amniotic fluid may detect increase in AFP prenatally.
• MRI, CT scan, ultrasonography, and myelography will evaluate brain and spinal cord involvement.

Nursing Interventions

Prevent Trauma and Infection Before Surgical Repair of the Defect

- Use sterile, saline-soaked, nonadhesive gauze or antibiotic-soaked gauze to keep the sac moist.
- Immediately report any seepage of clear fluid from the lesion because this could indicate an opening in the sac and provide a portal of entry for microorganisms.
- Position the infant in the prone position or supported on the side to avoid pressure on the sac.
- To keep the infant warm, place the infant in a warmer or Isolette to avoid the use of blankets which could exert too much pressure on the sac. Pay special attention while the infant is in a warmer or Isolette because the radiant heat can cause drying and cracking of the sac.
- Keep the lesion free of feces and urine to help avoid infection.
- Position the infant so that urine and feces flow away from the sac (e.g., prone position, or place a folded towel under the abdomen).
- Placing a piece of plastic wrap below the meningocele is another way of preventing feces from coming into contact with the lesion.
- After surgery, position the infant in the prone or side-lying position to allow the incision to heal. Continue with precautions to prevent urine or feces from coming into contact with the incision.

Promote Urinary and Bowel Elimination

- Children with myelomeningocele often have bladder and bowel incontinence, though some children may achieve normal urinary and some degree of bowel continence. The level of the lesion will influence the amount of dysfunction.
- Determine the child's pattern and success of toilet training, both for bladder and for bowel.
- Assess the child's cognitive/developmental level.
- Observe the genital area for dribbling of urine from the urethra, noting odor of urine if present.
- Note redness of the urethra or excoriation in the diaper area.
- Inspect the abdomen for scars from prior surgeries and the presence of urinary diversion or continent stoma.
- Palpate the abdomen for the presence of distended bladder, fecal mass, or enlarged kidneys.
- Determine the child's level of paralysis or paresthesia.
- Bowel training with the use of timed enemas or suppositories along with diet modifications can allow for defecation at predetermined times once or twice a day.

- Neurogenic bladder is common. Therefore, evaluation of renal function by a pediatric urologist should be performed on each child with myelomeningocele. Interventions for neurogenic bladder include the following:
  - Clean intermittent catheterization to promote bladder emptying
  - Medications such as oxybutynin chloride (Ditropan) to improve bladder capacity
  - Prompt recognition and treatment of infections
  - In some children, surgical interventions such as a continent urinary reservoir or vesicostomy to facilitate urinary elimination

Promote Adequate Nutrition

- The risk for altered nutrition, less than body requirements, related to the restrictions on positioning of the infant before and after surgery is another nursing concern.
- Assist the family in assuming as normal a feeding position as possible.
- Preoperatively, the risk of rupture may be too high to warrant holding. Therefore, the infant's head can be turned to the side or the infant can be placed in the side-lying position to facilitate feeding.
- If the infant is held, special care needs to be taken to avoid pressure on the sac or postoperative incision.
- Encourage the parents to interact as much as possible with the infant by talking to and touching the infant during feeding to help promote intake.
- If the mother was planning on breast-feeding the infant, assist her in meeting this goal, if possible. If the infant can be held, encourage her to do this, or assist her in pumping and saving breast milk to be given to the infant via bottle until the infant can be held.
- Feeding an infant in an unusual position can be difficult, and it is the nurse's role to provide support, education, and modeling for the parents and family when needed.

Prevent Latex Allergic Reaction

- A latex-free environment should be created for all procedures performed on children with myelomeningocele to prevent latex allergy.
- Children who are at a high risk for latex sensitivity should wear medical alert identification.
- Children with a known latex allergy must be identified and managed in a latex-free environment.
- Be familiar with those products and equipment at your facility that contain latex and those that are latex free. Each hospital should have a list readily available to healthcare professionals. For an updated list of latex-containing products and other helpful information for parents regarding consumer products, contact the Spina Bifida Association of America at http://www.sbaa.org.

- Education programs regarding latex sensitivity and ways to prevent it need to be directed at those who care for high-risk children, including teachers, school nurses, relatives, babysitters, and all healthcare professionals.

Maintain Skin Integrity

- Ensure that the infant is kept as clean and dry as possible. This is made more difficult because diapering may be contraindicated preoperatively to avoid pressure on the sac and by the constant dribbling of stool and urine that may be present. The prone position puts constant pressure on the knees and elbows, therefore special precautions need to be taken.
- Placing a pad beneath the diaper area and changing it frequently are important.
- Perform meticulous skin care.
- Place the infant on a special care mattress and place synthetic sheepskin under the infant to help reduce friction.
- Special attention to the infant's legs is needed when positioning them because paralysis may be present. Using a folded diaper between the legs can help reduce pressure and friction from the legs rubbing together.

Educate the Child and Family

- Adjusting to the demands this condition places on the child and family is difficult. Parents may need time to accept their infant's condition, but as soon as possible they should be involved in the infant's care.
- Teaching should begin immediately and include positioning, preventing infection, feeding, promoting urinary elimination through clean intermittent catheterization, preventing latex allergy, and the signs and symptoms of complications such as increased ICP.
- Because of the chronic nature of this condition, long-term planning needs to begin in the hospital.
- These children usually require multiple surgical procedures and hospitalizations, and this can place stress on the family and their finances.
- The nurse has an important role in providing ongoing education about the illness and its treatment and the plan of care.
- As the family becomes more comfortable with the condition, they will become the experts in the child's care.
- Respect and recognize the family's changing needs. Providing intense daily care can take its toll on a family, and continual support and encouragement are needed.
- Referral to the Spina Bifida Association and a local support group for families of children with myelomeningocele is appropriate.

- Teach parents and the child the technique of clean intermittent catheterization via the urethra, unless a urinary diversion or continent stoma has been created (see Teaching Guideline 2.18). Children with normal intelligence and upper extremity motor skills usually learn to self-catheterize at the age of 6 or 7 years (Zak & Chan, 2014).

Teaching Guidelines 2.18
CLEAN INTERMITTENT CATHETERIZATION

- Wash hands with soap and water or use waterless antibacterial cleanser.
- Have supplies within reach and place child on his or her back on toilet or in wheelchair.
- Clean genitalia with a washcloth or disposable wipe (in girls, separate labia and wipe front to back; in boys, clean the tip of the penis; if uncircumcised, pull back foreskin so that the tip of penis is visible).
- Apply generous amount of water-based lubricant to catheter.
- Perform catheterization. Insert catheter only as far as needed to obtain urine flow (about 2–3 inches for females, about 4–6 inches for males). Hold catheter there until urine flow stops. Move catheter slightly, press on lower abdomen, or have child lean forward to tense abdominals in order to ensure no more urine is in the bladder.
- Wash reusable catheter after use with soapy water inside and out; rinse well (a syringe can be used to flush the catheter) and allow to dry.
- When dry, store in zip-top plastic bag or other clean storage container.
- Sterilize daily (time frames and procedure may vary on the basis of institution policy and procedures), soak the catheter in a 1:1 vinegar and water solution for about 30 minutes, rinsing well before next use, or place the catheter in boiling water for 10 minutes. Allow to dry very well before storing.
- Replace the catheter when it becomes cloudy, stiff, rough, cracked, or damaged.
- When developmentally ready, teach the child to self-catheterize.

Adapted from Bozic, D., & Daniels, C. (2009a). AboutKidsHealth. Clean intermittent catheterization (CIC): Step by step instructions for boys. Retrieved on October 10, 2015, from http://www.aboutkidshealth.ca/en/healthaz/testsandtreatments/medicaldevices/pages/clean-intermittent-catheterization-cic-step-by-step-instructions-for-boys.aspx; Bozic, D., & Daniels, C. (2009b). AboutKidsHealth clean intermittent catheterization (CIC): Step by step instructions for girls. Retrieved October 10, 2015, from http://www.aboutkidshealth.ca/En/HealthAZ/TestsAndTreatments/Medical Devices/Pages/Clean-Intermittent-Catheterization-CIC-Step-By-Step-Instructions-for-Girls.aspx

MUSCULAR DYSTROPHY

Description

- Muscular dystrophy refers to a group of inherited conditions that result in progressive muscle weakness and wasting, primarily the skeletal (voluntary) muscles.
- The skeletal muscle fibers are affected, yet there are no structural abnormalities in the spinal cord or the peripheral nerves.
- Nine types of muscular dystrophy exist, and they are most often diagnosed in childhood and affect a variety of muscle groups. Duchenne muscular dystrophy is the most common neuromuscular disorder and is discussed here.
- There is no cure and it is universally fatal (Zak & Chan 2014).
- Additional complications include pulmonary, urinary, or systemic infections, depression, learning or behavioral disorders, aspiration pneumonia (as oropharyngeal muscles become affected), cardiac dysrhythmias, and eventually respiratory insufficiency and failure (as weakness of the chest muscles and diaphragm progresses).

Pathophysiology

- The gene mutation in Duchenne muscular dystrophy results in the absence of dystrophin, a protein that is critical for maintenance of muscle cells.
- The gene is X-linked recessive, meaning that mainly boys are affected and they receive the gene from their mothers (women are carriers but have no symptoms).
- Absence of dystrophin leads to generalized weakness of voluntary muscles; the weakness progresses over time. The hips, thighs, pelvis, and shoulders are affected initially.
- As the disease progresses, all voluntary muscles as well as cardiac and respiratory muscles are affected.

Therapeutic Management

- The use of corticosteroids may slow the progression of the disease (Muscular Dystrophy Association, 2011; Zak & Chan, 2014). It is thought that prednisone helps by protecting muscle fibers from damage to the sarcolemma (defective in the absence of dystrophin).
- Calcium and vitamin D supplements are prescribed to prevent osteoporosis,
- Antidepressants may be helpful when depression occurs related to the chronicity of the disease and/or as an effect of corticosteroid use (Muscular Dystrophy Association, 2011)
- Medications to decrease the workload of the heart, such as beta-blockers and ACE (Angiotensin-converting enzyme) inhibitors may be prescribed.
- Braces or orthoses and mobility and positioning aids are necessary.

- Contractures may require surgical tendon release.
- Surgical spinal fixation with rod implantation is often required by adolescence due to spinal curvatures that result over time (Muscular Dystrophy Association, 2011).

Assessment Findings

Health History of the Undiagnosed Child

- Family history of neuromuscular disorders
- Pregnancy problem or birth trauma
- Late to learn to walk or unable to walk
- Pseudohypertrophy (enlarged appearance) of the calves
- Frequent falling and clumsiness
- Difficulty climbing stairs and running; cannot get up from the floor in the usual fashion
- Walks on the toes or balls of the feet with a rolling or waddling gait
- Significantly disturbed balance; child's belly may stick out when the shoulders are pulled back to stay upright and keep from falling over
- Difficulty in raising the arms
- Loss of the ability to ambulate sometime between 7 and 12 years of age and assistance or support required for any activity of the arms, legs, or trunk by the teen years (Muscular Dystrophy Association, 2011)
- Specific learning disability (Sarant, 2007).

Health History of the Diagnosed Child

- Progression of disease
- Need for assistive or adaptive equipment such as braces or wheelchairs
- Determine skills related to activities of daily living
- History of cough or frequent respiratory infections, which occur as the respiratory muscles weaken
- Presence of psychosocial issues such as decreased self-esteem, depression, alterations in socialization, or altered family processes.

Physical Examination

- Presence of Gowers sign: the child cannot rise from the floor in standard fashion because of increasing weakness
- Altered gait
- Ineffective cough
- Note tachycardia, which develops as the heart muscle weakens
- Diminished breath sounds with decreasing respiratory function
- Decreased muscle strength with resistance testing
- Decreased muscle tone.

Laboratory and Diagnostic Tests

- Electromyography demonstrates that the problem lies in the muscles and not in the nerves.
- Serum creatine kinase levels are elevated early in the disorder, when significant muscle wasting is actively occurring.
- Muscle biopsy provides definitive diagnosis, demonstrating the absence of dystrophin.
- DNA testing reveals the presence of the gene.

Nursing Interventions

Promote Mobility

- Administer corticosteroids and calcium supplements as ordered.
- Encourage at least minimal weight bearing in a standing position to promote improved circulation, healthier bones, and a straight spine.
- Perform passive stretching or strengthening exercises as recommended by the physical therapist.
- Use orthotic supports such as hand braces or AFOs to prevent contractures of joints.
- Schedule activities during the part of the day when the child has the most energy.
- Teach parents the use of positioning, exercises, orthoses, and adaptive equipment.

Maintain Gas Exchange and Perfusion

- Assess respiratory rate, depth of respirations, and work of breathing.
- Auscultate the lungs to determine whether aeration is sufficient and to assess clarity of breath sounds.
- Position the child for maximum chest expansion, usually in the upright position.
- Teach the child and family deep breathing exercises to strengthen or maintain respiratory muscles and encourage coughing to clear the airways.
- Perform chest physical therapy or assist with chest percussion.
- Monitor the results of pulmonary function testing.
- Use of intermittent positive pressure ventilation and mechanically assisted coughing will become necessary in the teen years for some boys, possibly later for others.
- Teach parents monitoring and use of these modalities in conjunction with the respiratory therapist.
- Monitor cardiac status closely to identify heart failure early.
- Assess for edema, weight gain, or crackles.
- Strictly monitor fluid intake and output.

Maximize Quality of Life

- Long periods of bed rest may contribute to further weakness. Work with the child and family to develop a schedule for diversional activities that provide appropriate developmental stimulation but avoid overexertion or frustration (related to inability to perform the activity).
- Periods of adequate rest must be balanced with activities.
- Walking or riding a stationary bike is appropriate for the child who has upper extremity involvement. For the child with lower extremity involvement, a wheelchair may become necessary for mobility, and the child may participate in crafts, drawing, and computer activities.
- Participating in the Special Olympics may be appropriate for some children (www.specialolympics.org).
- Assess the child's educational status. Some children attend school, others may opt for home schooling.
- Administer antidepressants as ordered: Managing depression may increase the child's desire to participate in activities and self-care.

Educate the Child and Family

- Provide emotional support to the child and family.
- Long-term direct care is stressful for families and becomes more complex as the child gets older. Families often need respite from continual caregiving duties. When a child is hospitalized, the caregiver may feel comfortable allowing nurses and other healthcare professionals to assume more of the child's daily care; this can be an opportunity for the caregiver to obtain respite from daily care. Respite care may also be offered in the home by various community services, so explore these resources with families.
- Refer the child and family to the Muscular Dystrophy Association (www.mda.org), which provides multidisciplinary care via clinics located throughout the United States. The association is also a clearinghouse for resources for individuals with muscular dystrophy.
- Ensure that families receive genetic counseling for family planning purposes as well as determining which family members may be carriers for muscular dystrophy.

NEPHROTIC SYNDROME

Description

- Nephrotic syndrome occurs as a result of increased glomerular basement membrane permeability, which allows abnormal loss of protein in the urine.
- The most commonly occurring type is idiopathic nephrotic syndrome and is also called minimal change nephrotic syndrome (Lum, 2014).

- Complications include anemia, infection, poor growth, peritonitis, thrombosis, and renal failure. Children with nephrotic syndrome are at increased risk for clotting (thromboembolism) and development of serious infection, most commonly pneumococcal pneumonia, sepsis, or spontaneous peritonitis.

Pathophysiology
- Increased glomerular permeability results in the passage of larger plasma proteins through the glomerular basement membrane.
- This results in excess loss of protein (albumin) in the urine (proteinuria) and decreased protein and albumin (hypoalbuminemia) in the bloodstream.
- Hypoalbuminemia results in a change in osmotic pressure, and fluid shifts from the bloodstream into the interstitial tissue (causing edema).
- The decrease in blood volume triggers the kidneys to respond by conserving sodium and water, leading to further edema.
- The liver senses the protein loss and increases production of lipoproteins, with subsequent development of hyperlipidemia.

Therapeutic Management
- Medications such as corticosteroids or immunosuppressive therapy with cyclophosphamide, cyclosporine A, or mycophenolate mofetil may be used. Long-term therapy is usually required to induce remission.
- IV albumin and diuretics may be used in the edematous phase.

Assessment Findings

Health History
- Nausea or vomiting
- Recent weight gain
- Periorbital edema upon waking, progressing to generalized edema throughout the day
- Weakness
- Fatigue
- Irritability or fussiness.

Risk Factors
- Intrauterine growth retardation
- Young age (younger than 3 years)
- Male sex.

Physical Examination
- Edema (periorbital, generalized [anasarca], or abdominal ascites)
- Skin appears stretched and tight
- Pallor
- Skin breakdown related to significant edema
- Weight gain

- Increased work of breathing
- Usually normal or low blood pressure, although can be elevated
- Gallop, adventitious breath sounds.

Laboratory and Diagnostic Tests
- Urinalysis: marked proteinuria, mild hematuria (infrequent)
- Serum protein and albumin levels: low (often markedly so)
- Serum cholesterol and triglyceride levels: elevated
- Serum creatinine and BUN: elevated (with progression of disease).

Nursing Interventions
- Administer corticosteroids as ordered (tapering or weaning doses are required when the time comes to stop corticosteroid therapy).
- Administer diuretics if ordered, usually furosemide (Lasix). Administer potassium supplementation or a diet higher in potassium-containing foods if hypokalemia develops.
- Monitor urine output and the amount of protein in the urine (by dipstick).
- Weigh the child daily on the same scale, either naked or wearing the same amount of clothing.
- Assess for resolution of edema. Measure pulse rate and blood pressure every 4 hours to detect hypovolemia resulting from excessive fluid shifts.
- Enforce oral fluid restrictions if ordered.
- If ordered, administer IV albumin, followed by a diuretic.
- Monitor the child's temperature.
- Administer pneumococcal vaccine and prophylactic antibiotics as prescribed.
- Teach parents that if the child is unimmunized and is exposed to chickenpox, the pediatrician or nephrologist should be notified immediately so that the child may receive VZIG.
- Encourage a nutrient-rich diet within prescribed restrictions.
- Provide support and education to the family. Teach families monitoring of urine dipsticks.

NEUROBLASTOMA

Description
- Neuroblastoma is the most common extracranial solid tumor in children and the second most frequently occurring solid tumor in children (Hendershot, 2010).
- Ninety percent of cases are diagnosed before the age of 5 years (Graham et al., 2014).
- Survival and prognosis depend upon age at diagnosis, tumor location, and the extent and location of metastasis (Hendershot, 2010).

Pathophysiology

- Neuroblastoma arises from embryonic neural crest cells.
- It most frequently occurs in the abdomen, mainly in the adrenal gland, but it may occur anywhere along the paravertebral sympathetic chain in the chest or retroperitoneum (Hendershot, 2010).
- Usually by the time of diagnosis, the neuroblastoma has already metastasized.

Therapeutic Management

- The neuroblastoma must be removed surgically.
- Radiation and chemotherapy are administered to all children with neuroblastoma except those with stage I disease, in whom the tumor is completely resected.

Assessment Findings

Health History

- Swollen or asymmetric abdomen
- Alteration in bowel or bladder dysfunction
- Neurologic symptoms (brain metastasis)
- Bone pain (bone metastasis)
- Anorexia, vomiting, or weight loss.

Physical Examination

- Neck or facial swelling
- Bruising above the eyes or edema around the eyes (metastasis to skull bones)
- Skin pallor or bruising (bone marrow metastasis)
- Cough, difficulty breathing, wheezing
- Cervical lymphadenopathy
- Firm and nontender abdominal mass
- Hepatomegaly or splenomegaly.

Laboratory and Diagnostic Tests

- CT scan or MRI: to determine the site of tumor and evidence of metastasis
- Chest radiographs, bone scan, and skeletal survey: to identify metastasis
- Bone marrow aspiration and biopsy: to determine metastasis to the bone marrow
- Twenty-four-hour urine collection for homovanillic acid (HVA) and vanillylmandelic acid (VMA); levels will be elevated.

Nursing Interventions

- Provide routine care after abdominal surgery. Refer to the section on leukemia for information related to caring for a child receiving chemotherapy.

• Provide emotional support and possible referrals to help children and families cope with a potentially poor prognosis (due to the fact that the disease has often metastasized significantly by the time of diagnosis).

Atraumatic Care

The child with cancer often undergoes a large number of painful procedures related to laboratory specimens and treatment protocols. To assist the child to cope with these procedures, provide distraction in the form of reading a favorite book or playing a favorite movie or musical selection.

OBSTRUCTIVE UROPATHY

Description
• Obstructive uropathy is an obstruction at any level along the upper or lower urinary tract.
• Common sites for congenital obstructive uropathy are ureteropelvic junction obstruction, ureterovesical junction obstruction, ureterocele, and posterior urethral valves (occurs in males only).

Pathophysiology
• The obstruction is a congenital malformation.
• The defect may be unilateral or bilateral and can cause partial or complete obstruction of urine flow, resulting in dilation of the affected kidney (hydronephrosis).
• Complications include recurrent UTI, renal insufficiency, and progressive damage to the kidney resulting in renal failure.

Take Note!

Children with renal malformations are at increased risk for latex allergy.

Therapeutic Management
• Surgical correction is specific to the type of obstruction and generally consists of removal of the obstruction, reimplantation of the ureters as necessary, and occasionally creation of a urinary diversion.

Assessment Findings

Health History
• Recurrent UTI
• Incontinence
• Fever
• Foul-smelling urine
• Flank pain

- Abdominal pain
- Urinary frequency or urgency
- Dysuria or blood in the urine.

Risk Factors
- Prune belly syndrome
- Chromosome abnormalities
- Anorectal malformations
- Ear defects.

Physical Examination
- Abdominal mass (hydronephrotic kidney)
- Elevated blood pressure if renal insufficiency present.

Laboratory and Diagnostic Tests
- Prenatal or kidney ultrasonography may reveal the anomaly.

Nursing Interventions
- Postoperatively, assess urine output via vesicostomy, nephrostomy, suprapubic tube, or urethral catheter for color, clots, clarity, and amount.
- Encourage fluids once the child can tolerate them orally.
- Administer analgesics and/or antispasmodics as needed for bladder spasms.
- Teach parents care of vesicostomy or drainage tubes, with which the child may be discharged.

Take Note!
Upon return from surgery, most children have IV fluids without added potassium infusion. Potassium is withheld from the IV fluid until adequate urine output is established postoperatively to avoid the development of hyperkalemia should the kidneys fail to function properly (Browne, Flanigan, McComiskey, & Pieper, 2013).

ORAL CANDIDIASIS (THRUSH)

Description
- Oral candidiasis (thrush) is a fungal infection of the oral mucosa, most common in newborns and infants.
- It appears as white patches on the tongue and oral mucosa.

Pathophysiology
- Fungal overgrowth occurs on the oral mucosa in the young infant or child with an altered immune status (immunodeficiency, use of inhaled corticosteroids or chemotherapeutic drugs, or antibiotic use).

Therapeutic Management
- Oral antifungal agents such as nystatin or fluconazole.

Assessment Findings

Risk Factors
- Young age
- Immunosuppression
- Antibiotic use or the use of corticosteroid inhalers
- Presence of fungal infection in the mother.

Physical Examination
- Thick white patches on the tongue, mucosa, or palate, resembling curdled milk that do not easily wipe off with a swab or washcloth
- Candidal diaper rash (beefy-red rash with satellite lesions).

Laboratory and Diagnostic Tests
- Careful scraping of the lesions can be sent out for fungal culture.

Nursing Interventions
- Ensure appropriate administration of oral antifungal agents.
- Administer nystatin suspension four times per day following feeding to allow the medication to remain in contact with the lesions. In the younger infant, apply nystatin to the lesions with a cotton-tipped applicator.
- If the mother is also infected, she must receive antifungal treatment as well.
- Stress appropriate handwashing and keeping bottle nipples, pacifiers, and toys clean.

> *Take Note!*
>
> Geographic tongue is a benign, noncontagious condition. A reduction in the filiform papillae (bumps on the tongue) occurs in patches that migrate periodically, thus giving a map-like appearance to the tongue, with darker and lighter, higher and lower patches. Do not confuse the lighter patches of geographic tongue with the thick white plaques that form on the tongue with thrush.

OTITIS MEDIA

Description
- Otitis media is defined as inflammation of the middle ear with the presence of fluid.
- Categories are acute otitis media ([AOM]; an acute infectious process of the middle ear) and otitis media with effusion ([OME];

a collection of fluid in the middle ear space without signs and symptoms of infection).

Pathophysiology

- Fluid and pathogens travel upward from the nasopharyngeal area, invading the middle ear space.
- Fluid has difficulty draining back out toward the nasopharyngeal area because of the horizontal positioning of the eustachian tube.
- In AOM, fever and pain occur acutely, as well as increased pressure behind the tympanic membrane, which may lead to perforation.
- Most commonly caused by viral pathogens, *S. pneumoniae, H. influenzae,* and *Moraxella catarrhalis.*
- After clearance of the infection, fluid remains in the middle ear space behind the tympanic membrane, sometimes for several months (OME).

Therapeutic Management

- AOM is treated according to the severity of illness and the child's age (Table 2.11).

Assessment Findings

Health History

- Rapid onset of ear pain
- Fever (may be low grade or higher)
- Fussiness, irritability, or crying inconsolably
- Batting or tugging at the ears, rolling the head from side to side
- Poor feeding or loss of appetite
- Lethargy, difficulty sleeping or awakening, and crying in the night.

Physical Examination

- Fluid draining from the ear
- Complaints of pain upon otoscopy
- Otoscopic examination: dull, opaque, bulging, or red, immobile tympanic membrane. Pus may be present.
- Possible cervical lymphadenopathy.

Take Note!

Evaluation of hearing is recommended when OME lasts 3 months or more if language delay, hearing loss, or a learning problem is suspected.

Laboratory and Diagnostic Tests

- With OME, tympanometry reveals limited tympanic membrane mobility.

| TABLE 2.11 | TREATMENT RECOMMENDATIONS FOR ACUTE OTITIS MEDIA |

Age	Unilateral or Bilateral AOM?	Severe Signs & Symptoms?[a]	Otorrhea Present?	Treatment
6 months to 2 years	Either		Yes	Antibiotics
6 months to 2 years	Either	Yes		Antibiotics
6 months to 2 years	Bilateral	No	No	Antibiotics
6 months to 2 years	Unilateral	No	No	Antibiotics or Observation[b]
>2 years	Either		Yes	Antibiotics
>2 years	Either	Yes		Antibiotics
>2 years	Bilateral	No	No	Antibiotics or Observation[b]
>2 years	Unilateral	No	No	Antibiotics or Observation[b]

[a]Severe illness is defined as temperature 39°C (102.2°F) or higher or moderate to severe otalgia or otalgia for at least 48 hours. Nonsevere illness is defined as mild otalgia for less than 48 hours and fever less than 39°C (102.2°F).

[b]Observation is appropriate when follow-up can be ensured in order that antibiotic therapy may begin if the child fails to improve or worsens within 48 to 72 hours.

Adapted from American Academy of Pediatrics. (2013). Clinical practice guideline: The diagnosis and management of acute otitis media. *Pediatrics*, *131*, e964–e999.

Nursing Interventions

- Administer analgesics (acetaminophen, ibuprofen) or numbing ear drops (benzocaine) as ordered (American Academy of Pediatrics, 2013).
- Apply heat, or cold compress, to help relieve pain.
- Administer antibiotics if ordered.
- Explain rationale for watchful waiting if this is determined to be the appropriate course of treatment.
- Encourage the family to return for reevaluation if the child is not improving or if the AOM progresses to severe illness.
- Educate about the importance of completing the entire course of antibiotics.
- Inform families that follow-up for resolution of AOM is necessary for all children and the physician or nurse practitioner will determine the timing of that follow-up. Emphasize the importance of follow-up to the parents, educating them about OME and its potential impact on hearing and speech (AAP, 2013).
  - Prevent otitis media:
    - Encourage mothers to breast-feed at least 6 to 12 months (Friedman, Scholes, & Yoon, 2014).
    - Avoid excess exposure to individuals with URIs.
    - Prevent exposure to secondhand smoke.
    - Encourage immunization with Prevnar and influenza vaccine.
    - Older children may chew xylitol-containing gum (Klein & Pelton, 2015).

PNEUMONIA

Description

- Pneumonia is an inflammation of the lung parenchyma caused by a virus, bacteria, *Mycoplasma,* fungus, or aspiration of foreign material.
- Viral pneumonia is usually better tolerated in children of all ages, whereas children with bacterial pneumonia are more apt to present with a toxic appearance.
- Potential complications of pneumonia include bacteremia, pleural effusion, empyema, lung abscess, pneumatocele, and pneumothorax.

Take Note!

Community-acquired pneumonia (CAP) refers to pneumonia in a previously healthy person that is contracted outside of the hospital setting (Barson, 2013).

Pathophysiology

- Respiratory viruses, *S. pneumoniae,* or *Mycoplasma pneumoniae* invade the lower respiratory tract from either the upper respiratory tract or the bloodstream.
- Viral pneumonia usually results in an inflammatory reaction limited to the alveolar wall.
- In bacterial pneumonia, mucous stasis occurs as a result of vascular engorgement. Cellular debris accumulates in the alveolar space. Relative hyperexpansion with air trapping follows. Inflammation of the alveoli results in atelectasis, so gas exchange becomes impaired.
- Secondary bacterial infection often occurs following viral or aspiration pneumonia and requires antibiotic treatment.

Therapeutic Management

- Antipyretics, adequate hydration, and close observation for less severely ill children
- Antibiotics (oral or IV) in bacterial pneumonia
- Hospitalization if child has tachypnea, significant retractions, poor oral intake, or lethargy in order that supplemental oxygen or IV hydration may be administered.

Assessment Findings

Health History

- Antecedent viral URI
- Fever
- Cough
- Increased respiratory rate
- History of lethargy, poor feeding, vomiting, or diarrhea in infant
- Chills, headache, dyspnea, chest pain, abdominal pain, and nausea or vomiting in older children.

Risk Factors

- Prematurity
- Malnutrition
- Passive smoke exposure
- Low socioeconomic status
- Daycare attendance
- Underlying cardiopulmonary, immune, or nervous system disease (John & Brady, 2013b).

Physical Examination

- Cyanosis (particularly with coughing spells)
- Ill appearance
- Tachypnea

- Nasal flaring
- Wheezing, rales, and diminished breath sounds.

Laboratory and Diagnostic Tests

- Oxygen saturation decreased or normal per pulse oximetry.
- Chest radiographs may show bilateral air trapping and perihilar infiltrates in infants and younger children, or lobar consolidation in older children.
- Sputum culture may determine causative bacteria.
- Elevated WBC count.

Nursing Interventions

- Ensure adequate hydration by encouraging oral fluid intake in the child whose respiratory status is stable.
- Administer IV fluids if needed.
- Allow and encourage the child to assume a position of comfort, usually with the head of the bed elevated to promote aeration of the lungs.
- Administer antibiotics as ordered and analgesics as prescribed for pain related to prolonged coughing.
- Provide supplemental oxygen to the child with respiratory distress or hypoxia as needed.

PRECOCIOUS PUBERTY

Description

- The child develops sexual characteristics before the usual age of pubertal onset.
- Typically, puberty occurs around 10 to 12 years of age for girls and 11 to 14 years of age for boys.
- In precocious puberty, secondary sex characteristics develop in girls before the age of 8 years and in boys younger than 9 years (Saenger, 2015).
- The disorder is more common in females. The majority of the time the cause is unknown in females, while in males the majority of the time a structural CNS abnormality is present (Garibaldi & Chemaitilly, 2011). Other causes include benign hypothalamic tumor, brain injury or radiation, a history of infectious encephalitis, meningitis, CAH, and tumors of the ovary, adrenal gland, pituitary gland, or testes.

Pathophysiology

- Central precocious puberty, the most common form, develops as a result of premature activation of the hypothalamic–pituitary–gonadal

axis that results in the production of gonadotropin-releasing hormone (GnRH), which stimulates the pituitary to produce luteinizing hormone (LH) and follicle-stimulating hormone (FSH).
- These hormones in turn stimulate the gonads to secrete the sex hormones (estrogen or testosterone).
- The child develops sexual characteristics, shows increased growth and skeletal maturation, and has reproductive capability.
- Peripheral precocious puberty presents with no early secretion of gonadotropin or maturation of gonads but rather early overproduction of sex hormones. The condition results in increased end-organ sensitivity to low levels of circulating sex hormones and leads to premature pubic hair and breast development.

Therapeutic Management
- The clinical treatment of precocious puberty first involves determining the cause. For example, if the etiology is a tumor of the CNS, the child undergoes surgery, radiation therapy, or chemotherapy.
- The treatment of central precocious puberty involves administering a GnRH analogue. This is available as a subcutaneous injection given daily, an intranasal compound given two or three times each day, a depot injection given every 3 to 4 weeks, a depot injection given four times a year, or a subcutaneous implant yearly.
- This analogue stimulates gonadotropin release initially but when given on a long-term basis will suppress gonadotropin release.
- With this treatment, the growth rate slows and secondary sexual development stabilizes or regresses.
- Medroxyprogesterone injections (Depo-Provera) or tablets (Cycrin) reduce secretion of gonadotropins and prevent menstruation.
- When treatment is discontinued, puberty resumes according to appropriate developmental stages.

Assessment Findings

Health History
- Complaints of headaches, nausea, vomiting, and visual difficulties due to the circulating hormones.
- Psychosocial development is typical for the child's age, but the child may show emotional lability, aggressive behavior, and mood swings.

Risk Factors
- Exposure to exogenous hormones
- History of CNS trauma or infection
- Family history of early puberty

Physical Examination
- Acne and an adult-like body odor.
- Accelerated rate of growth.
- The Tanner staging of breasts, pubic hair, and genitalia reveals advanced maturation for the child's age, but the child does not typically display sexual behavior.

Laboratory and Diagnostic Tests
- Radiologic examinations and pelvic ultrasonography identify advanced bone age, increased uterus size, and development of ovaries consistent with the diagnosis of precocious puberty.
- Screening radioimmunoassays for LH, FSH, estradiol, or testosterone.
- The child's response to GnRH stimulation confirms the diagnosis of central precocious puberty versus gonadotropin-independent puberty. This test involves administering synthetic GnRH intravenously and drawing serial blood levels, about every 2 hours, of LH, FSH, and estrogen or testosterone. A positive result is defined as pubertal or adult levels of these hormones in response to the GnRH administration.
- CT scan, MRI, or skull radiography reveals any lesions in the CNS or tumors or cysts present in abdomen, pelvic area, or testes.

Nursing Interventions
- Assess and document the physical changes the child is experiencing.
- Administer medications as ordered.
- Demonstrate correct administration of medication and observing for potential adverse effects (teach this information to the family as well).
- Encourage the family to comply with follow-up appointments, which typically occur every 6 months and include scheduled stimulation tests.
- Help the child to deal with self-esteem issues related to the accelerated growth and development of secondary sexual characteristics:
  - The goal is for the child to exhibit normal psychosocial development and understand the physical and emotional changes that occur with early onset of puberty.
  - Communicate with the child on an age-appropriate level, even when physical characteristics make the child appear older.
  - Maintain a calm, supportive atmosphere and provide for privacy during examinations.
  - Encourage the child to express his or her feelings about the changes he or she is experiencing and use role-playing to show the child how to handle teasing from other children.
  - Let the child know that everyone develops sexual characteristics in time.

- Educate and support the child and family:
  - Teach correct procedure for administering medication and potential adverse effect.
  - Inform families that pharmacologic intervention stops when the child reaches the age appropriate for pubertal development.
  - Provide appropriate sex education. Reassure parents that precocious puberty does not usually involve precocious sexual behavior, but that it may be seen, especially in boys (Dowshen, 2015).
  - Refer the child and family for counseling as needed.

RETINOBLASTOMA

Description
- Retinoblastoma is a highly malignant tumor of the eye and accounts for 5% of cases of blindness in children (Graham et al., 2014).
- Most children have a diagnosis by age 3, and the overall survival rate is 90% (Graham et al., 2014).

Pathophysiology
- Retinoblastoma arises from embryonic retinal cells.
- The tumor may grow forward into the vitreous cavity of the eye or extend into the subretinal space, causing retinal detachment.
- It may extend into the choroid, the sclera, and the optic nerve.

Therapeutic Management
- Retinoblastoma may be treated with radiation, chemotherapy, laser surgery, cryotherapy, or a combination of these treatments.
- Moderate vision may be preserved for most children without advanced disease.
- In advanced disease or in the case of a massive tumor with retinal detachment, enucleation (removal of the eye) is necessary.

Assessment Findings

Health History
- Parental identification of the "cat's eye reflex" or "whitewash glow" to the child's affected pupil
- Strabismus
- Orbital inflammation
- Vomiting
- Headache

Risk Factors
- Family history of retinoblastoma or other cancer
- Presence of chromosomal anomalies

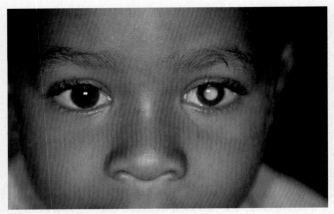

FIGURE 2.20 **Leukocoria.**

Physical Examination
- Leukocoria in the affected eye (see Fig. 2.20)
- Orbital inflammation or erythema
- Hyphema

Laboratory and Diagnostic Tests
- Diagnostic evaluation includes an ophthalmologic examination under anesthesia.
- CT scan, MRI, or ultrasound of the head and eyes will help to visualize the tumor.
- The infant or toddler may also undergo lumbar puncture and bone marrow aspiration to determine the presence and extent of metastasis.

Nursing Interventions
- Provide routine postoperative care to the infant or toddler.
- If the eye is enucleated, observe the large pressure dressing on the eye socket for bleeding.
- Provide dressing changes to the socket with sterile saline rinses and/or antibiotic ointment application.
- Monitor for side effects of chemotherapy if ordered (see the leukemia section).
- Instruct parents to comply with follow-up eye examinations every 3 to 6 months until age 6 and then annually to check for further tumor development.
- Teach families use of the prosthetic eye if needed.
- Provide parents with support and encouragement.

- Refer the family for genetic counseling (Kaufman, Kim, & Berry, 2015).

> *Take Note!*
>
> Educate parents about protecting vision in the remaining eye: routine eye checkups, protection from accidental injury, use of safety goggles during sports, and prompt treatment of eye infections. Generally, children with one eye should not participate in contact sports.

SCOLIOSIS

Description
- Scoliosis is a lateral curvature of the spine that exceeds 10 degrees.
- It may be congenital, associated with other disorders or idiopathic.
- Idiopathic scoliosis, with the majority of cases occurring during adolescence, is the most common form of scoliosis and is discussed here (Spiegel & Dormans, 2011).
- Early screening and detection of scoliosis result in improved outcomes.

Pathophysiology
- The etiology of idiopathic scoliosis is not known, but genetic factors, growth abnormalities, and bone, muscle, disk, or CNS disorders may contribute to its development.
- In the rapidly growing adolescent, the involved vertebrae rotate around a vertical axis, resulting in lateral curvature. The vertebrae rotate to the convex side of curve, with the spinous processes rotating toward the concave side.
- Wedge-shaped vertebral bodies and disks develop because growth is suppressed on the concave side of the curve (Haut, 2014).
- As the curve progresses, the shape of the thoracic cage changes and respiratory and cardiovascular compromise may occur (the main complications of severe scoliosis).

Therapeutic Management
- Treatment of scoliosis is aimed at preventing progression of the curve and decreasing the impact on pulmonary and cardiac function.
- Treatment is based on the age of the child, expected future growth, and severity of the curve.
- Observation with serial examinations and spine x-rays is used to monitor curve progression.
- For curves of 25 to 40 degrees, bracing may be sufficient to decrease progression of the curve (Haut, 2014). The choice of

brace will depend on the location and severity of the curve. Some curves will progress despite appropriate bracing and compliance.
- Surgical correction is often required for curves >45 degrees; it is achieved with rod placement and bone grafting (Grewal & Ahier, 2010; Spiegel & Dormans, 2011).
  - Partial spinal fusion accompanies many of the corrective surgeries.
  - Multiple surgical approaches and techniques with various instrumentation methods exist for fusion and rod placement.
  - The surgical approach may be anterior, posterior, or both.
  - Traditional rod placement (Harrington rod) involved a single rod fused to the vertebrae, resulting in not only curve correction but also a flat-backed appearance.
  - Newer rod instrumentations allow for scoliosis curve correction with maintenance of normal back curvature. The rods are shorter, and several rods are wired or grafted to the appropriate vertebrae to achieve correction.

Assessment Findings

Health History
- Mild discomfort or back pain, depending on the severity of the curve associated with idiopathic scoliosis
- Asymmetry in the hips or shoulders (noticed by the family or after being screened for scoliosis at school).

Risk Factors
- Family history of scoliosis
- Recent growth spurt
- Physical changes related to puberty.

Physical Examination
- Poor posture
- Asymmetries such as shoulder elevation, prominence of one scapula, uneven curve at the waistline, or a rib hump on one side
- Difference between the height of the high and low shoulder
- Difference between heights of anterior and posterior iliac spines
- Abnormalities in the spinal curve
- Asymmetry of the back (pronounced hump on one side)
- Leg-length discrepancy
- Normal balance, motor strength, sensation, and reflexes
- Compromise of heart and lungs related to severe curvature.

Laboratory and Diagnostic Tests
- Full-spine radiographs will determine the degree of curvature. The radiologist will determine the extent of the curve on the basis of specific formulas and techniques of measurement.

Nursing Interventions

Encourage Compliance With Bracing

- Explain to the child and family that the brace must be worn 23 hours/day to prevent curve progression.
- Inspect the skin for evidence of rubbing by the brace that may impair skin integrity. Teach families appropriate skin care and recommend they check the brace daily for fit and breakage.
- Encourage the teen to shower during the 1 hour/day that the brace is off and to ensure that the skin is clean and dry before putting the brace back on. Wearing a cotton T-shirt under the brace may decrease some of the discomfort associated with brace wear.
- Encourage the child to perform exercises to strengthen back muscles, which may prevent muscle atrophy from prolonged bracing and maintain spine flexibility.

Promote a Positive Body Image

- Encourage the teen to express his or her feelings or concerns about wearing the brace.
- Give the teen ways to explain scoliosis and its treatment to his or her peers.
- Wearing stylish baggy clothes may help the teen to conceal the brace if desired.

Provide Preoperative Teaching

- Teach the teen the importance of turning, coughing, and deep breathing in the postoperative period.
- Explain the tubes and catheters that will be present immediately after the surgery.
- Review positioning guidelines: back flexion or extension will not be allowed.
- Introduce the child to the patient-controlled analgesia (PCA) pump and explain pain scales.
- There is a high risk for significant blood loss with spinal fusion and instrumentation, so if possible arrange for preoperative autologous blood donation.

Avoid Complications in the Postoperative Period

- Perform neurovascular checks with each set of vital signs.
- When turning the child, use the logroll technique to avoid flexion of the back.
- Provide proper pain management and medicate for pain before repositioning and ambulation.
- Administer prophylactic IV antibiotics if ordered.
- Assess for drainage from the operative site and for excess blood loss via the Hemovac or other drainage tube.

- Maintain Foley patency, as the child will be confined to bed for the first couple of days.
- Maintain strict recording of fluid intake and output.
- Administer transfusions of PRBCs if ordered.
- Ambulation, once ordered, should be done slowly to avoid orthostatic hypotension.

Educating the Child and Family
- Teach families ways to encourage compliance with bracing (see earlier).
- Assist the family with arrangements to continue the teen's schoolwork while hospitalized and/or arrange for home tutoring during the several-week recovery period.
- Refer teens and their families to the National Scoliosis Foundation (www.scoliosis.org) for additional support.

SEPSIS

Description
- Systemic overresponse to infection results from bacteria and viruses, which are the most common, as well as fungi, viruses, rickettsial bacteria, or parasites.
- Cause may be unknown, but common causative organisms in infants less than 3 months old include *Escherichia coli,* group B *Streptococcus, S. aureus,* enteroviruses, and herpes simplex virus and common causative organisms in children include *Neisseria meningitides, S. pneumoniae,* and *S. aureus* (Pomerantz & Weiss, 2015).

Pathophysiology
- Sepsis results in systemic inflammatory response syndrome (SIRS) due to infection.
- Complex process results from the effects of circulating bacterial products or toxins, mediated by cytokine release, occurring as a result of sustained bacteremia.
- Impaired pulmonary, hepatic, or renal function may result from excessive cytokine release.

Therapeutic Management
- Neonates and infants with sepsis or even suspected sepsis are treated in the hospital.
- The infant is admitted for close monitoring along with antibiotic therapy.
- IV antibiotics are started immediately after the blood, urine, and CSF cultures have been obtained.

- The length of therapy and the specific antibiotic used will be determined on the basis of the source of the positive culture and the results of the culture and sensitivity.
- If final culture reports are negative and symptoms have subsided, antibiotics may be discontinued (usually after 72 hours of treatment).
- If the child is not responding to therapy and symptoms worsen, sepsis may be progressing to shock. Management of the child with septic shock is usually done in the intensive care unit.

Assessment Findings

Health History
- Child just does not look or act right
- Crying more than usual, inconsolable
- Weak cry
- Fever
- Hypothermia (in neonates and those with severe disease)
- Lethargic and less interactive or playful
- Increased irritability
- Poor feeding or poor suck
- Rash (e.g., petechiae, ecchymosis, diffuse erythema)
- Difficulty breathing
- Nasal congestion
- Diarrhea
- Vomiting
- Decreased urine output
- Hypotonia
- Changes in mental status (confused, anxious, excited)
- Seizures
- Older child may complain of heart racing.

Risk Factors
- Prematurity
- Lack of immunizations
- Immunocompromise
- Exposure to communicable pathogens

In neonates and young infants, seek pregnancy and labor risk factors such as:
- Premature rupture of membranes or prolonged rupture
- Difficult delivery
- Maternal infection or fever, including sexually transmitted infections
- Resuscitation and other invasive procedures
- Positive maternal group β-streptococcal vaginosis

Sepsis may occur in the hospitalized child. Assess for risk factors such as:
- Intensive care unit stay
- Presence of central line or other invasive lines or tubes
- Immunosuppression.

Physical Examination
- Lethargic and pale
- Weak cry, lack of smile or facial expression, or lack of responsiveness.
- Presence of petechiae or other skin lesions.
- Tachypnea and increased work of breathing, such as nasal flaring, grunting, and retractions.
- Elevation in temperature or hypothermia in the young infant.
- Tachypnea or tachycardia in the child or apnea or bradycardia in the infant.
- Hypotension, especially when accompanied by signs of poor perfusion, can be a sign of worsening sepsis with progression to shock.

Take Note!
Listen to the parents' descriptions of the neonate's or infant's behavior and appearance, as well as changes they have observed. Many times they are the first to notice when their child is not acting right, even before clinical signs of infection are seen.

Laboratory and Diagnostic Tests
- CBC count: WBC levels will be elevated; in severe cases, they may be decreased (this is an ominous sign).
- CRP: elevated
- Blood culture: positive
- Urine culture: may be positive
- CSF: may reveal increased WBCs and protein and low glucose levels
- Stool culture: may be positive
- Culture of tubes, catheters, or shunts suspected to be infected: The fluid inside these tubes may be tested for bacteria or fungus.
- Chest radiographs: may reveal signs of pneumonia.

Nursing Interventions
- Monitor closely for changes in condition, especially the development of signs of shock.
- Administer antibiotics as ordered.
- Prevent infection:
  - Practice *strict* handwashing.

- Minimize environmental sources of infection by cleaning equipment and disposing of soiled linens and dressings properly and adhering to proper aseptic technique with all invasive procedures.
- Encourage recommended immunizations.
- Educate the child and family:
  - Explain that early recognition of the signs of sepsis is essential in preventing morbidity and mortality.
  - Educate parents about the importance of fever, especially in neonates and infants younger than 3 months.
  - Instruct parents to contact their physician or nurse practitioner if their infant or neonate has a fever. A physician or nurse practitioner should see any child with a fever accompanied by lethargy, poor responsiveness, or lack of facial expressions.
  - Explain that signs and symptoms of sepsis can be vague and vary from child to child.
  - Encourage parents to contact their physician or nurse practitioner if they feel their febrile child is "just not acting right."

SICKLE CELL DISEASE

Description
- Sickle cell disease (hemoglobin SS disease) is an inherited hemoglobinopathy in which the RBCs carry a less effective type of hemoglobin than does the normal adult hemoglobin.
- Sickle cell anemia is a severe chronic blood disorder that occurs once in every 2,000 newborns in the United States each year (Chandrakason & Kamat, 2013)
- It is most common in individuals of African, Mediterranean, Middle Eastern, and Indian decent. One in 400 African Americans has sickle cell anemia (Ambruso et al., 2014).
- Complications of sickle cell anemia include recurrent vaso-occlusive pain crises, stroke, sepsis, acute chest syndrome, splenic sequestration, reduced visual acuity related to decreased retinal blood flow, chronic leg ulcers, cholestasis and gallstones, delayed growth and development, delayed puberty, priapism, enuresis, and for some children eventual multiple organ dysfunction.

Pathophysiology
- Instead of hemoglobin AA, people with sickle cell anemia have hemoglobin SS. In hemoglobin S, glutamic acid is replaced with valine in the hemoglobin molecule. This results in an elongated RBC with a shortened life span. The elongated cell is more rigid than a normal cell and becomes sickled in shape (Fig. 2.21).

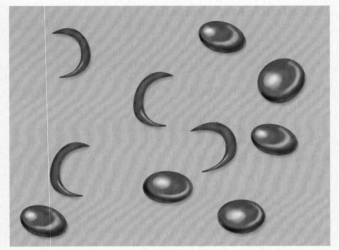

FIGURE 2.21 This peripheral blood smear demonstrates the elongated sickle-shaped RBC seen in sickle cell disease.

- Sickling may be triggered by any stress or traumatic event, such as infection, fever, acidosis, dehydration, physical exertion, excessive cold exposure, or hypoxia (Ambruso et al., 2014).
- As the cells sickle, the blood becomes more viscous because the sickled cells clump together and prevent normal blood flow to the tissues of that area.
- This vaso-occlusive process leads to local tissue hypoxia followed by ischemia and may result in infarction. Pain crisis results, as circulation is decreased to the area.
- Clumping of cells in the lungs (acute chest syndrome) results in decreased gas exchange, producing hypoxia, which leads to further sickling.
- Sequestration of blood in the spleen leads to splenomegaly and abdominal pain. Hemolysis follows sickling and leads to further anemia.
- The increased activity of the spleen related to RBC hemolysis leads to splenomegaly and then fibrosis and atrophy.
- Functional asplenia may develop as early as 6 months of age and occurs by 9 years of age in 90% of children with sickle cell disease (Pitts & Record, 2010).

Therapeutic Management

- Therapeutic management of children with sickle cell anemia focuses on preventing sickling crisis and infection as well as other complications.
- Prophylactic antibiotics in young children and appropriate immunization in all children with sickle cell anemia can reduce the risk of serious infection (Pitts & Record, 2010).
- Hydroxyurea administration, cholecystectomy, splenectomy, or HSCT may be used in some children.
- Treatment of sickle cell crisis focuses on pain control. Oxygen administration and adequate hydration are key. Transfusion of PRBCs may be necessary.

Assessment Findings

Health History

- Delayed growth and development
- History of vaso-occlusive crises
- Note past hospitalizations, treatment of pain crises, previous blood transfusions, and/or history of recurrent infections.
- For the current illness event, note the precipitating factor, location, onset, character, and quality of pain.
- Determine immunization history, particularly pneumococcal, influenza, and meningococcal vaccinations.

Risk Factors

- Stress
- Exposure to cold
- Hypoxia
- Infection
- Dehydration.

Physical Examination

- Pale conjunctivae, palms, or soles
- Lesions or ulcers on the skin
- Sticky or dry oral mucosa
- Jaundice
- Icteric sclerae
- Fever
- Decreased blood pressure
- Altered LOC
- Heart murmur
- Tachycardia
- Adventitious breath sounds
- Warm, tender joints with decreased range of motion
- Hepatomegaly
- Splenomegaly
- Abdominal pain.

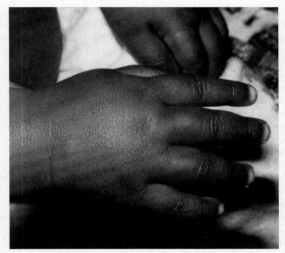

FIGURE 2.22 Swelling of the hands and feet (dactylitis) in a toddler.

Take Note!

Immediately report symmetric swelling of the hands and feet in the infant or toddler. Termed dactylitis, aseptic infarction occurs in the metacarpals and metatarsals. (Fig. 2.22).

Laboratory and Diagnostic Tests

- Hemoglobin electrophoresis shows the presence of hemoglobin S and hemoglobin F in the young infant and hemoglobin SS in the older infant or child.
- CBC count will reveal baseline hemoglobin of 7 to 10 mg/dL (significantly lower with splenic sequestration, acute chest syndrome, or aplastic crisis), greatly elevated reticulocyte count, presence of sickle-shaped cells and target cells on peripheral smear, and increased platelet count.
- ESR and bilirubin will be elevated.
- X-ray studies or other scans may be performed to determine the extent of organ or tissue damage resulting from vaso-occlusion.

Nursing Interventions

- Administer prophylactic penicillin V potassium to the infant or young child as ordered. Teach families how to administer this medication.

- Ensure appropriate immunization per the current recommended schedule. The 23-valent pneumococcal conjugate vaccine annually after 2 years of age, as well as meningococcal vaccination and influenza immunization annually before the onset of influenza season (after 6 months of age; Pitts & Record, 2010).
- Monitor growth and development as well as school performance.
- Initially, teach the family about the genetics of the disease and encourage family members to be tested for carrier status.
- Educate families about the disease process and emphasize the importance of regularly scheduled health maintenance visits and immunizations.
- Encourage families to seek medical evaluation urgently for any febrile illness.
- Educate families about how to prevent and recognize vaso-occlusive events (Teaching Guidelines 2.19).
- Teach the child age-appropriate distraction and coping skills to assist the child to relieve stress related to his or her disease and/or recurrent crises.
- Initiate pain assessment with a standardized pain scale upon admission.
- To bring the pain under control, initially administer analgesics routinely rather than on an "as needed" (PRN) basis. Once the pain is better managed, medications may be moved to PRN status.
- Monitor PCA in the child or adolescent.
- Use nonpharmacologic pain management techniques such as relaxation or hypnosis, music, massage, play, guided imagery, therapeutic touch, or behavior modification to augment the pain medication regimen.

Teaching Guidelines 2.19
PREVENTION OR EARLY RECOGNITION OF VASO-OCCLUSIVE EVENTS

- Seek immediate attention for *any* febrile illness.
- Obtain vaccinations and penicillin prophylaxis.
- Encourage adequate fluid intake daily.
- Avoid temperatures that are too hot or too cold.
- Avoid overexertion or stress.
- Have 24-hour access to medical provider or facility familiar with sickle cell care.
- Contact medical provider promptly if you suspect a pain crisis is developing.

- Seek medical attention immediately if any of the following develops:
  - Child is pale and listless
  - Abdominal pain
  - Limp or swollen joints
  - Cough, shortness of breath, chest pain
  - Increasing fatigue
  - Unusual headache, loss of feeling, or sudden weakness
  - Sudden vision change
  - Painful erection that won't go down (priapism).

Take Note!

Avoid repeated use of meperidine for pain management during sickle cell crisis because it has been associated with an increased risk of seizures when used in children with sickle cell anemia (Sickle Cell Information Center [SCIC], 2011).

- Provide 150 mL/kg of fluids per day or as much as double maintenance, either orally or intravenously.
- Frequently evaluate respiratory and circulatory status. Administer supplemental oxygen if the pulse oximetry reading is ≤92% to promote adequate oxygenation (SCIC, 2011).
- Monitor LOC and immediately report changes.
- Maintain the child's temperature as close to normal as possible without the use of cooling mattresses.
- Refer families to a regional sickle cell disease center for multidisciplinary care.

PREPARING THE CHILD AND FAMILY FOR SURGERY

- If the child is to undergo a surgical procedure, special interventions are necessary. Allow parents to stay with the child until surgery begins. In addition, allow parents to be with the child when he or she wakes up in the postanesthesia recovery area. Good preparation provides reassurance and comfort to the child and allows him or her to know what will happen and what is expected of him or her.
- Preoperative care for the child who is to undergo surgery is similar to that for an adult. The major difference is that the preparation and teaching must be geared to the child's age and developmental level. For example, when teaching a toddler or preschooler about breathing exercises, have the child blow a pinwheel or cotton balls across the table through a straw. The child will enjoy the activity while also reaping the respiratory benefits of the activity.

- Allow the child to role-play various experiences with dolls. Dolls designed to simulate surgical experiences have been developed. The dolls were developed to help children cope with their illness or disease and send the message that it is okay to be different. These dolls also provide the child with a companion to talk to.
- Table 2.12 discusses strategies for preoperative teaching. Many facilities offer special programs, such as presurgical preparation, or

TABLE 2.12	STRATEGIES FOR PREOPERATIVE TEACHING BASED ON DEVELOPMENTAL LEVEL
Developmental Level	**Implications for Teaching**
Infants and toddlers	Encourage parents to use a soft tone of voice and stroking and secure, comfortable holding positions to promote calm. Remind parents to use positive facial expressions. Encourage the parent or caregiver to stay with the child as much as possible. Use terms that the child and parents can understand. For toddlers, provide information as close to the day of surgery as possible to prevent undue anxiety.
Preschoolers and school-aged children	Provide factual explanations using terms the child and parents can understand. Incorporate photographs and other visual aids in explanation. Tailor the timing of education to meet the child's learning needs, allowing enough time for the child to ask questions. For preschoolers, provide information 1–2 days before surgery. For school-aged children, provide information 3–5 days before surgery.
Adolescents	Provide detailed explanations of the procedure at least 7–10 days beforehand. Answer questions honestly, ensuring privacy at all times. Remain available for questions or concerns arising before or after surgery.

books, videos, and tours to help prepare children and families for the surgical experience. Child and family teaching is essential. Like any intervention, adapt the teaching to the child's developmental level.

THALASSEMIA MAJOR

Description

- Thalassemia major is an autosomal recessive genetic disorder that most often affects those of African descent, but it also affects individuals of Caribbean, Middle Eastern, South Asian, and Mediterranean descent (Bryant, 2010).
- It results in reduced production of normal hemoglobin.

Pathophysiology

- The beta-globulin chain in hemoglobin synthesis is reduced or entirely absent. A large number of unstable globulin chains accumulate, causing the RBCs to be rigid and hemolyzed easily, resulting in severe hemolytic anemia and chronic hypoxia. Erythroid activity increases, causing massive bone marrow expansion and thinning of the bony cortex. Growth retardation, pathologic fractures, and skeletal deformities (frontal and maxillary bossing) result.
- Hemosiderosis (excessive supply of iron) occurs as a result of rapid hemolysis of RBCs, decrease in hemoglobin production, and increased absorption of dietary iron in response to the severely anemic state. The excess iron is deposited in body tissues, causing bronze pigmentation of the skin, bony changes, and altered organ function, particularly in the cardiac system.

Therapeutic Management

- Chronic blood transfusions at regular intervals and chelation therapy are necessary to increase life expectancy beyond the teen years (Ambruso et al., 2014).

Assessment Findings

Health History

- Pallor
- Jaundice
- Failure to thrive
- Hepatosplenomegaly
- Chronic transfusion/chelation therapy.

Physical Examination

- Pallor of the skin, oral mucosa, conjunctivae, soles, and/or palms
- Icteral sclerae or jaundice of the skin

- Delayed growth and development
- Low oxygen saturation via pulse oximetry
- Altered LOC
- Hepatosplenomegaly
- Frontal bossing (prominent forehead; Fig. 2.23).

Laboratory and Diagnostic Tests

- Hemoglobin electrophoresis shows the presence of hemoglobin F and hemoglobin A_2 only.
- CBC count and peripheral smear show significantly decreased hemoglobin and hematocrit, prominence of target cells, hypochromia, microcytosis, and extensive anisocytosis and poikilocytosis (variation in the size and shape of the RBCs, respectively).
- Iron and bilirubin levels are elevated.

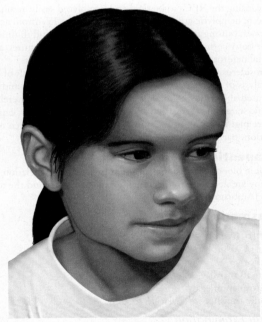

FIGURE 2.23 Iron overload related to thalassemia leads to bony changes such as frontal bossing and maxillary prominence.

Nursing Interventions
- Administer PRBC transfusions as prescribed. Monitor for reactions to the transfusions.
- Administer the chelating agent deferoxamine (Desferal) with the transfusion.
- Provide oral deferasirox (EXJADE) if also prescribed.
- Educate the child and family about the recommended regimen. Ensure that families understand that adhering to the prescribed blood transfusion and chelation therapy schedule is essential to the child's survival.
- Teach family members to administer deferoxamine subcutaneously with a small battery-powered infusion pump over a period of several hours each night (usually while the child is sleeping).
- If oral deferasirox is prescribed, instruct the family to dissolve the tablet in juice or water and administer it once daily.
- Refer the family for genetic counseling and family support as needed.

Atraumatic Care

When a child is receiving blood transfusion every few weeks, he or she must experience at least 2 venipunctures each time, one for the type and cross-match and other relevant laboratory tests on the day before transfusion, and the IV insertion for the actual transfusion. Minimize trauma by teaching the parent to apply EMLA cream at home just before leaving for the blood draw or transfusion appointment.

TRACTION

Traction is a common method of immobilization and may be used to reduce and/or immobilize a fracture, to align an injured extremity, and to allow the extremity to be restored to its normal length. Traction may also reduce pain by decreasing the incidence of muscle spasm.

Caring for the Child in Traction

Nursing care of the child in any type of traction focuses on the following:
- Providing appropriate application and maintenance of traction. Whether skin or skeletal traction is used, be sure that constant and even traction is maintained.
  - In skin traction:
    - Apply skin traction over intact skin only so that the pull of the traction is effective.

- Prepare the skin with an appropriate adhesive before applying the traction tapes to ensure that the tapes adhere well, preventing skin friction.
- After application of the traction tapes, apply the elastic bandage or use the foam boot.
- Attach the traction spreader block and then apply the prescribed amount of weight via a rope attached to the spreader block.
- Ensure that the rope moves without obstruction and that the weights hang freely without touching the floor.
- In skeletal traction:
  - Apply weight via ropes attached to the skeletal pins.
  - The pin sites should be treated as surgical wounds with routine pin site care provided.
  - Protect the exposed ends of the pins to avoid injury.

Take Note!

Avoid sudden bumping or movement of the bed: This can disturb traction alignment and cause additional pain to the child as the weights are jostled.

- Promoting normal growth and development:
  - Place age-appropriate toys within the child's reach.
  - Encourage visits from friends.
  - Provide diversional activities such as drawing, coloring, or video games.
- Preventing complications:
  - Provide appropriate pain management.
  - Promote skin integrity.
  - Prevent contractures and atrophy that may result from disuse of muscles; ensure that unaffected extremities are exercised. Assist the child to exercise the unaffected joints and to use the unaffected extremity if this does not disrupt traction alignment.
  - Promote use of a trapeze if not contraindicated to involve the child in repositioning and assist with movement.
  - Encourage deep breathing exercises to prevent the pulmonary complications of long-term immobilization.

Take Note!

Ongoing, careful neurovascular assessments are critical in the child with a cast or in skeletal traction. Notify the physician or nurse practitioner immediately if these signs of compartment syndrome occur: extreme pain (out of proportion to the situation), pain with passive range of motion of digits, distal extremity pallor, inability to move digits, or loss of pulses.

TRISOMY 21 (DOWN SYNDROME)

Description

- Trisomy 21 is a genetic disorder caused by the presence of all or part of an extra chromosome 21.
- It is the most common chromosomal abnormality associated with intellectual disability (Ostermaier, 2015a).
- It is associated with some degree of intellectual disability, characteristic facial features (e.g., slanted eyes and depressed nasal bridge), and other health problems (e.g., cardiac defects, visual and hearing impairment, intestinal malformations, and an increased susceptibility to infections). The severity of these problems varies.
- The prognosis has been improving over the past few decades. Fundamental changes in the care of these children have resulted in longer life expectancy (around 55 to 56 years of age) and an improved quality of life (Ostermaier, 2015b).

Pathophysiology

- Caused by nondisjunction (an error in cell division) prior to or at conception. Each egg and sperm cell normally contains 23 chromosomes. When they join, this results in 23 pairs or 46 chromosomes. Sometimes, due to nondisjunction, a cell contributes an extra critical portion of chromosome number 21, resulting in an embryo with three copies of chromosome 21 in all cells.
- This results in the characteristic features and birth defects of Down syndrome. This error in cell division and the presence of three copies of chromosome 21 in all cells is responsible for the majority of cases of Down syndrome (Bull & the Committee on Genetics, 2011).
- In a small percentage of cases of Down syndrome, the nondisjunction occurs after fertilization and a mixture of two cell types is seen (Bull & the Committee on Genetics, 2011). In these cases, some cells have 47 chromosomes (due to three copies of chromosome 21) whereas others have the normal 46 chromosomes (with the normal two copies of chromosome 21 present). This is referred to as the mosaic form of Down syndrome.
- Other cases of Down syndrome involve a translocation, in which part of chromosome 21 breaks off during cell division prior to or at conception and attaches to another chromosome. The cells will remain with 46 chromosomes, but this extra portion of chromosome 21 results in the clinical findings of Down syndrome.

Therapeutic Management

- Management of Down syndrome will involve multiple disciplines, including a primary physician, specialty physicians such as a cardiologist, an ophthalmologist, and a gastroenterologist, nurses, physical therapists, occupational therapists, speech therapists, dietitian, psychologist, counselors, teachers, and of course the parents.

- There is no standard treatment option for all children, and there is no cure or prevention. Treatment is mainly symptomatic and supportive.
- The overall focus of therapeutic management will be to promote the child's optimal growth and development and function within the limits of the disease.
- Children with Down syndrome need the usual immunizations, well-child care, and screening recommended by the American Academy of Pediatrics.
- Because of their increased risk for certain congenital anomalies and diseases, children with Down syndrome will need to be monitored closely, and regular medical care is essential.
- Therapeutic management will focus on complications associated with Down syndrome, including the following (Bull & the Committee on Genetics, 2011):
  - CHD occurs often in children with Down syndrome. Cardiac problems vary from minor defects that respond to medication therapy to major defects that require surgical intervention.
  - Children with Down syndrome also have an increased incidence of GI disorders. These disorders vary from those that can be managed by dietary manipulation, such as celiac disease and constipation, to intestinal malformations such as Hirschsprung disease and imperforate anus, which require surgical intervention.
  - Hearing and vision impairments also are common. So, regular evaluation of vision and hearing is essential.
  - Obstructive sleep apnea is present in many children with Down syndrome. Often parents are unaware that their child is having sleep disturbances, so baseline testing in young children may be warranted.
  - Children with Down syndrome have a higher incidence of thyroid disease, which can affect growth and cognitive function. Most of these children have hypothyroidism (an underactive thyroid), but sometimes hyperthyroidism (an overactive thyroid) occurs. Periodic thyroid testing may be warranted.
  - Children with Down syndrome are at a higher risk for obesity and malocclusions.
  - Atlantoaxial instability (increased mobility of the cervical spine at the first and second vertebrae) is seen in some children with Down syndrome. In most cases, these children are asymptomatic,

but symptoms may appear if spinal cord compression occurs. Screening for atlantoaxial instability may be appropriate, especially if the child is involved in sports.

Take Note!

If neck pain, unusual posturing of the head and neck (torticollis), change in gait, loss of upper body strength, abnormal reflexes, or change in bowel or bladder functioning is noted in the child with Down syndrome, immediate attention is required.

- Children with Down syndrome are at an increased risk for certain hematologic problems, such as anemia, transient leukemia (mostly during the newborn period), leukemia (later onset) and polycythemia during infancy
- Children with Down syndrome also have a higher susceptibility to infection and a higher mortality rate from infectious diseases. Therefore, precautions to prevent and monitor for infection are needed.
- Other potential complications include alopecia, communication disorders, and seizures.
- Early intervention therapy can help in the development of gross and fine motor skills, language, and social and self-care skills.
  - Early intervention refers to a variety of specialized programs and resources available to young children with developmental delay or other impairment.
  - These programs may involve an array of healthcare professionals such as physical, occupational, and speech therapists, special educators, and social workers.
  - The programs focus on providing stimulation and encouragement to children with Down syndrome. They help encourage and accelerate development and may help to prevent some developmental delays.
  - The earlier the intervention can begin, the more beneficial it will be. The programs are individualized to meet the specific needs of each child.
  - Children with Down syndrome progress through the same developmental stages as typical children, but they do so on their own timetable (Table 2.13).
  - Parents also benefit from early intervention programs in terms of support, encouragement, and information. Early intervention programs teach parents how to interact with their child while meeting the child's specific needs and encouraging development.

TABLE 2.13	AVERAGE AGE OF SKILL ACQUISITION IN CHILDREN WITH DOWN SYNDROME	
Developmental Milestone	Average Age of Acquisition, Children With Down Syndrome (months)	Average Age of Acquisition, Typical Children (months)
Smile	2	1
Roll over	6	4
Sit alone	9	7
Crawl	11	9
Walk	21	13
Speak words	14	10
Speak in sentences	24	21
Feed self with fingers	12	8
Use spoon	20	13
Bladder training	48	32
Bowel training	42	29
Undress	40	32
Put on clothes	58	47

Adapted from Pueschel, S. M. (2011). *A parent's guide to Down syndrome: Toward a brighter future* (rev. ed.). Baltimore: Paul H. Brookes Publishing Company, Inc.

Assessment Findings

Health History of the Undiagnosed Infant

- Down syndrome is often diagnosed prenatally, using perinatal screening and diagnostic tests.
- If not diagnosed prenatally, most cases are diagnosed in the first few days of life on the basis of the physical characteristics associated with Down syndrome.
- High-risk deliveries should be identified.

Health History of the Diagnosed Infant or Child

- The older infant or child known to have Down syndrome is often admitted to the hospital for corrective surgeries or other complications of the disease, such as infections.

- In an infant or child returning for a clinic visit or hospitalization, the health history should include questions related to the following:
  - Cardiac defects or disease (treatment regimen, surgical repair)
  - Hearing or vision impairment (last hearing and vision evaluation, any corrective measures)
  - Developmental delays (speech, gross and fine motor skills)
  - Sucking or feeding problems
  - Cognitive abilities (degree of intellectual disability)
  - GI disorders such as vomiting or absence of stools (special dietary management, surgical interventions)
  - Thyroid disease
  - Hematologic problems, such as anemia, leukemia
  - Atlantoaxial instability
  - Seizures
  - Infections such as recurrent or chronic respiratory infections, otitis media
  - Growth (height and weight changes, feeding problems, unexplained weight gain)
  - Signs and symptoms of sleep apnea, such as snoring, restlessness during sleep, daytime sleepiness
  - Any other changes in physical state or medication regimen

Risk Factors
- Lack of prenatal care
- Abnormal prenatal screening or diagnostic tests for Down syndrome (e.g., fetal nuchal translucency, triple/quadruple screen, ultrasonography, amniocentesis)
- Maternal age greater than 35 years

Physical Examination
- Certain physical features characteristic of Down syndrome may be noted (see Box 2.6).
- Lack of muscle tone and loose joints; this is usually more pronounced in infancy, and the infant has a floppy appearance.
- Delayed growth and development:
  - Plot growth on appropriate growth charts. Because children with Down syndrome grow at a slower rate, special growth charts have been developed (see http://thepoint.lww.com for an example).
  - Assess developmental milestones. It may be more useful to look at the sequence of milestones rather than the age at which they were achieved. Each milestone represents a skill that is needed for the next stage of development.
  - Hearing problems.
  - Vision problems, especially cataracts.

BOX 2.6

COMMON CLINICAL MANIFESTATIONS OF DOWN SYNDROME

- Hypotonia
- Short stature
- Flattened occiput
- Small (brachycephalic) head
- Flat facial profile
- Depressed nasal bridge and small nose
- Oblique palpebral fissures (an upward slant to the eyes)
- Brushfield spots (white spots on the iris of the eye)
- Low-set ears
- Abnormally shaped ears
- Small mouth
- Protrusion of tongue; tongue is large compared to mouth size
- Arched palate
- Hands with broad, short fingers
- A single deep transverse crease on the palm of the hand (simian crease)
- Congenital heart defect
- Short neck, with excessive skin at the nape
- Hyperflexibility and looseness of joints (excessive ability to extend the joints)
- Dysplastic middle phalanx of fifth finger (one flexion furrow instead of two)
- Epicanthal folds (small skin folds on the inner corner of the eyes)
- Excessive space between large and second toe

Adapted from Summar, K. & Lee, B. (2011). Chapter 76.2: Down syndrome and other abnormalities of chromosome number. In R. M. Kleigman, B.F. Stanton, J.W. St. Geme III, N.F. Schor & R.E. Behrman (Eds.), *Nelson textbook of pediatrics* (19th ed., pp. 399–403). Philadelphia, PA: Saunders; Bull, M.J. & the Committee on Genetics (2011). From the American Academy of Pediatrics: Clinical Report: Health supervision for children with Down syndrome. *Pediatrics, 128*(2), 393–406. Retrieved February 17, 2015, from http://pediatrics. aappublications.org/content/128/2/393.full

---

- Murmurs and pulmonary changes, which can indicate CHD.
- Chronic or recurrent respiratory infections, such as pneumonia and otitis media.

Laboratory and Diagnostic Tests
- Echocardiography: to detect cardiac defects
- Vision and hearing screening: to detect vision and hearing impairments
- Thyroid hormone level: to detect thyroid disease

- Cervical radiography: to assess for atlantoaxial instability
- Ultrasonography: to assess GI malformations.

Nursing Interventions

Promoting Growth and Development

- Children with Down syndrome tend to grow more slowly, learn more slowly, have shorter attention spans, and have trouble with reasoning and judgment.
- Their personality tends to be one of genuine warmth and cheerfulness along with patience, gentleness, and a natural spontaneity.
- Nurses play a key role in connecting families with appropriate resources that can facilitate the child's growth and development.
- The sooner early intervention programs can begin, the better for the child (see the earlier discussion on early intervention).
- Speech and language therapy, occupational therapy, and physical therapy will be important in promoting the child's growth and development.
- Special education should fit the child's individual needs, and the child should be integrated into mainstream education whenever possible.

Preventing Complications

- Children with Down syndrome are at risk for certain health problems (see earlier).
- Even though most nurses will encounter a child with Down syndrome in their practice, only a few nurses will become experts in their care.
- The needs of these children are complex, and the American Academy of Pediatrics has developed guidelines that can help the nurse care for these children and their families (these guidelines can be accessed at http://pediatrics.aappublications.org/content/128/2/393/T2.large.jpg).
- Nurses also play a key role in educating parents and caregivers about how to prevent the complications of Down syndrome (see Teaching Guidelines 2.20).

Teaching Guidelines 2.20
HEALTH GUIDELINES FOR CHILDREN WITH DOWN SYNDROME

Have your child evaluated by a pediatric cardiologist, including an echocardiogram.
- Take your child for routine vision and hearing tests. By 6 months have your child seen by a pediatric ophthalmologist.

- Make sure your child gets regular medical care, including recommended immunizations and a thyroid test at 6 and 12 months and then yearly.
- Have your child follow a regular diet and exercise routine.
- Make sure all family members perform proper hand hygiene to prevent infection.
- Monitor for signs and symptoms of respiratory infections, such as pneumonia and otitis media.
- Discuss with your physician the use of pneumococcal, respiratory syncytial virus, and influenza vaccines.
- Begin early interventions, therapy, and education as soon as possible.
- Make sure your child brushes his or her teeth regularly. He or she should visit the dentist every 6 months.
- Make sure the child gets a cervical radiograph between 3 and 5 years of age to screen for atlantoaxial instability. Report any changes in gait or use of arms and hands, weakness, changes in bowel or bladder function, complaints of neck pain or stiffness, head tilt, torticollis, or generalized changes in function. Ensure cervical spine positioning precautions (to avoid over extending or flexing of the neck) are utilized during procedures, such as those involving anesthetic, surgery, or radiographs.

Adapted from Bull, M. J. & the Committee on Genetics (2011). From the American Academy of Pediatrics: Clinical Report: Health supervision for children with Down syndrome. *Pediatrics, 128*(2), 393–406. Retrieved February 17, 2015, from http://pediatrics.aappublications.org/content/128/2/393.full

Promoting Nutrition

- Children with Down syndrome may have difficulty sucking and feeding due to lack of muscle tone. They tend to have small mouths; a smooth, flat, large tongue; and because of the underdeveloped nasal bone, chronically stuffy noses. This may lead to poor nutritional intake and problems with growth. These problems usually improve as the child gains tongue control.
- Use of a bulb syringe, humidification, and changing the infant's position can lessen the problem.
- Breast-feeding a baby with Down syndrome is usually possible, and the antibodies in breast milk can help the infant fight infections. The caregiver's hand can be used to provide additional support to the chin and throat.
- Speech or occupational therapists can work on strengthening muscles and assisting in feeding accommodations. Other feeding problems and failure to thrive can be related to cardiac defects and

usually improve after medical management is initiated or corrective surgery is performed.

- Children with Down syndrome do not need a special diet unless underlying GI disease is present, such as celiac disease. A balanced, high-fiber diet and regular exercise are important.
- Research has suggested that children with Down syndrome have lower basal metabolic rates, which can lead to problems with obesity, so it is important in the early years to develop appropriate eating habits and a regular exercise routine.
- High fiber intake is important for children with Down syndrome because their lack of muscle tone may decrease gastric motility, leading to constipation.

Educating and Supporting the Child and Family

- Down syndrome is a lifelong disorder that can result in health problems and cognitive disability.
- The diagnosis is usually made prenatally or shortly after birth. Parents and caregivers will need support and education during this difficult time.
- The range of mental impairment varies from mild to moderate; severe deficits occur occasionally.
- Evaluate how the family defines and manages this experience. Base the plan of care on each individual family's values, beliefs, strengths, and resources.
- Family members may have trouble meeting the demands of caring for a child with Down syndrome. These children have complex medical needs, which place strain on the family and its finances.
- From the time of diagnosis, the family should be involved in the child's care. Include parents in planning interventions and care for the child. In most cases, they are the primary caregivers and will provide daily care as well as assisting the child in the development of functioning and skills. They can provide essential information to the healthcare team and will be advocates for their child throughout his or her life.
- As the child grows, the needs of the family and child will change. Recognize and respect these needs and provide ongoing education and support to the child and family.
- Children with Down syndrome will need meaningful education programs. Many children with Down syndrome begin formal education in infancy and continue through high school.
- Be familiar with local and national resources for families of children with Down syndrome so that you can help them fulfill their potential.

TUBERCULOSIS INFECTION IN CHILDREN

- Children infected with tuberculosis can be asymptomatic or exhibit a broad range of symptoms. Symptoms may include fever, malaise, weight loss, anorexia, pain and tightness in the chest, and, rarely, hemoptysis.
- Cough might or might not be present and usually progresses slowly over several weeks to months. As tuberculosis progresses, the respiratory rate increases and the lung on the affected side is poorly expanded. Dullness to percussion might be present, as well as diminished breath sounds and crackles. Fever persists and pallor, anemia, weakness, and weight loss are present.
- Diagnosis is confirmed with a positive Mantoux test, positive gastric washings for acid-fast bacillus, and/or a chest radiograph consistent with tuberculosis.
- Antitubercular medication is required for all infected children.

URINARY TRACT INFECTION (UTI)

Description
- UTI occurs most often as a result of bacteria ascending to the bladder via the urethra. The short urethra in the infant and young child places the child at increased risk for infection (Lum, 2014).

Pathophysiology
- *E. coli* most commonly causes UTI, as it is usually found in the perineal and anal region, close to the urethral opening. Other organisms include *Klebsiella, S. aureus, Proteus, Pseudomonas,* and *Haemophilus.*
- Urinary stasis contributes to the development of a UTI once the bacteria have gained entry, as does decreased fluid intake.

Therapeutic Management
- Treatment includes oral or IV antibiotics, depending on the severity of the infection.
- Adequate fluid intake and fever management are also important.

Assessment Findings

Health History
- Fever
- Nausea or vomiting
- Chills
- Abdomen, back, or flank pain
- Lethargy
- Jaundice (in the neonate)

- Poor feeding or "just not acting right" (in the infant)
- Urinary urgency or frequency
- Burning or stinging with urination (the infant may cry with urination, the toddler may grab the diaper)
- Foul-smelling urine
- Poor appetite (child), enuresis, or incontinence in a previously toilet-trained child or blood in the urine.

Risk Factors
- Previous UTI
- Obstructive uropathy
- Inadequate toileting hygiene (often occurs with preschool girls)
- Vesicoureteral reflux (VUR)
- Constipation
- Urine holding or dysfunctional voiding
- Neurogenic bladder
- Uncircumcised male
- Sexual intercourse
- Pregnancy
- Chronic illness.

Physical Examination
- Jaundice or increased respiratory rate (in the neonate or young infant)
- Perineal redness or irritation
- Urine with visible blood, cloudiness, dark color, sediment, mucus, or foul odor
- Pallor, edema, or elevated blood pressure
- Distended bladder, abdominal mass, or tenderness, particularly in the flank area.

Laboratory and Diagnostic Tests
- Urinalysis (clean-catch, suprapubic, or catheterized): may be positive for blood, nitrites, leukocyte esterase, WBCs, or bacteria
- Urine culture: will be positive for infecting organism
- Renal ultrasonography: may show hydronephrosis if child also has a structural defect
- Voiding cystourethrography (VCUG): not usually performed until the child has been treated with antibiotics for at least 48 hours, as infected urine tends to reflux up the ureters anyway. VCUG performed once the urine has regained sterility may be positive for VUR.

Nursing Interventions
- Administer antibiotics as ordered (IV or oral). Urge the parent to complete the entire course of oral antibiotic at home, even though the child is feeling better.

- Administer IV fluids as ordered or encourage generous oral fluid intake.
- Administer antipyretics such as acetaminophen or ibuprofen to reduce fever.
- Apply a heating pad or warm compress to help relieve abdomen or flank pain.
- If the child is afraid to urinate due to burning or stinging, encourage voiding in a warm sitz or tub bath.
- Encourage the parents to return as ordered for a repeat urine culture after completion of the antibiotic course to ensure eradication of bacteria.
- Refer to Teaching Guidelines 2.21 for information on preventing UTI.

Teaching Guidelines 2.21
PREVENTING URINARY TRACT INFECTION IN FEMALES

- Drink enough fluid (to keep urine flushed through bladder).
- Drink cranberry juice to acidify the urine. Avoid colas and caffeine, which irritate the bladder.
- Urinate frequently and do not "hold" urine (to discourage urinary stasis).
- Avoid bubble baths (they contribute to vulvar and perineal irritation).
- Wipe from front to back after voiding (to avoid contaminating the urethra with rectal material).
- Wear cotton underwear (to decrease the incidence of perineal irritation).
- Avoid wearing tight jeans or pants.
- Wash the perineal area daily with soap and water.
- While menstruating, change sanitary pads frequently to discourage bacterial growth.
- Void immediately after sexual intercourse.

VOMITING

Description
- Vomiting is the forceful expulsion of gastric contents through the mouth.
- It occurs as a reflex with three different phases: nausea, retching, and then vomiting.

Pathophysiology
- Vomiting may result from a variety of causes including infectious processes (viral, bacterial, or parasitic), intestinal obstruction, genitourinary alteration, endocrine or metabolic alteration, GERD, or increased ICP.

Therapeutic Management
- Slow oral rehydration or IV fluid
- At times, administration of antiemetics.

Assessment Findings

Health History
- Infectious exposure or symptoms of other illnesses
- Associated diarrhea or pain
- Character and contents of the vomitus may include the following:
  - Effortless (as with gastroesophageal disease)
  - Projectile (as in pyloric stenosis)
  - Long periods after meals may occur with delayed gastric emptying
  - Upon awakening may occur with increased ICP
  - Bloody (GI bleeding)
  - Bilious (intestinal obstruction) (Hoffenberg et al., 2014).

Physical Examination
- Altered hydration status
- Normoactive, hypoactive, or hyperactive bowel sounds
- Abdominal mass or tenderness.

Laboratory and Diagnostic Tests
- Abdominal ultrasonography, upper GI series, or plain abdominal radiographs may reveal cause of the vomiting.

Nursing Interventions
- Teach the primary caregiver about oral rehydration therapy (refer to Teaching Guidelines 2.9).
- In the child with mild to moderate dehydration resulting from vomiting, withhold oral feeding for 1 to 2 hours after emesis, after which time oral rehydration can begin.
- Give the infant or child 0.5 to 2 ounces of oral rehydration solution every 15 minutes, depending on the child's age and size.
- As the child improves, larger amounts will be tolerated.
- Administer antiemetics and IV fluids if ordered.

Take Note!

Homemade oral rehydration solution can be made by combining 1 quart of water (can be water poured from cooking rice if desired), 8 teaspoons sugar, and 1 teaspoon salt.

WILMS TUMOR

Description

- Wilms tumor is the most common renal tumor in children and the fourth most common solid tumor in children (Hendershot, 2010).
- Peak incidence occurs between 2 and 3 years of age (Hendershot, 2010), and it usually affects only one kidney (Fig. 2.24).
- The prognosis depends on staging at diagnosis and the extent of metastasis, but the overall survival rate is about 90%.

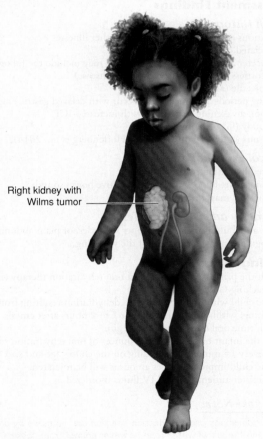

Right kidney with
Wilms tumor —

FIGURE 2.24 Wilms tumor.

- Complications include metastasis or complications from radiation therapy such as liver or renal damage, female sterility, bowel obstruction, pneumonia, or scoliosis.

Pathophysiology

- The etiology of Wilms tumor is unknown, but some cases occur via genetic inheritance.
- It demonstrates rapid growth and is usually large at diagnosis.
- Metastasis occurs via direct extension or through the bloodstream.

Therapeutic Management

- Surgical removal of the tumor and affected kidney (nephrectomy) is the treatment of choice and also allows for accurate staging and assessment of tumor spread.
- Radiation or chemotherapy may be administered either before or after surgery.

Assessment Findings

Health History

- Parental identification of a swollen abdomen or visible mass
- Abdominal pain
- Constipation
- Vomiting
- Anorexia
- Weight loss
- Difficulty breathing.

Risk Factors

- Hemihypertrophy of the spine
- Beckwith–Wiedemann syndrome
- Genitourinary anomalies
- Absence of the iris
- Family history of cancer.

Physical Examination

- Elevated blood pressure (in 25% of cases)
- Asymmetric abdomen
- Visible mass
- Adventitious breath sounds
- Lymphadenopathy.

Take Note!

Avoid palpating the abdomen after the initial assessment preoperatively. Wilms tumor is highly vascular and soft, so excessive handling of the tumor may result in tumor seeding and metastasis.

Laboratory and Diagnostic Tests

- Renal ultrasonography is used to assess the tumor and contralateral kidney.
- CT scan or MRI of the abdomen and chest determines local spread to lymph nodes or adjacent organs, as well as any distant metastasis.
- Urinalysis may reveal hematuria or leukocytes.
- Twenty-four-hour urine collection for HVA and VMA is done to distinguish the tumor from neuroblastoma (levels will not be elevated with Wilms tumor).

Nursing Interventions

- Provide routine postoperative care for abdominal surgery.
- Assess kidney function via urine output and serum BUN and creatinine.
- Monitor for effects of chemotherapy (see leukemia section).

Take Note!

To avoid injuring the remaining kidney, children with a single kidney should not play contact sports.

VISUAL OR HEARING IMPAIRMENT

The Child With a Visual Impairment

- Use the child's name to gain attention.
- Identify yourself and let the child know you are there before you touch the child.
- Encourage the child to be independent while maintaining safety.
- Name and describe people/objects to make the child more aware of what is happening.
- Discuss upcoming activities with the child.
- Explain what other children or individuals are doing.
- Make directions simple and specific.
- Allow the child additional time to think about the response to a question or statement.
- Use touch and tone of voice appropriate to the situation.
- Use parts of the child's body as reference points for the location of items.
- Encourage exploration of objects through touch.
- Describe unfamiliar environments and provide reference points.
- Use the sighted-guide technique when walking with a visually impaired child. (Delta Gamma Center for Children with Visual Impairments, 2011).

The Child with a Hearing Impairment

- Determine child's level of hearing difficulty.
- Always ensure the child can see you when you are speaking.
- Utilize the child's preferred form of communication (American sign language, cued speech, augmented communication). Access an interpreter if needed.
- If the child uses a communication device, ensure it is present with the child in the hospital.
- For older children who can read, ensure closed-caption option is functional on hospital room television.
  - For children with hearing aids:
  - Clean daily with damp cloth.
  - Change batteries weekly.
  - When inserting the aid, the volume should be turned down and then adjusted to the appropriate level after insertion.

REFERENCES

Abed, R., & Grimer, R. (2010). Surgical modalities in the treatment of bone sarcoma in children. *Cancer Treatment Reviews, 36*(4), 342–347.

Alemzadeh, R., & Ali, O. (2011). Section 6: Diabetes mellitus in children. In R. M. Kleigman, B. F. Stanton, J. W. St. Geme III, N. F. Schor, & R. E. Behrman (Eds.), *Nelson textbook of pediatrics* (19th ed., pp. 1968–1997). Philadelphia, PA: Saunders.

Ambruso, D. R., Nuss, R., & Wang, M. (2014). Hematologic disorders. In W. W. Hay, M. J. Levin, R. R. Deterding, & M. J. Abzug, (Eds.), *Current pediatric diagnosis and treatment* (22nd ed.). New York, NY: McGraw-Hill.

American Academy of Allergy, Asthma and Immunology. (2011). Asthma action plan. Retrieved October 10, 2015, from http://www.aaaai.org/professionals/asthma-action-plan.pdf

American Academy of Pediatrics. (2011). Update of newborn screening and therapy for congenital hypothyroidism. *Pediatric, 117*(6), 2290–2303. Retrieved October 10, 2015, from http://pediatrics.aappublications.org/content/117/6/2290.full

American Academy of Pediatrics. (2013). Clinical practice guideline: The diagnosis and management of acute otitis media. *Pediatrics, 131*, e964–e999.

American Academy of Pediatrics. (2015). Meningococcal vaccines: What you need to know (VIS). Healthy Children. Retrieved October 10, 2015, from http://www.healthychildren.org/English/safety-prevention/immunizations/pages/Meningococcal-Vaccines-What-You-Need-to-Know.aspx

American Diabetes Association. (2014). Standards of medical care in diabetes—2014. *Diabetes Care, 37*(Suppl 1), S14–S80.

American Heart Association. (2011). *Pediatric advanced life support provider manual.* Dallas, TX: Author.

Atkinson, W., Wolfe, S., & Hamborsky, J. (Eds.). (2012). *Epidemiology and prevention of vaccine-preventable diseases* (12th ed.). Washington, DC: Public Health Foundation.

Baddour, L. M. (2015). *Impetigo.* Retrieved October 10, 2015 from http://www.uptodate.com/contents/impetigo.

Beke, D. M., Braudis, N. J., & Lincoln, P. (2005). Management of the pediatric postoperative cardiac surgery patient. *Critical Care Nursing Clinics of North America, 17*(4), 405–416.

Bichet, D. G. (2013a). Treatment of central diabetes insipidus. UpToDate. Retrieved on January 13, 2015, from http://www.uptodate.com/contents/treatment-of-central-diabetes-

insipidus?source=machineLearning&search=diabetes+insipidus&selectedTitle=2~150&
sectionRank=1&anchor=H10#H10

Bichet, D. G. (2013b). Clinical manifestations and causes of central diabetes insipidus.
UpToDate. Retrieved on January 13, 2015, from http://www.uptodate.com/contents/
clinical-manifestations-and-causes-of-central-diabetes-insipidus?source=see_link

Bowden, V. R., & Greenberg, C. S. (2012). Pediatric nursing procedures (3rd ed.).
Philadelphia, PA: Lippincott Williams & Wilkins.

Bozic, D., & Daniels, C. (2009a). AboutKidsHealth. Clean intermittent catheterization
(CIC): Step by step instructions for boys. Retrieved on June 28, 2015, from http://
www.aboutkidshealth.ca/en/healthaz/testsandtreatments/medicaldevices/pages/
clean-intermittent-catheterization-cic-step-by-step-instructions-for-boys.aspxhttp://
www.aboutkidshealth.ca/HealthAZ/Clean-Intermittent-Catheterization-CIC-Step-
By-Step-Instructions-for-Boys.aspx?articleID=10379&categoryID

Bozic, D., & Daniels, C. (2009b). AboutKidsHealth clean intermittent catheterization
(CIC): Step by step instructions for girls. Retrieved June 28, 2015, from http://www.
aboutkidshealth.ca/En/HealthAZ/TestsAndTreatments/MedicalDevices/Pages/Clean-
Intermittent-Catheterization-CIC-Step-By-Step-Instructions-for-Girls.aspx

Breault, D. T., & Majzoub, J. A. (2011). Chapter 552: Diabetes insipidus. In R. M.
Kleigman, B. F. Stanton, J. W. St. Geme III, N. F. Schor, & R. E. Behrman (Eds.),
Nelson textbook of pediatrics (19th ed., pp. 1881–1884). Philadelphia, PA: Saunders.

Browne, N. T., Flanigan, L. M., McComiskey, C. A., & Pieper, P. (2013). Nursing care
of the pediatric surgical patient (3rd ed.). Burlington, MA: Jones & Bartlett Learning.

Bryant, R. (2010). Anemias. In D. Tomlinson & N. E. Kline (Eds.), Pediatric oncology
nursing (2nd ed., pp. 142–171). New York, NY: Springer.

Bull, M. J. & the Committee on Genetics (2011). From the American Academy of
Pediatrics: Clinical Report: Health supervision for children with Down syndrome.
Pediatrics, 128(2), 393–406. Retrieved February 17, 2015, from http://pediatrics.
aappublications.org/content/128/2/393.full

Burstein, A., Talmi, A., Stafford, B., & Kelsay, K. (2014). Child & adolescent psychiatric
disorders & psychosocial aspects of pediatrics. In W. W. Hay, M. J. Levin, R. R.
Deterding, & M. J. Abzug, (Eds.), Current pediatric diagnosis and treatment (22nd ed.).
New York, NY: McGraw-Hill.

Centers for Disease Control and Prevention. (2015). Epilepsy: Frequently asked questions. Retrieved October 10, 2015, from http://www.cdc.gov/epilepsy/basics/faq.htm

Centers for Disease Control and Prevention. (2014a). Meningitis: Bacterial meningitis.
Retrieved Ocotber 10, 2015, from http://www.cdc.gov/meningitis/bacterial.html

Cervasio, K. (2011). Lower extremity orthoses in children with spastic quadriplegic
cerebral palsy: Implications for nurses, parents, and caregivers. Orthopaedic Nursing,
30(3), 155–159.

Chandrakasan, S., & Kamat, D. (2013). An overview of hemoglobinopathies and the
interpretation of newborn screening results. Pediatric Annals, 42(12), 502–508.

Chiesa, A., & Sirotnak, A. P. (2014). Child abuse & neglect. In W. W. Hay, M. J. Levin,
R. R. Deterding, & M. J. Abzug, (Eds.), Current pediatric diagnosis and treatment
(22nd ed.). New York, NY: McGraw-Hill.

Child Trends Databank. (2014). Unintentional injuries. Retrieved on October 10, 2015,
from http://www.childtrends.org/?indicators=unintentional-injuries

Child Welfare Information Gateway. (2014). Mandatory reporters of child abuse and
Neglect: Summary of state laws. Retrieved October 10, 2015, from https://www.
childwelfare.gov/topics/systemwide/laws-policies/statutes/manda/

Children's Hospital of Boston. (2012). Diabetes insipidus in children. Retrieved October
10, 2015, http://www.childrenshospital.org/conditions-and-treatments/conditions/
diabetes-insipidus

Christian, C. & Endom, E. E. (2014). Child abuse: Evaluation and diagnosis of abusive
head trauma in infants and children. UpToDate. Retrieved October 10, 2015, from

http://www.uptodate.com/contents/child-abuse-evaluation-and-diagnosis-of-abusive-head-trauma-in-infants-and-children

Committee on Obstetric Practice. (2013). *Committee Opinion Number 550: Maternal–Fetal Surgery for Myelomeningocele.* Retrieved October 10, 2015 from, http://www.acog.org/Resources-And-Publications/Committee-Opinions/Committee-on-Obstetric-Practice/Maternal-Fetal-Surgery-for-Myelomeningocele

Cook, E. H., & Higgins, S. S. (2010). Chapter 21: Congenital heart disease. In P. J. Allen, J. A. Vessey, & N. A. Schapiro (Eds.), *Primary care of the child with a chronic condition* (5th ed., pp. 385–404). St. Louis, MO: Mosby.

Covar, R. A., Fleischer, D. M., Cho, C., & Boguniewicz, M. (2014). Allergic disorders. In W. W. Hay, M. J. Levin, R. R. Deterding, & M. J. Abzug, (Eds.), *Current pediatric diagnosis and treatment* (22nd ed.). New York, NY: McGraw-Hill.

Curtin, G., & Boekelheide, A. (2010). Chapter 19: Cleft lip and cleft palate. In P. J. Allen, J. A. Vessey, & N. A. Schapiro (Eds.), *Primary care of the child with a chronic condition* (5th ed., pp. 347–363). St. Louis, MO: Mosby.

Cystic Fibrosis Foundation. (n. d.). About cystic fibrosis. Retrieved October 10, 2015, from https://www.cff.org/What-is-CF/About-Cystic-Fibrosis/

Dabelea, D., Mayer-Davis, E. J., Saydah, S., Imperatore, G., Linder, B., Divers, J., …, Hamman, R. F. (2014). Prevalence of type 1 and type 2 diabetes among children and adolescents from 2001 to 2009. *JAMA, 311*(17), 1778–1786.

Darst, J. R., Collins, K. K., & Miyamoto, S. D. (2014). Cardiovascular diseases. In W. W. Hay, M. J. Levin, R. R. Deterding, & M. J. Abzug, (Eds.), *Current pediatric diagnosis and treatment* (22nd ed.). New York, NY: McGraw-Hill.

Delta Gamma Center for Children with Visual Impairments. (2011). *Interacting with visually impaired.* Retrieved October 10, 2015, from http://dgckids.org/resources/interacting-with-visually-impaired/

DeNicola, L. K. Maraqua, N. F., Udeani, J., & Custodio, H. T. (2015). Bronchiolitis. Retrieved October 10, 2015, from http://emedicine.medscape.com/article/961963-overview

Dowshen, S. (2015). Precocious puberty. Retrieved October 10, 2015, from http://kidshealth.org/parent/medical/sexual/precocious.html

Doyle, T., Kavanaugh-McHugh, A., & Fish, F. A. (2015). Management and outcome of tetralogy of Fallot. Retrieved October 10, 2015, from http://www.uptodate.com/contents/management-and-outcome-of-tetralogy-of-fallot

Dunn, A. (2013). Elimination patterns. In C. Burns, A. Dunn, M. Brady, N. B. Starr, & C. Blosser (Eds.), *Pediatric primary care* (5th ed.). Philadelphia, PA: Saunders.

Endom, E. E. (2015). Medical child abuse (Munchausen syndrome by proxy). Retrieved October 10, 2015, from http://www.uptodate.com/contents/medical-child-abuse-munchausen-syndrome-by-proxy

Engorn, B., & Flerlage, J. (2015). *The Harriet Lane handbook* (20th ed.). Philadelphia, PA: Saunders.

Fahrner, R., & Romano, S. (2010). HIV infection and AIDS. In P. J. Allen, J. A. Vessey, & N. A. Schapiro (Eds.), *Primary care of the child with a chronic condition* (5th ed., pp. 527–545). St. Louis, MO: Mosby.

Federico, M. J., Baker, C. D., Balasubramaniam, V., Beboer, E. M., Deterding, R. R., …, Zemarick, E. T. (2014). Respiratory tract & mediastinum. In W. W. Hay, M. J. Levin, R. R. Deterding, & M. J. Abzug, (Eds.), *Current pediatric iagnosis and treatment* (22nd ed.). New York, NY: McGraw-Hill.

Fisher, R. S., Acevedo, C., Arzimanoglou, A., Bogacz, A., Cross, J. H., Elger, C. E., …, Wiebe, S. (2014). ILAE Official Report: A practical clinical definition of epilepsy. *Epilepsia, 55*(4):475–482.

Fleisher, G. R. (2014). Evaluation of diarrhea in children. Retrieved October 10, 2015, from http://www.uptodate.com/contents/evaluation-of-diarrhea-in-children

Ford, D. M. (2014). Fluid, electrolyte, and acid-base disorders & therapy. In W. W. Hay, M. J. Levin, R. R. Deterding, & M. J. Abzug, (Eds.), *Current pediatric diagnosis and treatment* (22nd ed.). New York, NY: McGraw-Hill Companies, Inc.

Foote, J. M., Brady, L. H., Burke, A. L., Cook, J. S., Dutcher, M. E., Gradoville, K. M., …, Phillips, K. T. (2011). Development of an evidence-based clinical practice guideline on linear growth measurement of children. *Journal of Pediatric Nursing, 26*(4), 312–324.

Francis, G. S., Wilson Tang, W. H., & Walsh, R. A. (2011). Pathophysiology of heart failure. In V. Fuster, R. A. Walsh, & R. A. Harrington (Eds.), *Hurst's the heart* (13th ed.). New York, NY: McGraw-Hill Companies, Inc.

Freedman, S. (2015). Oral rehydration therapy. Retrieved October 10, 2015, from http://www.uptodate.com/contents/oral-rehydration-therapy

Friedman, N. R., Scholes, M. A., & Yoon, P. J. (2014). Ear, nose, & throat. In W. W. Hay, M. J. Levin, R. R. Deterding, & M. J. Abzug, (Eds.), *Current pediatric diagnosis and treatment* (22nd ed.). New York, NY: McGraw-Hill.

Garibaldi, L. & Chemaitilly, W. (2011). Chapter 556: Disorders of pubertal development. In R. M. Kleigman, B. F. Stanton, J. W. St. Geme III, N. F. Schor & R. E. Behrman (Eds.), *Nelson textbook of pediatrics* (19th ed., pp. 1886–1895). Philadelphia: Saunders.

Garzon, D. L. (2013). Coping and stress tolerance: Mental health and illness. In C. E. Burns, A. M. Dunn, M. A. Brady., N. B. Starr, & C. G. Blosser. *Pediatric primary care* (5th ed.). Philadelphia, PA: Saunders.

Gaylord, N. M., & Petersen-Smith, A. M. (2013). Genitourinary disorders. In C. Burns, A. Dunn, M. Brady, N. B. Starr, & C. Blosser (Eds.), *Pediatric primary care* (5th ed.). Philadelphia, PA: Saunders.

Graham, D. K., Craddock, J. A., Quinones, R. R., Keating, A. K., Maloney, K., Foreman, N. K., Giller, R. H., & Greffe, B. S. (2014). Neoplastic disease. In W. W. Hay, M. J. Levin, R. R. Deterding, & M. J. Abzug, (Eds.), *Current pediatric diagnosis and treatment* (22nd ed.). New York, NY: McGraw-Hill.

Grossman, S. (2014). Chapter 58: Disorders of musculoskeletal function: Developmental and metabolic disorders. In S. Grossman & C. M. Porth (Eds.), *Porth's Pathophysiology: Concepts of altered health states* (9th ed., pp. 489–574). Philadelphia, PA: Wolters Kluwer Health/Lippincott Williams & Wilkins.

Haemer, M., Primark, L. E., & Krebs, N. R. (2012). Normal childhood nutrition and its disorders. In W. W. Hay, M. J. Levin, R. R. Deterding, & M. J. Abzug, (Eds.), *Current pediatric diagnosis and treatment* (22nd ed.). New York, NY: McGraw-Hill.

Haut, C. M. (2014). Chapter 54: Pediatric orthopedic disorders. In S. M. Nettina (Ed.), *Lippincott manual of nursing practice* (10th ed., pp. 1743–69). Philadelphia, PA: Wolters/Kluwer Health: Lippincott Williams & Wilkins.

Hazle, L. A. (2010). Cystic fibrosis. In P. J. Allen, J. A. Vessey, & N. A. Schapiro (Eds.), *Primary care of the child with a chronic condition* (5th ed., pp. 405–426). St. Louis, MO: Mosby.

Hendershot, E. (2010). Solid tumor. In D. Tomlinson & N. E. Kline (Eds.), *Pediatric oncology nursing* (2nd ed., pp. 60–127). New York, NY: Springer.

Hoffenberg, E., Brumbaugh, D., Furuta, G. T., Kobak, G., Liu, E., Soden, J., & Kramer, R. (2014). Gastrointestinal tract. In W. W. Hay, M. J. Levin, R. R. Deterding, & M. J. Abzug, (Eds.), *Current pediatric diagnosis and treatment* (22nd ed.). New York, NY: McGraw-Hill.

iCommunicate Therapy. (2015). Hearing problems, hearing impairment, and being deaf. Retrieved October 10, 2015, from http://www.icommunicatetherapy.com/child-speech-language/child-speech-language-hearing-literacy-communication-disorders-delays/hearing-problems-hearing-impairment-being-deaf/

John, R. M. & Brady, M. A. (2013a). Atopic and rheumatic disorders. In C. E. Burns, A. M. Dunn, M. A. Brady, N. B. Starr, & C. G. Blosser (Eds.), *Pediatric primary care* (5th ed.). Philadelphia, PA: Elsevier Saunders.

John, R. M. & Brady, M. A. (2013b). Respiratory disorders. In C. E. Burns, A. M. Dunn, M. A. Brady, N. B. Starr, & C. G. Blosser (Eds.), *Pediatric primary care* (5th ed.). Philadelphia, PA: Elsevier Saunders.

Johnston, M. V. (2011). Chapter 591: Encephalopathies. In R. M. Kleigman, B. F. Stanton, J. W. St. Geme III, N. F. Schor, & R. E. Behrman (Eds.), *Nelson textbook of pediatrics* (19th ed., pp. 2061–2069). Philadelphia, PA: Saunders.

Jones, K. B., & Higgins, G. C. (2010). Juvenile rheumatoid arthritis. In P. J. Allen, J. A. Vessey, & N. A. Schapiro (Eds.), *Primary care of the child with a chronic condition* (5th ed., pp. 587–606). St. Louis, MO: Mosby.

Karp, S., & Riddell, J. P. (2010). Bleeding disorders. In P. J. Allen, J. A. Vessey, & N. A. Schapiro (Eds.), *Primary care of the child with a chronic condition* (5th ed., pp. 243–261). St. Louis, MO: Mosby.

Kaufman, P. L., Kim, J., & Berry, J. L. (2015). Overview of retinoblastoma. Retrieved June 27, 2015, from http://www.uptodate.com/contents/overview-of-retinoblastoma

Kinsman, S. L., & Johnston, M. V. (2011). Chapter 585: Congenital anomalies of the central nervous system. In R. M. Kleigman, B. F. Stanton, J. W. St. Geme III, N. F. Schor, & R. E. Behrman (Eds.), *Nelson textbook of pediatrics* (19th ed., pp. 1998–2013). Philadelphia, PA: Saunders.

Klein, J. O., & Pelton, S. (2015). Acute otitis media: Prevention of recurrence. Retrieved June 27, 2015, from http://www.uptodate.com/contents/acute-otitis-media-in-children-prevention-of-recurrence

Klein, M. S. (2010). Chapter 32: Kidney disease, chronic. In P. J. Allen, J. A. Vessey, & N. A. Schapiro (Eds.), *Primary care of the child with a chronic condition* (5th ed., pp. 607–626). St. Louis, MO: Mosby.

Kline & O'Hanlon-Curry. (2010). Central nervous system tumors. In D. Tomlinson & N. E. Kline (Eds.), *Pediatric oncology nursing* (2nd ed., pp. 129–141). New York, NY: Springer.

Ko, D. Y. (2015). *Seizures and epilepsy.* Retrieved October 10, 2015, from http://emedicine.medscape.com/article/1184846-overview

Kyle, T., & Carman, S. (2017). *Essentials of pediatric nursing* (3rd ed) Philadelphia, PA: Wolters Kluwer.

Lafranchi, S. (2011). Section 2: Disorders of the thyroid gland. In R. M. Kleigman, B. F. Stanton, J. W. St. Geme III, N. F. Schor, & R. E. Behrman (Eds.), *Nelson textbook of pediatrics* (19th ed., pp. 1894–1916). Philadelphia, PA: Saunders.

LaFranchi, S. (2014). Treatment and prognosis of congenital hypothyroidism. UpTo-Date. Retrieved on January 14, 2015, from http://www.uptodate.com/contents/treatment-and-prognosis-of-congenital-hypothyroidism?source=machineLearning&search=congenital+hypothyroidism&selectedTitle=2~63&anchor=H2&sectionRank=1#H2

Lum, G. M. (2014). Kidney & urinary tract. In W. W. Hay, M. J. Levin, R. R. Deterding, & M. J. Abzug, (Eds.), *Current pediatric diagnosis and treatment* (22nd ed.). New York, NY: McGraw-Hill.

MacNeil, J. & Cohn, A. (2011). Chapter 8: Meningococcal disease. In Centers for disease control and prevention. *Manual for the surveillance of vaccine-preventable diseases.* Atlanta, GA: Author.

March of Dimes. (2015). *Newborn screening.* Retrieved October 10, 2015, from http://www.marchofdimes.org/baby/newborn-screening-tests-for-your-baby.aspx

McFarland, E. J. (2014). Human immunodeficiency virus infection. In W. W. Hay, M. J. Levin, R. R. Deterding, & M. J. Abzug, (Eds.), *Current pediatric diagnosis and treatment* (22nd ed.). New York, NY: McGraw-Hill.

Mikati, M. A. (2011). Chapter 586. Seizures in childhood. In R. M. Kleigman, B. F. Stanton, J. W. St. Geme III, N. F. Schor, & R. E. Behrman (Eds.), *Nelson textbook of pediatrics* (19th ed., pp. 2013–2039). Philadelphia, PA: Saunders.

Morelli, J. G., & Prok, L. D. (2014). Skin. In W. W. Hay, M. J. Levin, R. R. Deterding, & M. J. Abzug, (Eds.), *Current pediatric diagnosis and treatment* (22nd ed.). New York, NY: McGraw-Hill.

Mount Nittany Medical Center. (n. d.). *When your son needs surgery for hypospadias.* Retrieved October 10, 2015, from http://www.mountnittany.org/articles/healthsheets/11970

Muscular Dystrophy Association. (2011). Facts about Duchenne and Becker muscular dystrophies. Retrieved October 10, 2015, http://www.mda.org/publications/PDFs/FA-DMD.pdf

National Asthma Education and Prevention Program. (2007). *Expert panel report 3: Guidelines for the diagnosis and management of asthma (NIH Publication No. 07–4051).* Bethesda, MD: National Institutes of Health, National Heart, Lung and Blood Institute.

National Diabetes Information Clearinghouse (NDIC). (2013). What I need to know about diabetes medicines: Types of Insulin. Retrieved October 10, 2015 from http://www.niddk.nih.gov/health-information/health-topics/Diabetes/diabetes-medicines/Pages/insert_C.aspx

National Hemophilia Foundation. (2009). Fast facts. Retrieved October 10, 2015, from http://www.hemophilia.org/walk/docs/FastFacts.pdf

National Institute of Neurological Disorders and Stroke (NINDS). (2015). *NINDS cerebral palsy information page.* Retrieved December 7, 2014, from http://www.ninds.nih.gov/disorders/cerebral_palsy/cerebral_palsy.htm#What_research_is_being_done

Nelson-Tuttle, C (2014). Chapter 50: Pediatric metabolic and endocrine disorders. In S. M. Nettina (Ed.), *Lippincott manual of nursing practice* (10th ed., pp. 1657–1678). Philadelphia, PA: Wolters/Kluwer Health: Lippincott Williams & Wilkins.

Nixon, C. (2010). Blood transfusion therapy. In D. Tomlinson & N. E. Kline (Eds.), *Pediatric oncology nursing* (2nd ed., pp. 546–558). New York, NY: Springer.

Ostermaier, K. K. (2015a). Down syndrome: Clinical features and diagnosis. UpToDate. Retrieved on October 10, 2015, from http://www.uptodate.com/contents/down-syndrome-clinical-features-and-diagnosis

Ostermaier, K. K. (2015b). Down syndrome: Management. UpToDate. Retrieved on October 10, 2015, from http://www.uptodate.com/contents/down-syndrome-management

Parks, J. S., & Felner, E. I. (2011). Hypopituitarism. In R. M. Kleigman, B. F. Stanton, J. W. St. Geme III, N. F. Schor, & R. E. Behrman (Eds.), *Nelson textbook of pediatrics* (19th ed., pp. 1876–1881). Philadelphia, PA: Saunders.

Pfeil, M., & Lindsay, B. (2010). Hypospadias repair: An overview. *International Journal of Urological Nursing, 4*(1), 4–12.

Pitts, R. H., & Record, E. O. (2010). Sickle cell disease. In P. J. Allen, J. A. Vessey, & N. A. Schapiro (Eds.), *Primary care of the child with a chronic condition* (5th ed., pp. 772–794). St. Louis, MO: Mosby.

Pivalizza, P., & Lalani, S. R. (2014). *Intellectual disability (mental retardation) in children: Definition; diagnosis; and assessment of needs.* Retrieved October, 10, 2015 from http://www.uptodate.com/contents/intellectual-disability-mental-retardation-in-children-definition-diagnosis-and-assessment-of-needs

Pomerantz, W. J. & Weiss, S. L. (2015). Systemic inflammatory response syndrome (SIRS) and sepsis in children: Definitions, epidemiology, clinical manifestations, and diagnosis. UpToDate. Retrieved on October 10, 2015, from http://www.uptodate.com/contents/systemic-inflammatory-response-syndrome-sirs-and-sepsis-in-children-definitions-epidemiology-clinical-manifestations-and-diagnosis

Pueschel, S. M. (2011). *A parent's guide to Down syndrome: Toward a brighter future* (rev. ed.). Baltimore: Paul H. Brookes Publishing Company, Inc.

Quilty, J. (2010, May). Pediatric burn management. Presented at meeting of the Florida Chapter of the National Association of Pediatric Nurse Practitioners, Orlando, FL.

Ralston, S. L., Lieberthal, A. S., Meissner, C., Alverson, B. K., Baley, J. E., Gadomski, A. M., …, Hernandez-Cancio, S. (2014). Clinical practice guideline: The diagnosis, management, and prevention of bronchiolitis. *Pediatrics, 134,* e1474–e1502.

Robinson, R. (2011). Prenatal surgery to correct spina bifida found to improve fetal outcomes. *Neurology Today, 11*(6), 1–6,7. doi: 10.1097/01.NT.0000396251.38853.8d

Safe Kids. (2015). Choking and strangulation. Retrieved October 10, 2015, from http://www.safekids.org/safetytips/field_risks/choking-and-strangulation

Saenger, P. (2015). Definition, etiology, and evaluation of precocious puberty. UpToDate. Retrieved on October 10, 2015, from http://www.uptodate.com/contents/definition-etiology-and-evaluation-of-precocious-puberty

Sankar, W. N., Horn, B. D., Wells, L., & Dormans, J. P. (2011). Chapter 670: The hip. In R. M. Kleigman, B. F. Stanton, J. W. St. Geme III, N. F. Schor, & R. E. Behrman (Eds.), *Nelson textbook of pediatrics* (19th ed., pp. 2355–2365). Philadelphia, PA: Saunders.

Schweich, P. (2014). Patient information: Cast and splint care (beyond the basics). UpToDate. Retrieved on October 10, 2015, from http://www.uptodate.com/contents/cast-and-splint-care-beyond-the-basics

Sickle Cell Information Center. (2011). Care path: Inpatient management of vaso-occlusive pain. Retrieved October 10, 2015, from http://scinfo.org/care-paths-and-protocols-children-adolescents/care-path-inpatient-management-of-vaso-occlusive-pain

Simon, C. (2010). Pain in children with cancer. In D. Tomlinson & N. E. Kline (Eds.), *Pediatric oncology nursing* (2nd ed., pp. 529–545). New York, NY: Springer.

Sirivimonpan, S. (2013). Airway remodeling in asthma. Retrieved October 10, 2015, from http://www.slideshare.net/AllergyChula/airway-remodeling-in-asthma

Sloand, E., & Cashchera, J. (2010). Allergies. In P. J. Allen, J. A. Vessey, & N. A. Schapiro (Eds.), *Primary care of the child with a chronic condition* (5th ed., pp. 145–167). St. Louis, MO: Mosby.

Solomon, D. H. (2014). Patient information: Nonsteroidal anti-inflammatory drugs (NSAIDs) (beyond the basics). Retrieved October 10, 2015, from http://www.uptodate.com/contents/nonsteroidal-antiinflammatory-drugs-nsaids-beyond-the-basics

Sood, M. R. (2015). Constipation in infants and children: Evaluation. Retrieved October 10, 2015, from http://www.uptodate.com/contents/constipation-in-infants-and-children-evaluation.

Spiegel, D. A., & Dormans, J. P. (2011). Chapter 671: The spine. In R. M. Kleigman, B. F. Stanton, J. W. St. Geme III, N. F. Schor, & R. E. Behrman (Eds.), *Nelson textbook of pediatrics* (19th ed., pp. 2365–2377). Philadelphia, PA: Saunders.

Summar, K., & Lee, B. (2011). Chapter 76.2: Down syndrome and other abnormalities of chromosome number. In R. M. Kleigman, B. F. Stanton, J. W. St. Geme III, N. F. Schor, & R. E. Behrman (Eds.), *Nelson textbook of pediatrics* (19th ed., pp. 399–403). Philadelphia, PA: Saunders.

Starr, N. B., Fookson, M., Burns, C. D., & Bowman-Harvey, C. A. (2013). Cognitive perceptual disorders. In C. E. Burns, A. M. Dunn., M. A. Brady., N. B. Starr., & C. G. Blosser. *Pediatric primary care* (5th ed.). Philadelphia, PA: Saunders.

Sundel, R. (2015). Kawasaki disease: Clinical features and diagnosis. Retrieved October 10, 2015, from http://www.uptodate.com/contents/kawasaki-disease-clinical-features-and-diagnosis.

Tan, A. J. & Silverberg, M. A. (2015). Hemolytic uremic syndrome in emergency medicine. Retrieved October 10, 2015, from http://emedicine.medscape.com/article/779218-overview

UNAIDS. (2014). Children and HIV fact sheet. Geneva, Switzerland: World Health Organization.

Vernon, P., Brady, M. A., Starr, N. B., & Petersen-Smith, A. M. (2013). Dermatologic disorders. In C. Burns, A. Dunn, M. Brady, N. B. Starr, & C. Blosser (Eds.), *Pediatric primary care* (5th ed.). Philadelphia, PA: Saunders.

Wells, L., Sehgal, K., & Dormans, J. P. (2011). Chapter 675: Common fractures. In R. M. Kliegman, R. E. Behrman, H. B. Jenson, & B. F. Stanton. *Nelson's textbook of pediatrics* (19th ed., pp. 2387–2394). Philadelphia, PA: Saunders.

White, P. C. (2011). Section 4: Disorders of the adrenal glands. In R. M. Kliegman, B. F. Stanton, J. W. St. Geme III, N. F. Schor, & R. E. Behrman (Eds.), *Nelson textbook of pediatrics* (19th ed., pp. 1923–1943). Philadelphia, PA: Saunders.

Winter, H. S. (2015a). Clinical manifestations and diagnosis of gastroesophageal reflux disease in children and adolescents. Retrieved October 10, 2015, from http://www.uptodate.com/contents/clinical-manifestations-and-diagnosis-of-gastroesophageal-reflux-disease-in-children-and-adolescents.

Winter, H. S. (2015b). Gastroesophageal reflux in infants. Retrieved October 10, 2015, from http://www.uptodate.com/contents/gastroesophageal-reflux-in-infants.

Zak, M., & Chan, V. W. (2014). Chapter 46: Pediatric neurologic disorders. In S. M. Nettina (Ed.), *Lippincott manual of nursing practice* (10th ed., pp. 1545–1575). Philadelphia, PA: Wolters/Kluwer Health: Lippincott Williams & Wilkins.

Zupanec, S., & Tomlinson, D. (2010). Leukemia. In D. Tomlinson & N. E. Kline (Eds.), *Pediatric oncology nursing* (2nd ed., pp. 2–32). New York, NY: Springer.

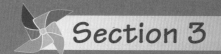

Common Laboratory and Diagnostic Tests and Nursing Procedures

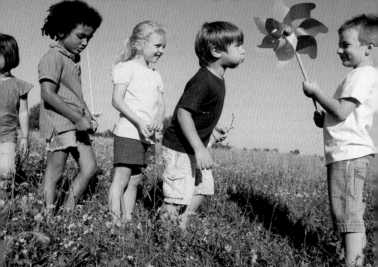

Overview of Laboratory and Diagnostic Tests and Nursing Procedures

- Children undergo numerous diagnostic tests and therapeutic procedures in a wide range of settings during their development.

OBTAINING CONSENT

- Generally, only people older than the age of majority (18 years of age) can legally provide consent for health care.
- Because children are minors, the process of consent involves obtaining written permission from a parent or legal guardian. Biologic or adoptive parents are usually considered to be the child's legal guardian.
- When divorce occurs, one or both parents may be granted custody of the child.
- In certain cases (such as child abuse or neglect, or during foster care), the courts may appoint a guardian *ad litem*.
- In cases requiring a signature for consent, usually the parent gives consent for care for children younger than 18 years except in certain situations (see "Exceptions to Parental Consent Requirement").

 Take Note!

Never assume that the adult accompanying the child is the parent or legal guardian. Always clarify the relationship of the accompanying adult.

Informed Consent

- Just as in adults, most care given in a healthcare setting is covered by the initial consent for treatment signed when the child becomes a patient at that office or clinic or by the consent to treatment signed upon admission to the hospital or other inpatient facility.
- Certain procedures, however, require a specific process of **informed consent**. Procedures that require informed consent include the following:
  - Major and minor surgery
  - Invasive procedures such as lumbar puncture or bone marrow aspiration
  - Treatments placing the child at higher risk, such as chemotherapy or radiation therapy procedures or treatments involving research
  - Photography involving children
  - Applying restraints to children

- The nurse's responsibility related to informed consent includes the following:
  - Determining that the parents or legal guardians understand what they are signing by asking them pertinent questions
  - Ensuring that the consent form is completed with signatures from the parents or legal guardians
  - Serving as a witness to the signature process.

Special Situations to Informed Consent

- If the parent is not available, then the person in charge (relative, babysitter, or teacher) may give consent for emergency treatment if that person has a signed form from the parent or legal guardian allowing him or her to do so.
- During an emergency situation, a verbal consent via the telephone may be obtained. Two witnesses must be listening simultaneously and will sign the consent form, indicating that consent was received via telephone.
- Healthcare providers can provide emergency treatment to a child without consent if they have made reasonable attempts to contact the child's parent or legal guardian (American Academy of Pediatrics [AAP], Committee on Pediatric Emergency Medicine [CPEM], 2011). In urgent or emergent situations, appropriate medical care should never be delayed or withheld because of an inability to obtain consent (AAP, CPEM, 2011).
- If a child is not living with his or her biologic or adoptive parents, such as a child living in foster care, with potential adoptive parents, or with a relative, the legally appointed guardian must provide consent. Verify authority and include documentation of legally appointed guardian in child's medical record.
- If a child's parents are divorced, the ability to give consent for healthcare rests with parent who has legal custody by divorce decree. Determine whether the parents have joint custody or whether there is sole custody by one parent. In cases of emergency, the parent with physical custody may give consent. If there is joint legal custody and the parents disagree on care, court involvement may be necessary.

Exceptions to Parental Consent Requirement

Mature Minor

- In some states, a **mature minor** may give consent to certain medical treatment. The physician or nurse practitioner must determine that the adolescent (usually older than 14 years) is sufficiently mature and intelligent to make the decision for treatment.
- The physician or nurse practitioner also considers the complexity of the treatment, its risks, and benefits and whether the treatment

is necessary or elective before obtaining consent from a mature minor (AAP, CPEM, 2011).

Emancipated Minor

- State laws vary in relation to the definition of an **emancipated minor** and the types of treatment that may be obtained by an emancipated minor (without parental consent). The nurse must be familiar with the particular state's law.
- Emancipation may be considered in any of the following situations, depending on the state's laws:
  - Membership in a branch of the armed services
  - Marriage
  - Court-determined emancipation
  - Financial independence and living apart from parents
  - Pregnancy
  - Mother younger than 18 years
- The emancipated minor is considered to have the legal capacity of an adult and may make his or her own healthcare decisions (AAP, CPEM, 2011).
- Depending on the state law, health care may be provided to minors for certain conditions, in a confidential manner, without including the parents.
- These types of care may include
  - pregnancy counseling
  - prenatal care
  - contraception
  - testing for and treatment of sexually transmitted infections and communicable diseases (including HIV); and
  - substance abuse and mental illness counseling and treatment (AAP, CPEM, 2011)
- Laws vary by state, so the nurse must be knowledgeable about the laws in the state where he or she is licensed to practice.

PROVIDING CARE DURING DIAGNOSTIC TESTS AND PROCEDURES

Regardless of the procedure to be performed and the setting, children, like adults, need thorough preparation before the diagnostic test or procedure and support during and after the diagnostic test or procedure, to promote the best outcome and to ensure atraumatic care.

Positioning

- Use positions that are comforting to the child during painful procedures (Fig. 3.1).

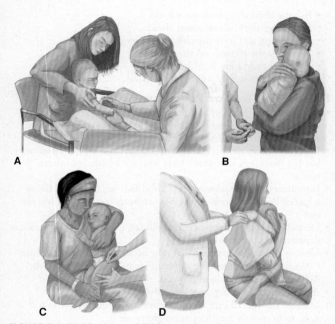

FIGURE 3.1 Positioning a child for comfort during a painful procedure. **A:** Sitting on the parent's lap while undergoing allergy testing provides this toddler with a sense of comfort. **B:** Position the infant cuddled over the parent's (preferable) or the nurse's shoulder when obtaining a heel stick. **C:** Use "therapeutic hugging" to maintain a child's position when the child is receiving an intramuscular injection. **D:** Use "therapeutic hugging" to position a child while the child is having an IV catheter inserted.

Take Note!

Make sure the parent understands his or her role and knows which body parts to hold still in a safe manner.

Distraction Methods

- Distraction or stimulation (such as with a toy) can help to gain the child's cooperation during tests and procedures.
- Distraction methods include the following:
  - Have the child point toes inward and wiggle them.

- Ask the child to squeeze your hand.
- Encourage the child to count aloud.
- Sing a song and have the child sing along.
- Point out the pictures on the ceiling.
- Have the child blow bubbles.
- Play music that is appealing to the child.

Before the Test or Procedure

- Provide a description of and the reason for the procedure using age-appropriate language ("the doctor will look at your blood to see why you are sick") See Table 3.1.
- Describe where the procedure will occur ("the x-ray department has big machines that won't hurt you; it's a little cold there too").
- Introduce strange equipment the child may see ("you will lie on a special bed that moves in the big machine, but you can still see out").
- Describe how long the procedure will last ("you will be in the x-ray department until lunchtime").
- Identify unusual sensations that may occur during the procedure ("you may smell something different" [e.g., alcohol smell], "the MRI machine makes loud noises").
- Inform the child if any pain is involved.
- Identify any special care required after the procedure ("you will need to lie quietly for 15 minutes afterward").

Take Note!

In the hospital, perform all invasive procedures in the treatment room or a room other than the child's room. The child's room should remain a safe and secure area.

- Incorporate play into the preparation.
- Consider the child's temperament, coping strategies, and previous experiences as well as developmental needs and cognitive abilities.
- Gain trust and provide support.
- Include the child's parents, because parents are usually the greatest source of comfort for the child.
- Be short, simple, and appropriate in explaining situations at the child's level of development.
- Explain what is to be done and what is expected of the child.
- Avoid terms that have double meanings or might be confusing.
- Watch for signs of anxiety or fear.

(text continues on page 334)

TABLE 3.1	ALTERNATIVES WORDS FOR CONFUSING OR MISUNDERSTOOD TERMS	
Terms to Avoid	**How Children Might Interpret It**	**Use These Terms Instead**
Catheter	Too technical	Tube
Deaden	Kill?	Make sleepy
Dye	"Die"	Special medicine to help the doctor see _____ (part of the body) better
Electrodes	Too technical	Stickers, ticklers, snaps
ICU	"I see you"	Special room with your own nurse
Incision, cut open, make a hole	Too explicit	Special or small opening
Monitor	Too technical	TV screen
Organ	Like a piano?	Special place in the body
Pain	May be too explicit	Child's word for hurt; "boo-boo"
Put to sleep, anesthesia	May confuse with putting a pet to sleep	Special kind of sleep
Shot	Children are scared of shots	Medication under the skin
Stool	Like you sit on?	"Poop" or child's word for it
Stretcher or gurney	"Stretch her"	Rolling bed or special bed on wheels
Take your temperature/ BP	Where are you going to "take" them?	See how warm you are/ hug your arm
Test	Like at school? (The child will need to perform)	See how your heart is working

(continued on page 334)

ALTERNATIVES WORDS FOR CONFUSING OR MISUNDERSTOOD TERMS *continued*		
Terms to Avoid	How Children Might Interpret It	Use These Terms Instead
Tourniquet	Too technical	Special kind of rubber band
Urine	"You're in?"	"Pee" or child's word for it
X-ray	Don't understand	Picture or big camera to take pictures of the inside of your body

Partially adapted from Florida Children's Hospital, Child Life Department. (n.d.). *Suggested vocabulary to use with children.* Orlando, FL: Author.

During the Procedure

- Use a firm, positive, confident approach that provides the child with a sense of security.
- Encourage cooperation by involving the child in decision making and allowing the child to select from a list or group of appropriate choices.
- Allow the child to express feelings of anger, anxiety, fear, frustration, or any other emotions.
- Tell the child that it is okay to scream or cry, but that it is very important to hold still.
- Use distraction methods such as those described earlier.

Take Note!

Toddlers and preschoolers often resist procedures despite preparation for them. Being held down or restrained is often more traumatizing to the young child than the procedure itself. Use alternative methods (positions that provide comfort for the child) to keep the child still during the procedure (refer to Fig. 3.1). The older child can be held while using a book or story for distraction.

After the Procedure

- Hold and comfort the child. Cuddle and soothe infants.
- Encourage children to express their feelings through play, such as dramatic play or use of puppets.

- Gross motor activities such as pounding or throwing are also helpful for children to discharge pent-up feelings and energy. School-aged children and adolescents may not outwardly demonstrate behavior indicating the need for comforting; however, provide them with opportunities to express their feelings and be comforted.
- Praise children for appropriate behavior during the procedure and after all interventions are completed.

 Take Note!
Remember to use the services of child life specialists when available.

Laboratory and Diagnostic Tests

ALLERGY SKIN TESTING

Description and Purpose
- Suggested allergen is applied to skin via scratch, pin, or prick to determine whether the child has a response.

Results
- A wheal response indicates allergy to the substance.

Nursing Considerations
- Discontinue antihistamines before testing to avoid inhibition of the test.
- Have epinephrine and emergency equipment readily available.
- Observe closely for risk of anaphylaxis.

α-FETOPROTEIN

Description and Purpose
- Measures level of α-fetoprotein (AFP) in the blood and is used to determine tumor burden.
- AFP is normally produced by the fetal liver and yolk sac.

Results
- Normally decreases to very low levels by 1 year of age
- May be elevated in Hodgkin disease and other cancers.

Nursing Considerations
• No food or fluid restriction required.

Description and Purpose
• Enzyme-linked assay testing for the presence of autoantibodies that react against cellular nuclear material.

Results
• Results may be weakly positive in about 20% of healthy people.
• Steroid use can give a false-negative result.
• Positive result is with many autoimmune diseases such as systemic lupus erythematosus.

Nursing Considerations
• Check for signs of infection at venipuncture site.

Description and Purpose
• Invasive method (requires blood sampling) of measuring arterial pH, partial pressure of oxygen and carbon dioxide, and base excess in blood.
• Usually reserved for severe illness, the intubated child, or suspected carbon dioxide retention.

Results
• May indicate normal oxygenation and ventilation:
  • pH: 7.35 to 7.45
  • pO_2: 80 to 100 mm Hg
  • pCO_2: 35 to 45 mm Hg
  • Base excess: −2 to +2 mmol/L
• Abnormal results indicate acidosis or alkalosis that is metabolic or respiratory in nature.

Nursing Considerations
• Hold pressure for several minutes after a peripheral arterial stick to avoid bleeding.
• Radial arterial sticks are common and can be very painful.
• Note if the child is crying excessively during the blood draw, as this affects the carbon dioxide level.

ARTERIOGRAM

Description and Purpose

- Radiopaque contrast solution is injected through a catheter and into the circulation. X-rays are then taken to visualize the structure of the heart and blood vessels.
- Allows for observation of blood flow to parts of body and detect lesions.
- May be used to confirm a diagnosis or to remove plaques.

Results

- The report will indicate any abnormalities of the heart chambers or vessels that are noted during the test.

Nursing Considerations

- Before the procedure:
  - Make sure the parent signs a consent form.
  - Obtain child's weight to determine amount of dye needed.
  - Keep the child NPO before the procedure according to institutional protocol.
  - Administer premedication as ordered.
- After the procedure:
  - Maintain the child on bed rest.
  - Observe the puncture site for bleeding.
  - Monitor vital signs frequently and check the pulse distal to the site.

ARTHROGRAPHY

Description and Purpose

- Multiple radiographic images of a joint after direct injection with a radiopaque substance.
- Used to assess ligaments, muscles, tendons, and cartilage, particularly after injury.

Results

- Normal result shows normal filling of the structures of the joint including the joint space, articular cartilage, ligaments, bursae, and menisci.

Nursing Considerations

- Do not perform this test if joint infection is present.
- Rest the joint for 12 hours after the test.
- Apply cold therapy after the test and assess for swelling and pain.

• Assess for crepitus, which may be present in the joint for 1 to 2 days after the test.

BARIUM ENEMA

Description and Purpose
• Fluoroscopy is used to visualize the colon after instillation of barium via the rectum.
• It is used to evaluate children with constipation, rectal prolapse, bleeding, or suspected intussusception.

Results
• May reveal mass, obstruction, or other abnormality.

Nursing Considerations
• Bowel preparation prior to examination may be ordered.
• Stool will be light colored because of barium for a few days.

BARIUM SWALLOW/UPPER GASTROINTESTINAL SERIES (WITH OR WITHOUT SMALL BOWEL FOLLOW-THROUGH)

Description and Purpose
• Child ingests barium and then undergoes fluoroscopy.
• Visualizes the form, position, mucosal folds, peristaltic activity, and motility of the esophagus, stomach, and upper gastrointestinal (GI) tract.
• Small bowel follow-through allows visualization of the small intestine contour, position, and motility.

Results
• May reveal the presence of foreign body; determine the source of abdominal pain or vomiting such as obstruction or the source of dysphagia.
• Small bowel follow-through may reveal obstruction, malrotation, intussusception, or bowel wall thickening.

Nursing Considerations
• Infants and children are usually NPO for several hours prior to procedure.
• Infants may need to be given barium via syringe if they refuse to drink it.
• Females of reproductive age must be screened for pregnancy.

- Encourage large amounts of water/fluids after the test to avoid barium-induced constipation.
- Stool will be light colored because of barium for a few days.

BLOOD CULTURE AND SENSITIVITY

Description and Purpose
- Deliberate growing of microorganism in a solid or liquid medium.
- Once the microorganism has grown, it is tested against various antibiotics to determine which antibiotics will kill it.
- Used to detect the presence of bacteria or yeast, which may have spread from a certain site in the body into the bloodstream. Also used to determine antibiotic sensitivity of the bacteria or yeast.
- The specimen for testing is obtained via venipuncture.

Results
- Normal result is negative for pathogens.

Nursing Considerations
- Follow aseptic technique and hospital protocol to prevent contamination.
- Preferably, take two cultures obtained from two different sites.
- Ideally, obtain specimens before administering antibiotics; if client is taking antibiotics, notify laboratory and draw specimen shortly before the next dose.
- Draw below intravenous (IV) line, if possible, to prevent dilution of sample.
- Deliver specimen to the laboratory immediately (within 30 minutes).

BLOOD TYPE AND CROSS-MATCH

Description and Purpose
- Blood sample is obtained to determine ABO blood type and the presence of antigens in preparation for possible blood transfusion.
- Cross-match is performed on red blood cell (RBC)-containing products to avoid transfusion reaction.

Results
- Child's blood type, Rh factor, and blood antigens are reported.

Nursing Considerations
- Appropriately sign and date specimen.
- Apply "type and cross" or "blood band" to child at the time of blood draw if indicated by the institution.
- Most type and cross-match specimens expire after 48 to 72 hours.

BONE AGE RADIOGRAPH

Description and Purpose

- Radiographic study of wrist or hand to determine bone maturation compared with national standards.
- Used to determine whether bone age is consistent with chronologic age to rule out growth hormone (GH) deficiency or excess, or hypothyroidism.

Results

- Normal result is no difference in child's bone age and child's chronologic age.

Nursing Considerations

- Explain the procedure to the child because the child must hold still for the radiography.
- Allow the family to accompany the child.
- Enlist the family's help if needed to calm the child during radiography.

BONE MARROW ASPIRATION AND BIOPSY

Description and Purpose

- A needle is inserted through the cortex of the bone into the bone marrow (most often the iliac spine), bone marrow is aspirated, and the cells are evaluated for the presence of leukemic cells or metastasis of other cancers to bone marrow.
- Multiple cell and chromosome tests may be performed to determine specific genetics of the particular leukemia in order to guide treatment.

Results

- Results will reveal the type and genetics of leukemic cells and whether or not metastasis from other cancers has entered the bone marrow.

Nursing Considerations

- Apply EMLA cream 1 to 3 hours prior to the procedure in order to decrease associated pain.
- Lidocaine may also be injected just prior to the procedure to decrease pain.
- Observe closely if performed under conscious (or moderate) sedation.
- Apply a pressure dressing to arrest bleeding.
- Assess for tenderness or erythema.
- Administer mild analgesia for postprocedure pain as needed.

BONE SCAN

Description and Purpose
- Administration of IV radionuclide material, which is taken up by the bone and is visible on the scans.
- May identify metastasis to the bones.

Results
- Normal result would show bone free from metastasis.

Nursing Considerations
- Requires patent IV for injection of radionuclide material.
- Encourage fluid intake after injection to increase uptake of injected radionuclide.
- Scan will be performed 1 to 3 hours after injection.

CEREBRAL ANGIOGRAPHY

Description and Purpose
- X-ray study of cerebral blood vessels.
- Involves injection of a contrast medium and use of fluoroscopy.
- Used to assess for vessel defects or space-occupying lesions.

Results
- Normal result shows normal cerebral blood vessels.

Nursing Considerations
- Children may be afraid during this test; allow a parent or family member to accompany the child.
- Restraint may be necessary if the child is unable or unwilling to stay still for radiography.
- Limit the time of restraint to the amount of time needed for radiography.
- Assess for allergy to contrast medium.
- Push fluids following the procedure, if not contraindicated, to help flush out contrast medium.

CLOTTING STUDIES

Description and Purpose
- Blood sample to measure prothrombin time (PT), partial thromboplastin time (PTT), activated partial thromboplastin time (aPTT), and international normalized ratio (INR).

Results

• PT, PTT, and/or INR may be elevated in children with clotting disorders or disseminated intravascular coagulation.

Nursing Considerations

• Apply pressure to venipuncture site after specimen withdrawal.
• Assess for bleeding (bleeding gums, bruising, blood in urine).

COAGULATION FACTOR CONCENTRATION

Description and Purpose

• Measures concentration of specific coagulating factors in the blood (i.e., factor VIII, von Willebrand factor, etc.).

Results

• These factors may be decreased in hemophilia or disseminated intravascular coagulation.

Nursing Considerations

• Apply pressure to venipuncture site.
• Deliver specimen to laboratory as soon as possible (unstable at room temperature).
• Assess for bleeding (gums, bruising, blood in urine or stool).

COMPLETE BLOOD CELL COUNT

Description and Purpose

• To evaluate hemoglobin and hematocrit, white blood cell count (particularly the percentage of individual white cells) and platelet count.
• Obtained via venipuncture, finger stick, or heel stick.
• Used to detect the presence of inflammation, infection, anemia, polycythemia, or thrombocytopenia.

Results

• Normal values vary according to age and gender.
• Myelosuppressive drugs may affect results.
• White blood cell count differential is helpful in differentiating source of infection.

Nursing Considerations

• Specimen may be obtained quickly via capillary puncture.
• False elevations in hemoglobin and hematocrit values may occur with dehydration.
• Overhydration can alter results and lead to false lower counts.

- Children with significantly depressed white blood cell counts should be protected from the possibility of infection.

COMPUTED TOMOGRAPHIC (CT) SCAN

Description and Purpose
- Noninvasive x-ray study that looks at tissue density and structures.
- Multiple images taken in successive layers to provide a three-dimensional view of the body part being scanned.
- Can be performed with or without the use of oral or IV contrast medium.
- Used to diagnose and evaluate congenital or structural abnormalities, hemorrhage, tumors, fractures, demyelinization, and inflammation.

Results
- Normal result shows normal tissue density and structures without evidence of fracture, tumor, or other pathology.

Nursing Considerations
- When contrast is ordered, notify physician if the child has iodine or shellfish allergy.
- Maintain the child on NPO status for several hours if contrast is used (contrast may cause nausea).
- Reassure the child; the machine is large and can be frightening.
- Keep the child still during the sometimes-lengthy procedure. If unable to do so, sedation may be necessary.
- Encourage fluids post procedure if not contraindicated to facilitate excretion of contrast dye.

C-REACTIVE PROTEIN

Description and Purpose
- Nonspecific test that measures a type of protein produced in the liver that is present during episodes of acute inflammation.
- Obtained via venipuncture, finger stick, or heel stick.
- Used to detect the presence of infection; C-reactive protein is a more sensitive and rapidly responding indicator than erythrocyte sedimentation rate (ESR).

Results
- Normal value is less than 1 mg/dL.
- Abnormal value is an elevated level.
- Presence of an intrauterine device may cause positive test results because of tissue inflammation.

- Exogenous hormones, such as oral contraceptives, may cause increased levels.
- Nonsteroidal anti-inflammatory drugs, salicylates, and steroids may cause decreased levels.

Nursing Considerations

- Explain to the child and family that fasting may be required.
- Send sample to laboratory immediately. If allowed to stand for longer than 3 hours, it may result in falsely low result.

CREATINE KINASE (CK); CREATINE PHOSPHOKINASE (CKP)

Description and Purpose

- A venous blood sample that reflects muscle damage (especially to the myocardium and skeletal muscles); it leaks from muscle into plasma as muscles deteriorate.
- Determining the specific isoenzyme which is high, helps the physician or nurse practitioner determine which tissue has been damaged.
- Used to diagnose acute myocardial infarction, muscular dystrophy, spinal muscular atrophy.

Results

- Normal results vary on the basis of age, gender, and method of testing.
- Increased levels also seen in central nervous system injury, dermatomyositis, Reye syndrome, Rocky Mountain spotted fever, cerebrovascular accidents, seizures, subarachnoid hemorrhage, muscle, and carbon monoxide poisoning.

Nursing Considerations

- Draw sample before electromyography or muscle biopsy, as these tests may lead to release of creatine kinase (CK).
- Strenuous exercise and surgical procedures that damage skeletal muscle may cause increased levels of CK.

CREATININE CLEARANCE

Description and Purpose

- A 24-hour urine collection is evaluated for the presence of creatinine and then compared with the serum creatinine level to determine creatinine clearance.

Results
- Alterations in creatinine clearance may indicate impaired renal function.

Nursing Considerations
- Discard the first void and then begin the 24-hour urine collection.
- Keep the specimen on ice during the collection period.
- Collect *all* urine passed in the 24-hour period.
- Ensure that a venous blood sample is drawn during the 24-hour period.
- The urine specimen should be sent promptly to the laboratory at the end of the 24-hour period.

CULTURE (WOUND, SKIN, OR OTHER DRAINAGE)

Description and Purpose
- Specimen is plated on culture media in the laboratory and evaluated daily for bacterial growth organism identification.

Results
- Specific bacteria will be identified if present.
- Sensitivities to specific antibiotics are usually reported.

Nursing Considerations
- Carefully obtain specimen with a sterile cotton-tipped applicator or culturette, taking care not to contaminate by touching anything other than the specimen fluid.
- Obtain specimen prior to introduction of antibiotic therapy if at all possible.

CYSTOSCOPY

Description and Purpose
- Endoscopic visualization of the urethra and bladder.
- Used to evaluate hematuria and recurrent urinary tract infection.

Results
- May determine the presence of ureteral reflux and abnormality or capacity of the bladder.

Nursing Considerations
- After the procedure:
  - Encourage fluids.
  - Monitor vital signs.

- Child may feel burning with voiding.
- Pink tinge to urine is common.

DYSTROPHIN

Description and Purpose
- A normal intracellular plasma membrane protein in the muscle made by the dystrophin gene.
- Assists in determination of specific type of muscular dystrophy.
- Performed via muscle biopsy or genetic blood test.

Results
- Absence of the protein found in Duchenne muscular dystrophy.
- Deficiency of the protein noted in Becker muscular dystrophy.

Nursing Considerations
- Provide appropriate patient education, support, and resource referral, as diagnosis is a progressive, lifelong disorder.
- Referral to genetic counseling may be appropriate.

ECHOCARDIOGRAM

Description and Purpose
- Noninvasive ultrasound procedure is used to assess heart wall thickness, size of heart chambers, motion of valves and septa, and relationship of great vessels to other cardiac structures.

Results
- Allows for specific diagnosis of structural defects.
- Determines hemodynamics and detects valvular defects.

Nursing Considerations
- Assure the child that the echocardiogram does not hurt.
- Instruct the child about electrocardiogram lead placement and use of gel on the scope's wand during the procedure.
- Encourage the child to lie still throughout the test.

ELECTROCARDIOGRAM (ECG OR EKG)

Description and Purpose
- A graphic record produced by an electrocardiograph (device used to record the electrical activity of the myocardium to detect transmission of the cardiac impulse through the conductive tissues of the muscle).

- Facilitates evaluation of the heart rate, rhythm, conduction, and musculature.

Results
- Detects heart rhythm and chamber overload.
- Also serves as a baseline for measuring postoperative complications.

Nursing Considerations
- Assure the child that monitoring is a painless procedure.
- Place electrodes in the appropriate location.
- The child must lie still during the ECG recording period (usually about 5 minutes).
- Wipe electrode paste or jelly off after procedure.

ELECTROENCEPHALOGRAM (EEG)

Description and Purpose
- Measures and records electrical activity of the brain.
- Used to diagnose epilepsy, investigate seizures, evaluate brain tumors, brain abscesses, subdural hematomas, cerebral infarcts and intracranial hemorrhages, and brain death.

Results
- Normal result shows normal symmetrical patterns of electrical brain activity.

Nursing Considerations
- Keep the child still. If unable to do so, sedation may be necessary but should be avoided if possible because sedatives can alter the **electroencephalogram** (EEG) reading.
- Inform technician of what anticonvulsants the child is taking.
- Hold morning anticonvulsants, if necessary.

ELECTROLYTES AND BLOOD CHEMISTRY

Description and Purpose
- Blood sample to determine serum levels of sodium, potassium, CO_2, chloride, blood urea nitrogen (BUN), and creatinine.
- Many institutions also include glucose and calcium on the basic electrolyte panel.

Results
- Levels may reveal hypernatremia, hyponatremia, hypokalemia, hyperkalemia, hypercalcemia, hypocalcemia, hyperglycemia,

hypoglycemia, acidosis, alkalosis, and renal insufficiency or failure or may indicate dehydration.

Nursing Considerations

- BUN may be elevated with high-protein diet or dehydration and may be decreased with overhydration or malnutrition.
- Creatinine is less affected by high-protein diet, and elevations are more indicative of renal dysfunction.
- Sodium, potassium, chloride, and CO_2 levels can be greatly affected with dehydration.
- Evaluate the child with increased or decreased potassium levels for cardiac arrhythmias. Immediately notify physician or nurse practitioner of critically high potassium levels.
- Avoid prolonged tourniquet use with venipuncture and squeezing with capillary puncture, as hemolysis may occur resulting in falsely elevated potassium or calcium levels.

ELECTROMYOGRAM (EMG)

Description and Purpose

- A recording electrode is placed in the skeletal muscle and electrical activity is recorded.
- Differentiates muscular disorders from those that are neurologic in origin.

Results

- Normal result shows normal electrical activity.

Nursing Considerations

- Requires insertion of short needles into the muscles.
- Sedation or analgesia may be ordered.

LOWER ENDOSCOPY (COLONOSCOPY)

Description and Purpose

- Allows visualization and biopsies of the lower GI tract from the anus to the terminal ileum utilizing a fiberoptic instrument.

Results

- May reveal the presence of tumor or foreign body or determine cause of rectal bleeding or lower abdominal pain.

Nursing Considerations

- The child must undergo a bowel cleansing prior to the examination. Encourage fluids to prevent dehydration.

- Provide conscious (moderate) sedation or postanesthesia care.
- Monitor for possible complications of perforation, bleeding, and increased abdominal pain.

ERYTHROCYTE SEDIMENTATION RATE (ESR)

Description and Purpose
- Nonspecific test used in conjunction with other tests to determine the presence of infection or inflammation.
- Obtained via venipuncture, finger stick, or heel stick.

Results
- Normal value in children is 0 to 10 mm/hour.

Nursing Considerations
- Send to laboratory immediately; specimens allowed to stand for longer than 3 hours may produce a falsely low result.

ESOPHAGEAL PH PROBE

Description and Purpose
- A single- or double-channeled probe is placed into the esophagus to monitor the pH of the contents that are regurgitated into the esophagus from the stomach.
- Used to determine source of vomiting, extent of gastroesophageal reflux, correlation of reflux events and high risk for problems, as in asthma, apparent life-threatening event, sinusitis, or choking/gagging episodes.

Results
- Acidic esophageal events are recorded in relation to their number, frequency, length, and severity over the 24-hour period.

Nursing Considerations
- Avoid antacid and histamine-2 blockers during the test.
- A special diet during the study may be prescribed.
- An accurate diary of symptoms and feedings during the study is essential.
- Assess for nasal irritation/sore throat as they may occur with this test.

FLUORESCENT ANTIBODY TESTING

Description and Purpose
- Nasopharyngeal secretion specimen is used to determine the cause of bronchiolitis.

Results

- May reveal the presence of respiratory syncytial virus, adenovirus, influenza virus, parainfluenza virus, or *Chlamydia*.

Nursing Considerations

- Instill 1 to 3 mL of sterile normal saline into one nostril.
- Aspirate the contents using a small sterile bulb syringe.
- Place the contents in a sterile container and immediately send them to the laboratory.

FLUOROSCOPY

Description and Purpose

- Radiographic examination that uses continuous x-rays to show live up-to-date images.
- Used to assess cervical spine for instability during movement.

Results

- Normal result shows normal bone and supporting tissue structures.

Nursing Considerations

- Children may be afraid.
- Allow a parent or family member to accompany the child.
- If the child is unable or unwilling to stay still for radiography, restraint may be necessary.
- The time of restraint should be limited to the amount of time needed for radiography.
- Child will need to cooperate with flexion and extension of neck.

GENETIC TESTING

Description and Purpose

- Tests for the presence of the gene either for the disease or for carrier status.
- It involves analysis of DNA, RNA, chromosomes, proteins, metabolites, and biochemical agents.
- Determination of disease or carrier status of inherited muscular disorder.
- To detect abnormalities that may indicate actual disease or predict future disease.
- Indicated in the evaluation of congenital anomalies, mental retardation, growth retardation, recurrent miscarriage to determine reason for the loss of a fetus and prenatal diagnosis of genetic disease.

Results
• Normal result shows normal genetic structure.

Nursing Considerations
• Encourage testing of the entire family, even those unaffected, to determine carrier status.
• Provide genetic counseling before and after testing.
• Provide support, information, and resources to family.

GLUCOSE MONITORING

Description and Purpose
• Finger-stick blood sample several times per day is used to monitor serum glucose level and glucose control.

Results
• Normal levels are as follows:
  • Nondiabetics: 70 to 110 mg/dL
  • Toddlers and children with type 1 diabetes mellitus (DM) younger than 6 years old: before meals 100 to 180 mg/dL; at bedtime 110 to 200 mg/dL
  • Children with type 1 DM, aged 6 to 12: before meals 90 to 180 mg/dL; at bedtime 100 to 180 mg/dL
  • Adolescents 13 to 19 years of age: before meals 90 to 130 mg/dL; at bedtime 90 to 150 mg/dL (American Diabetes Association, 2014)
• Target glucose levels will vary on the basis of individual differences.

Nursing Considerations
• Teach family appropriate procedure.
• Provide assessment of technique and education reinforcement at every visit.
• Refer family to sources for equipment and supplies.
• Assist family to develop a system of record keeping that works for them.

GROWTH HORMONE STIMULATION

Description and Purpose
• Stimulates release of GH in response to administration of insulin, arginine, clonidine, or glucagon.
• Used to evaluate and diagnose GH deficiency.

Results
- Normal result: GH levels not increased (no response or inadequate response) during GH stimulation.

Nursing Considerations
- Keep child NPO for specified time.
- Limit stress and physical activity at least 30 minutes before test.
- Obtain serial blood samples at specific times.
- Monitor blood glucose levels during study.
- Observe for signs of hypoglycemia, diaphoresis, and somnolence.
- Provide cookies and juice at end of the test.

HEMOCCULT

Description and Purpose
- Checks for occult blood in the stool.

Results
- May be positive when intestinal bleeding is present with Crohn disease, ulcerative colitis, malabsorption syndromes, diarrhea, or abdominal pain.

Nursing Considerations
- If performed in the laboratory, send a small stool specimen to the laboratory.
- If performed at bedside, apply a thin smear of stool on the paper inside the card windows (from different areas of the stool specimen).
- Wait 3 to 5 minutes and then apply two drops of developer to the paper on the back of the card.
- After 60 seconds, determine whether any trace of blue is present, indicating the presence of occult blood.

HEMOGLOBIN ELECTROPHORESIS

Description and Purpose
- Measures the percentage of normal and abnormal hemoglobin in the blood.

Results
- In the newborn, hemoglobin FA is normal; in the older infant, child, or adolescent, hemoglobin AA is normal.
- Sickle cell disease is indicated by hemoglobin SS; sickle cell trait by hemoglobin SA or AS.

- Evaluation of the globin chains is also reported; various alterations occur with thalassemia.

Nursing Considerations
- Blood transfusions within the previous 12 weeks may alter test results.

HIV ANTIBODIES

Description and Purpose
- Used to detect antibodies to HIV via enzyme-linked immunosorbent assay (ELISA) when HIV infection is suspected.

Results
- May remain negative for several weeks up to 6 months (false-negative).
- False-positive result may be obtained with autoimmune disease.
- Requires serial testing.
- HIV test results are confidential.

Nursing Considerations
- Positive results in the infant of mother with HIV are inconclusive, as maternal antibodies cross the placenta.
- Requires serial testing.
- HIV test results are confidential.

IMMUNOGLOBULIN ELECTROPHORESIS

Description and Purpose
- Determines the level of individual immunoglobulins (IgA, IgD, IgE, IgG, IgM) in the blood.

Results
- Normal levels vary with age.
- Depressed levels of IgG are found in primary immunodeficiency.
- IgE is often elevated in allergic or atopic disease.

Nursing Considerations
- Usually obtained via venipuncture.
- IV immunoglobulin administration and steroids alter levels.

INTRACRANIAL PRESSURE (ICP) MONITORING

Description and Purpose
- A sensing device (intraventricular catheter, subarachnoid screw or bolt, epidural sensor, or anterior fontanel pressure monitor) is placed in the head that monitors the pressure intracranially.

- Used to monitor increased intracranial pressure (ICP) resulting from hydrocephalus, acute head trauma, and brain tumors.
- Ventricular catheter also allows for draining of cerebrospinal fluid (CSF) to help reduce ICP.

Results
- Normal levels of ICP will depend on the age and position of the child during monitoring.

Nursing Considerations
- Usually monitored in critical care setting.
- Monitor for signs and symptoms of increased ICP.
- Monitor for infection.
- Keep head of bed elevated 15 to 30 degrees.
- Keep alarms for monitoring device on at all times.
- Reduce stimulation and avoid interventions that may cause pain or stress and result in an increased ICP.

IRON TESTS

Description and Purpose
- Serum blood test to evaluate iron metabolism (serum iron, total iron binding capacity [TIBC], transferrin, serum ferritin).

Results
- High, low, or normal results of iron, ferritin, TIBC, and transferrin may be reported.
- The combination of these results may lead to various medical diagnoses or occur with certain conditions such as chronic transfusion, hemolytic anemia, or chronic illness.
- Iron deficiency or iron overload may be identified.

Nursing Considerations
- Child should fast for 12 hours before the test.
- Avoid hemolysis (will falsely elevate result).
- Recent blood transfusions increase serum iron and ferritin levels.

JOINT FLUID ASPIRATION (ARTHROCENTESIS)

Description and Purpose
- Aspirated joint fluid is examined for the presence of pus and white blood cells.
- Culture is performed.
- Used to evaluate for septic arthritis.
- May also be used to relieve pressure in the joint space.

Results

- Normal result shows no presence of pus or white blood cells.
- Positive fluid culture indicates a bacterial infection in the joint.

Nursing Considerations

- Use cold therapy to decrease swelling after aspiration.
- Apply pressure dressing to prevent hematoma formation or fluid recollection.
- Assess for fever and joint pain or edema, which may indicate infection.

LEAD LEVEL

Description and Purpose

- Measures level of lead in blood.

Results

- Normal amount of lead in the blood is zero.

Nursing Considerations

- Elevated levels require observation and repeat measurements, as well as parent education related to decreasing lead exposure.
- If significant elevations occur, the child may require treatment of lead poisoning.

LIVER FUNCTION TESTS

Description and Purpose

- Serum blood test that measures enzymes (aspartate aminotransferase/alanine aminotransferase/γ-glutamyltransferase) that have high concentrations in the liver.

Results

- If elevated, it may indicate severity or extent of liver disease.

Nursing Considerations

- May be affected by drugs or viral illnesses.

LUMBAR PUNCTURE

Description and Purpose

- A spinal needle is placed by the physician or nurse practitioner in the subarachnoid space of the spinal column, below the base of the cord, to withdraw CSF for analysis.

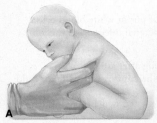
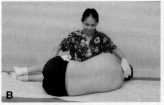

FIGURE 3.2 Proper positioning for a lumbar puncture. **A:** The newborn is positioned upright with head flexed forward. **B:** Child or older infant is positioned on the side with head flexed forward and knees flexed to abdomen.

- Used to measure spinal fluid pressure and to diagnose hemorrhage, infection, obstruction, malignancy, autoimmune disease, and multiple sclerosis.
- May also be used to administer intrathecal medications, in particular chemotherapy.

Results
- Normal CSF is virtually free of cells.
- Normal values vary.
- CSF culture should be negative; growth of organisms indicates infection.

Nursing Considerations
- Use EMLA cream 30 to 60 minutes before the procedure to reduce pain.
- May be performed under conscious (moderate) sedation.
- Position the child appropriately and help the child to remain still (Fig. 3.2).
- Use distraction techniques in the older child or teenager.
- Maintain strict asepsis.
- Assist with collection and transport of specimen.
- Encourage child to stay flat or recline for up to 12 hours after lumbar puncture (per orders).
- Encourage fluids postprocedure if not contraindicated.

LYMPHOCYTE IMMUNOPHENOTYPING T-CELL QUANTIFICATION

Description and Purpose
- Measures level of T cells (T-helper [CD4], T-suppressor [CD8]), B cells, and natural killer cells in the blood for ongoing.

monitoring of progressive depletion of CD4 T lymphocytes in HIV infection.

Results
- Results vary according to progression of disease.
- Generally, lower levels correlate with more severe disease.

Nursing Considerations
- Do not refrigerate the specimen.
- Steroids may elevate and immunosuppressive drugs may depress lymphocyte levels.

MAGNETIC RESONANCE IMAGING (MRI)

Description and Purpose
- Uses behavior of hydrogen atoms in a magnetic field when disturbed by radiofrequency signals to show different tissue compositions, presence of congenital abnormalities, tumors, and inflammation and identify normal versus abnormal organ tissues.
- Does not require ionizing radiation.
- Provides a three-dimensional view of the body part being scanned.
- Can be performed with or without the use of a contrast medium.

Results
- Normal result shows normal bones, joints, organs, nerves, and soft tissue structures.

Nursing Considerations
- Make sure the child does not have any metal devices, internal or external, while undergoing MRI; ensure hospital gown does not have metal snaps.
- Keep the child still during the often-lengthy procedure.
- Work to gain the child's cooperation, which may be difficult. Explain to the child that he or she is placed in a long narrow tube and the machine makes a booming noise during the procedure.
- Allow the child to use approved headphones with preferred music to decrease agitation and fear related to loud noise.
- Sedate the child, if necessary (if the child is unable to remain still).
- Assess for allergy if a contrast medium is used.
- Encourage fluids post procedure if not contraindicated.

MUSCLE BIOPSY

Description and Purpose
- Removal of a piece of muscular tissue either by needle biopsy or by open biopsy.

- Determination of the type of muscular dystrophy or spinal muscular atrophy.

Results
- Normal result shows normal muscle and related tissue anatomy.

Nursing Considerations
- Post biopsy care is similar to that for other types of biopsy.
- Involves a small incision with one or two sutures.

MYELOGRAM

Description and Purpose
- Radiographic study of the spinal cord allowing visualization of the cord, nerve roots, and surrounding meninges.
- This test involves injection of a contrast medium into the CSF via lumbar puncture. The most common contrast used is water-soluble iodine, but there is also an oil and air contrast.
- Used to detect space-occupying lesions of the spinal cord and to visualize neural tube defects.
- Used to evaluate traumatic injury.

Results
- Normal result shows normal lumbar, cervical, or thoracic structures.

Nursing Considerations
- Assess for allergies or sensitivities, especially to latex or iodine, and, if present, inform the radiology department.
- Determine which contrast medium was used, as this will guide postprocedure interventions.
- After the procedure, bed rest is necessary for 4 to 24 hours.
- Keep head of bed elevated for several hours.
- Encourage hydration.
- Observe for signs of meningeal irritation.

NERVE CONDUCTION VELOCITY

Description and Purpose
- Measures the speed of nerve conduction.
- Patch-like electrodes are attached to the skin at various nerve locations.
- Used for differentiation of muscular disorders.

Results
- Normal results vary on the basis of age.
- Decreased speed of nerve conduction indicates nerve disease.

Nursing Considerations
- Explain to the child that the test feels like mild electric shocks.
- Explain that it may be uncomfortable, depending on how strong the impulse is.
- Often followed by an **electromyogram** (EMG).

NEWBORN SCREENING

Description and Purpose
- Blood screening is performed shortly after birth.
- Every US state routinely screens all newborns, but each state dictates which disorders to screen for. Therefore, components of the screening vary from state to state.
- Used to identify many life-threatening genetic illnesses that have no immediate visible effects but can lead to physical problems, intellectual disability, and even death.
- Identification of newborns allows treatment to begin early in order to prevent impact of disorder, such as severe cognitive impairment or death.

Results
- Normal result is a negative newborn screen.

Nursing Considerations
- Refer to each state's protocol for fetal/newborn screening.
- Collect blood sample accurately.
- Collect the blood sample prior to blood transfusion if possible.
- Ideally performed after 24 hours of age.
- Obtain specimen as close to time of discharge from newborn or labor and delivery unit as possible and no later than 7 days of age.
- The test is less accurate if done before 24 hours of age and should be repeated by 2 weeks of age if the newborn is <24 hours old.
- Ensure screening is done for early discharges.
- Screening typically between 24 and 48 hours after birth (March of Dimes, 2015).
- Some states now require a repeat screen at 2 weeks of age.

PEAK EXPIRATORY FLOW

Description and Purpose
- Measures the maximum flow of air (in liters/second) that can be forcefully exhaled in 1 second.
- Daily use can indicate adequacy of asthma control.

Results
- Vary depending upon the child's "personal best" and extent of asthma control or exacerbation.

Nursing Considerations
- It is important to establish the child's "personal best" by taking twice-daily readings over a 2-week period while well. The average of these is termed "personal best."
- Charts based on height and age are also available to determine expected peak expiratory flow.

POLYMERASE CHAIN REACTION (PCR) FOR HIV

Description and Purpose
- A sensitive and specific blood test used to determine the viral load of HIV infection (the amount of HIV RNA and DNA).

Results
- In the noninfected child, the result is negative.
- Low viral loads indicate slow reproduction of the virus.
- High viral loads indicate viral reproduction and predict progression of disease.

Nursing Considerations
- Test of choice for diagnosis of HIV infection in children older than 1 month.
- Poor accuracy on samples obtained at birth.
- Sequential testing is used to determine perinatal transmission.

POSITRON EMISSION TOMOGRAPHY (PET)

Description and Purpose
- Similar to computed tomography (CT) or MRI, but a radioisotope is added.
- Measures physiologic function.
- Provides information on brain functional development.
- Used to assist in identifying seizure foci.
- Used to assess tumors and brain metabolism.

Results
- Normal result shows normal patterns of tissue metabolism and normal blood flow and tissue perfusion.

Nursing Considerations
- Keep the child still during the often-lengthy procedure. If unable to do so, sedation may be necessary.
- IV access will be needed for the procedure.
- Encourage fluids postprocedure, if not contraindicated, to help body eliminate radioisotopes.

POTASSIUM HYDROXIDE (KOH) PREP

Description and Purpose
- Specimen is placed on a microscope slide to determine fungal infection.

Results
- Reveals branching hyphae (fungus) when viewed under a microscope.

Nursing Considerations
- Place skin scrapings or vaginal secretions on a microscope slide and add KOH.

PULMONARY FUNCTION TESTS

Description and Purpose
- Measure respiratory flow and lung volumes.

Results
- Vary depending upon the extent of lung disease present in the child.

Nursing Considerations
- Usually performed by a respiratory therapist trained to do the full spectrum of tests.
- Assist the child to comply with the testing parameters.

PULSE OXIMETRY

Description and Purpose
- Noninvasive method of continuously (or intermittently) measuring oxygen saturation.
- Can be useful in any situation in which a child is experiencing respiratory distress.

Results
- Normal oxygen saturation is generally considered to be ≥94%.

Nursing Considerations
- Probe must be applied correctly to finger, toe, foot, hand, or ear in order for the machine to appropriately pick up the pulse and oxygen saturation.
- Allows evaluation of the child's color and work of breathing first, when the pulse oximeter alarms.

INTRAVENOUS PYELOGRAM

Description and Purpose
- Radiopaque contrast material is injected intravenously and filtered by the kidneys.
- X-rays are obtained at set intervals to show passage of the dye through the kidneys, ureters, and bladder.
- Used to detect urinary outlet obstruction, hematuria, trauma to the renal system, or suspected kidney tumor.

Results
- May show urinary outlet obstruction, trauma to the renal system, tumor, or reason for hematuria.

Nursing Considerations
- Contraindicated in children allergic to shellfish or iodine.
- If the dye infiltrates at the IV site, hyaluronidase may be used to speed absorption of the iodine.
- Ensure adequate hydration before and after the test.
- Some institutions require enema or laxative evacuation of the bowel prior to the study to ensure adequate visualization of the urinary tract.

RADIOALLERGOSORBENT TEST (RAST)

Description and Purpose
- Blood test that is used to diagnose allergies.
- Measures minute quantities of IgE in the blood.

Results
- Presence of immunoglobulin antibodies to particular foods; indicates food allergy.

Nursing Considerations
- Prepare the child for blood sample withdrawal.
- The test is usually sent out to a reference laboratory.

- It carries no risk of anaphylaxis but is not as sensitive as skin testing.

RANDOM SERUM HORMONE LEVELS

Description and Purpose
- Checking serum levels of various hormones.
- Immunoassay measures levels with very small amounts of blood.
- High or low levels are used to evaluate the function of a specific gland.

Results
- Normal results will vary on the basis of hormone tested.

Nursing Considerations
- May need to draw specimens at specific times.
- Keep child NPO after midnight before test if ordered.
- Diurnal variations and episodic secretion of many hormones may require special directions or further testing.

RAPID INFLUENZA TEST

Description and Purpose
- Rapid test for detection of influenza A or B.
- Done within first 24 hours of illness so that medication administration may begin.

Results
- A positive result indicates influenza infection.
- False-negative results are not frequent but may occur.

Nursing Considerations
- Have the child gargle with sterile normal saline and then spit into a sterile container.
- Send immediately to the laboratory.

RAPID STREP TEST

Description and Purpose
- Instant test for the presence of streptococcal A antibody in pharyngeal secretions.

Results

- Available within 5 to 10 minutes; if positive, indicate the presence of streptococcal infection.

Nursing Considerations

- Swab the nasopharynx well with two swabs at once.
- Negative tests should be backed up with throat culture.

RETICULOCYTE COUNT

Description and Purpose

- Measures the amount of reticulocytes (immature RBCs) in the blood, indicating the bone marrow's ability to respond to anemia with production of RBCs.

Results

- May be elevated with bleeding or hemolytic anemia.
- May be decreased with iron deficiency anemia, pernicious anemia, folic acid deficiency, bone marrow failure, or aplastic anemia.

Nursing Considerations

- Rises quickly in response to iron supplementation in the iron-deficient child, so may indicate compliance with therapy (iron and ferritin levels rise more slowly).

RHEUMATOID FACTOR

Description and Purpose

- Determines the presence of rheumatoid factor in the blood.

Results

- Positive in systemic lupus erythematosus and a particular type of juvenile idiopathic arthritis.

Nursing Considerations

- Chronic infectious disorders may also result in a positive rheumatoid factor.

STOOL CULTURE

Description and Purpose

- Stool is smeared on culture medium and assessed for growth of bacteria over a period of days.

- Indicated for children with diarrhea, fever, or abdominal pain to determine bacterial cause of illness.

Results

- Normal stool contains a variety of organisms.
- Pathogenic bacteria more commonly identified include *Escherichia coli* (*E. coli*) 0157:H7, *Campylobacter, Salmonella, Shigella,* and *Yersinia.*

Nursing Considerations

- A small amount of stool is collected.
- Stool must be free of urine, water, and toilet paper.
- Do not retrieve out of toilet water.
- Deliver to laboratory immediately.
- It requires minimum of 48 hours for growth and several days to weeks in some cases.

SINGLE-PHOTON EMISSION COMPUTED TOMOGRAPHY (SPECT)

Description and Purpose

- Use of radiopharmaceuticals to provide three-dimensional splices.
- Less expensive and more available than positron emission tomography.
- Used to detect brain death, presence of encephalitis, hydrocephalus, to localize epileptic foci, assess metabolic activity, evaluate brain tumors, assessment of childhood development disorders.

Results

- Normal result shows normal physiology or function.

Nursing Considerations

- Similar to PET; often combined with CT scan.
- Follow study-specific prep instructions from nuclear medicine department.
- In uncooperative children do not use sedation until after injection because it may affect brain activity.
- Secure child's head.
- Sudden distractions or loud noises can alter the distribution of radionuclide.

STOOL FOR OVA AND PARASITES (O&P)

Description and Purpose

- Checks for the presence of parasites or their eggs in the stool.

- May be ordered in children with diarrhea or continued abdominal pain.

Results
- Presence of parasites or their eggs in the stool indicates infestation.

Nursing Considerations
- Requires about two tablespoons of stool.
- Deliver to laboratory immediately.
- Mineral oil, barium, and bismuth interfere with the detection of parasites; specimen collection should be delayed for 7 to 10 days.
- Often a minimum of three specimens on 3 separate days is required for adequate examination because many parasites and worm eggs are shed intermittently.

SWEAT CHLORIDE TEST

Description and Purpose
- Collection of sweat on filter paper after stimulation of skin with pilocarpine.
- Measures concentration of chloride in the sweat.
- Used to diagnose cystic fibrosis.

Results
- Considered suspicious if the level of chloride in collected sweat is above 50 mEq/L and diagnostic if the level is above 60 mEq/L.

Nursing Considerations
- May be difficult to obtain sweat in a young infant because the young infant does not sweat as readily as the child.

THROAT CULTURE

Description and Purpose
- Tonsillar and posterior pharynx swabbing for bacterial culture (minimum of 24 to 48 hours required for results) in children with pharyngitis, tonsillitis, or fever of unknown origin.
- Most reliable method of detecting group A streptococcal pharyngitis.
- Will also detect *Bordetella pertussis* and *Corynebacterium diphtheriae*.

Results
- Normal result is negative for throat culture, with normal oral flora.
- Positive report indicates the presence of particular bacteria.

Nursing Considerations
- Ensure specimen is of secretions from the pharyngeal and tonsillar areas. Avoid touching the tongue or lips with swab.
- Can be obtained on separate swab at the same time as rapid strep test to decrease trauma to the child (swab both applicators at once).
- Do not perform immediately after the child has had medication or something to eat or drink.
- When performing on young children, have adult hold the child in lap.
- Stabilize the child's head by placing nondominant hand on the child's forehead.

TOXICOLOGY PANEL (BLOOD AND/OR URINE)

Description and Purpose
- Blood or urine sample used to determine the presence of most commonly abused mood-altering medications, as well as commonly ingested drugs.
- Used when drug abuse, overdose, or accidental ingestion is suspected.

Results
- Results should all be negative unless the child was using a prescription or illicit drug or substance.

Nursing Considerations
- Standard toxicology panel varies with the agency.
- Follow agency protocol; it may require special handling or labeling of specimen.
- Blood specimen is best for determining overdose or poisoning.

TUBERCULIN SKIN TEST

Description and Purpose
- Intradermal injection of purified protein derivative, also called the Mantoux test.

Results
- An induration of 5 to 10 mm in certain people (such as those recently immigrated or who have an immunodeficiency) and children younger than 4 years is considered positive.
- An induration of 15 mm in a person of any age is considered positive.

Nursing Considerations
- It must be given intradermally. It is not a valid test if injected incorrectly.

- Clearly document the location of injection and circle the area with a marker.
- Read the result 72 hours later in the hospitalized child.
- In the nonhospitalized child, instruct the parent to return for test reading in 72 hours.

ULTRASOUND

Description and Purpose

- Use of reflected sound waves to locate fluid, allow visualization of organs, presence of cysts or tumors, and the depth and structure within soft tissues.
- Head ultrasound is used to assess intracranial hemorrhage and ventricular size in newborns.
- Abdominal ultrasound is used to assess for pregnancy, origin of abdominal pain, or other suspected abnormalities in the abdomen.
- Renal ultrasound may be warranted in the child with renal dysfunction.
- Contrast is not required.

Results

- Normal result shows normal tissue and fluid, absence of fluid, cysts, and masses.

Nursing Considerations

- Fasting is required prior to abdominal ultrasound, rarely for renal ultrasound, and never for head ultrasound.
- The child should feel no discomfort during the procedure but will need to lie still for about 30 minutes or more.
- Better tolerated by nonsedated children than CT or MRI
- Can be performed portably at bedside

URINALYSIS

Description and Purpose

- Evaluates color, pH, specific gravity, and odor of urine
- Assesses for the presence of protein, glucose, ketones, blood, leukocyte esterase, red and white blood cells, bacteria, crystals, and casts.

Results

- In the child with urinary tract infection, the urinalysis may be positive for blood, nitrites, leukocyte esterase, white blood cells, or bacteria (these are indicators of infection but not diagnostic of infection).

- Blood may be present after accidental trauma, during menstruation, or if catheterization was traumatic.
- Protein and/or blood protein may be present in the child with a renal disorder.
- Transient or orthostatic proteinuria (benign events) may result in elevated protein levels.
- Glucose may be present in the child with diabetes.
- Elevated ketone levels occur with diabetes, high-protein carbohydrate-restricted diets, and malnutrition.

Nursing Considerations

- Obtained via clean-catch voided specimen (into a cup or urine bag), catheterization, or suprapubic tap (in the newborn or very young infant).
- At least 10 mL is preferred.
- Refrigerate specimen if not processed promptly.
- Be aware of the many drugs affecting urine color and notify laboratory if child is taking one.
- Notify laboratory if female is menstruating.

URINE CULTURE AND SENSITIVITY

Description and Purpose

- Urine is plated on culture media in the laboratory and evaluated daily for the presence of bacteria. It is indicated for children with fever of unknown origin, dysuria, frequency or urgency, or if urinalysis suggests infection.

Results

- Normal result is negative.
- Positive results identify the particular bacteria and the colony count.
- A final report is usually issued after 48 to 72 hours.
- Sensitivity testing is performed to determine the best choice of antibiotic.

Nursing Considerations

- Obtain culture specimen before starting antibiotics if at all possible.
- It may be obtained by catheterization, clean-catch specimen, or sterile urine bag (there is a high chance of contamination with this method; catheterization may be preferred).
- In some institutions, the physician or nurse practitioner performs the suprapubic tap in neonates and young infants.
- Avoid contamination with stool, vaginal secretions, hands, or clothing.
- Deliver to laboratory immediately (preferable) or refrigerate.

Atraumatic Care

When examining the genital area or performing urinary catheter-
ization of the young female, allow the girl to sit with her mother
on the examination table to decrease anxiety. Have the girl lie back
on her mother's chest, seated on the table between the mother's legs.
Encourage the mother to console and hug the girl while the invasive
examination or procedure is being performed.

VIDEO ELECTROENCEPHALOGRAM (VIDEO EEG)

Description and Purpose
- Measures electrical activity of the brain continuously along with recorded video of actions and behaviors.
- Can help determine precise localization of seizure area before surgery.
- Assists in diagnosis and management of seizures by correlating behaviors with abnormal EEG activity.

Results
- In seizure monitoring the expected outcome would be at least three typical recorded seizures. This may be different from what the child normally experiences because anticonvulsant medications may have been reduced.

Nursing Considerations
- Ensure that seizure precautions are in place.
- Parent or caregiver must be with the child at all times.
- Child's movements are limited and usually confined to the room.
- When the child changes position, ensure that he or she is still seen by the video camera.
- Boredom can be a problem.
- Must notify nurse if seizure activity occurs; push the alert button to highlight attack on EEG recording.
- If seizure activity occurs, go immediately to the room, expose as much of the child as possible (remove covers; if at night, turn on light), and avoid blocking the camera.
- Ask the child questions (i.e., what is your name, can you raise your left arm, remember the word banana) to help assess responsiveness more accurately.
- Stay with the child until full recovery has occurred.
- Ask the child what word you asked them to remember, and document all findings and time of the event.

VOIDING CYSTOURETHROGRAM

Description and Purpose
- The bladder is filled with contrast material via catheterization.
- Fluoroscopy is performed to demonstrate filling of the bladder and collapsing after emptying.

Results
- May reveal vesicoureteral reflux or structural anomalies.

Nursing Considerations
- Just prior to the test, insert the Foley catheter.
- Ensure that the adolescent female is not pregnant.
- After the test, encourage the child to drink fluids to prevent bacterial accumulation and aid in dye elimination.

WATER DEPRIVATION STUDY

Description and Purpose
- Child is deprived of fluids for several hours, and serum sodium and urine osmolality are monitored.
- Used to diagnose diabetes insipidus and distinguish among the major forms (cranial or nephrogenic).

Results
- Normal results will show decreased urine output, increased urine-specific gravity, and no change in serum sodium.

Nursing Considerations
- Stop test if child exhibits extreme weight loss or changes in vital signs or neurologic status.
- Weigh child before, during, and after the test.
- Rehydrate child after the test.
- Monitor for orthostatic hypotension.

X-RAY STUDIES

Description and Purpose
- Radiographic image without contrast media.
- Usually two views are obtained of the affected extremity or body area being evaluated (lateral and anteroposterior).
- Abdominal radiograph shows a flat (KUB) and upright view.
- To detect bone fracture or anomaly, organ abnormality, or to verify feeding tube, ventricular or central venous catheter placement.

Results
- Normal result shows normal bone and supporting tissue structures, as well as normal organs.
- Abnormal results include fracture, mass, defect, abnormal organ size, increased ventricular size, significant stool or air volume in intestines, pleural effusion, or hyperinflation, atelectasis, pneumonia, or foreign body in the lungs.
- Shows location and course of ventricular catheters and central venous catheters.
- Verifies location of distal end of feeding tube.
- Reveals information about increased ICP and skull defects.

Nursing Considerations
- Children may be afraid. Allow a parent or family member to accompany the child.
- Child must cooperate and hold still. If the child is unable or unwilling to stay still for radiography, restraint may be necessary.
- Limit the time of restraint to the amount of time needed for completion of radiography.
- For the chest x-ray, encourage the child to hold the breath as instructed to allow for radiography of expanded lungs.
- In the trauma victim, keep the cervical spine immobilized until cleared after cervical spine x-ray.

Nursing Procedures

CAPILLARY HEEL PUNCTURE

Purpose
- Used to obtain certain blood specimens such as a complete blood cell count, glucose testing, chemistries, and newborn screen, in neonates and infants younger than 6 months

Steps
1. Choose the collection site: the medial or lateral plantar heel. Avoid the posterior curvature of the heel (Fig. 3.3A).
2. Apply a commercial heel warmer or warm pack for several minutes prior to specimen collection.
3. Assemble equipment:
   - Gloves
   - Automatic lancet
   - Antiseptic wipe

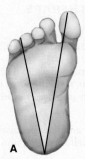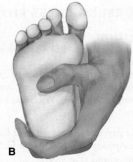

FIGURE 3.3 Capillary heel puncture. **A:** Selecting the medial or lateral plantar heel. **B:** Preparing to pierce the heel with the lancet by securing the dorsum of the foot with the nondominant hand.

- Cotton ball or dry gauze
- Capillary blood collection tube
- Band-aid
4. Don gloves. Remove the warm pack.
5. Cleanse the site with antiseptic prep pad and allow to dry.
6. Hold the dorsum of the foot with the nondominant hand; with the dominant hand, pierce the heel with the lancet (Fig. 3.3B).
7. Wipe away the first drop of blood with the cotton ball or dry gauze.
8. Collect the blood specimen with a capillary specimen collection tube. Avoid squeezing the foot during specimen collection if possible, as it may contribute to hemolysis of the specimen.
9. Hold dry gauze over the site until bleeding stops and then apply a Band-aid.

Nursing Considerations
- Explain procedure to the child and family in a developmentally appropriate manner.
- Do not choose a site that has previously been punctured.
- Do not penetrate deeper than 2 mm. The use of automatic lancet device is recommended.
- Do not perform in infants whose feet are edematous, injured, or infected.
- Provide atraumatic care by swaddling, holding by caregiver if possible, sucking on pacifier, or use of oral sucrose solution.

PERFORMING CHEST PHYSIOTHERAPY

Description

- Chest physiotherapy (CPT) involves percussion, vibration, and postural drainage.
- Physiotherapy may be performed several times daily to mobilize secretions from the lungs in any condition, resulting in an increase in mucous production or decrease in ability to move or expel mucus.

Steps

1. Provide percussion via a cupped hand or an infant percussion device. Appropriate percussion yields a hollow sound, not a slapping sound (Fig. 3.4).

(text continues on page 378)

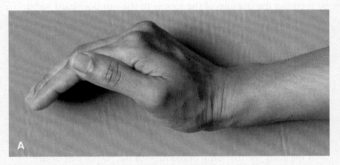

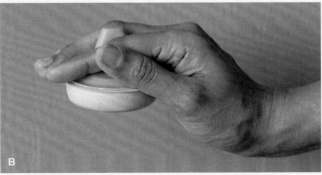

FIGURE 3.4 **Step 1:** Provide percussion via a cupped hand (**A**) or an infant percussion device (**B**). Appropriate percussion yields a hollow sound, not a slapping sound.

2. Percuss each segment of the lung for 1 to 2 minutes (Fig. 3.5).

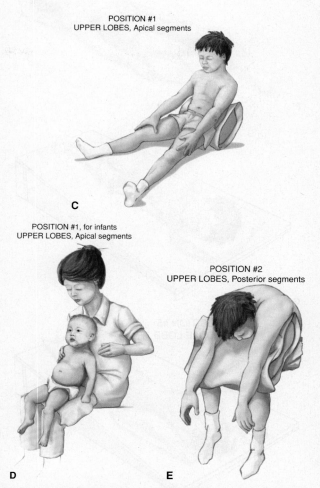

FIGURE 3.5 **Step 2:** Percuss each segment of the lung for 1 to 2 minutes: **C:** Position 1, upper lobes, apical segments. **D:** Position 1, for infants, upper lobes, apical segments. **E:** Position 2, upper lobes, posterior segments.

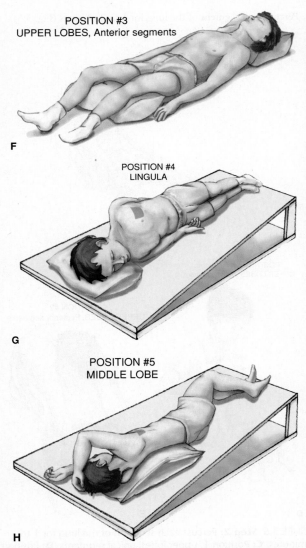

FIGURE 3.5 (*Continued*) **F:** Position 3, upper lobes, anterior segments. **G:** Position 4, lingual. **H:** Position 5, middle lobe.

POSITION #6
LOWER LOBES, Anterior basal segments

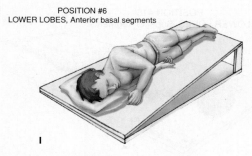

I

POSITION #7
LOWER LOBES, Posterior basal segments

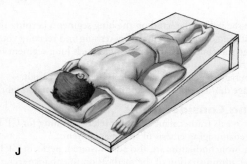

J

POSITION #8 & 9
LOWER LOBES, Lateral basal segments

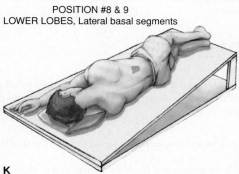

K

FIGURE 3.5 *(Continued)* **I:** Position 6, lower lobes, anterior basal segments. **J:** Position 7, lower lobes, posterior basal segments. **K:** Positions 8 and 9, lower lobes, lateral basal segments.

POSITION #10
LOWER LOBES, Superior segments

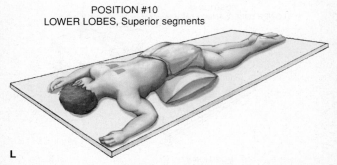

L

FIGURE 3.5 (*Continued*) **L:** Position 10, lower lobes, superior segments.

3. Place the ball of the hand on the lung segment, keeping the arm and shoulder straight. Vibrate by tensing and relaxing your arms during the child's exhalation. Vibrate each lung segment for at least five exhalations.
4. Encourage the child to take a deep breath and cough.
5. Change drainage positions and repeat percussion and vibration.

Nursing Considerations
- Before meals (rather than after) is preferred timing for CPT to avoid encouraging emesis of stomach contents.
- When bronchodilators are also administered, perform CPT during or after administration of the medication to enhance secretion mobilization.

DOUBLE DIAPERING

Purpose
- Double diapering is a method used to protect the urethra and stent or catheter after surgery, keeping the area clean and free from infection.

Steps
1. Cut a hole or a cross-shaped slit in the front of the smaller diaper (Fig. 3.6A).
2. Unfold both diapers and place the smaller diaper (with the hole) inside the larger one (Fig. 3.6B).
3. Place both diapers under the child.
4. Carefully bring the penis (if applicable) and catheter/stent through the hole in the smaller diaper and close the diaper (Fig. 3.6C).

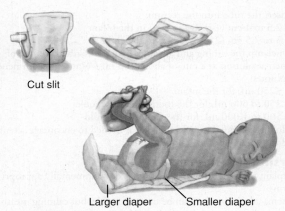

Cut slit

Larger diaper   Smaller diaper

FIGURE 3.6 Double diapering.

5. Close the larger diaper, making sure the tip of the catheter/stent is inside the larger diaper.

Nursing Considerations

- The inner diaper contains stool and the outer diaper contains urine, allowing separation between the bowel and bladder output.
- Change the outside (larger) diaper when the child is wet; change both diapers when the child has a bowel movement.

Adapted from Mount Nittany Medical Center. (2013). *When your son needs surgery for hypospadias.* Retrieved October 8, 2015, from http://www.mountnittany.org/articles/healthsheets/11970

ADMINISTERING AN ENEMA

Purpose
- Used to evacuate the colon of accumulated or impacted stool.

Steps
1. Gather supplies (enema bag, lubricant, enema solution).
2. Wash hands and put on gloves.
3. Position the child:
   - Infant or toddler on abdomen with knees bent
   - Child or adolescent on left side with right leg flexed toward chest
4. Clamp the enema tubing, remove the cap, and apply lubricant to the tip.

5. Insert the tube into the rectum:
   - 2.5 to 4 cm (1 to 1.5 inches) in the infant
   - 5 to 7.5 cm (2 to 3 inches) in the child
6. Unclamp the tubing and administer the prescribed volume of enema solution at a rate of about 100 mL/minute. Recommended volumes:
   - ≤250 mL for the infant
   - 250 to 500 mL for the toddler or preschooler
   - 500 to 1,000 mL for the school-aged child
7. Hold the child's buttocks together if needed to encourage retention of the enema for 5 to 10 minutes.

Nursing Considerations
- Explain the procedure to the child in developmentally appropriate terms.
- Enema administration can be uncomfortable, but calming measures, such as distraction and praise, provide a comforting environment.
- If multiple enemas are required for bowel cleansing, monitor for signs of electrolyte imbalance.
- After the impaction is removed, promote regular bowel habits to keep the impaction from recurring.

USING THE EPIPEN® OR EPIPEN Jr®

Purpose
- The EpiPen® or EpiPen Jr® is a single-dose injection pen of epinephrine that the allergic child who tends toward anaphylaxis (or his parent) carries at all times.
- It is used when the child is suspected to have come into contact with the critical allergen.

Steps
1. Grasp the EpiPen® or EpiPen Jr® with the black tip pointing downward, forming a fist (Fig. 3.7A).
2. With the other hand, pull off the gray safety release.
3. Swing and jab the EpiPen® firmly into the outer thigh at a 90-degree angle and hold firmly there for 10 seconds (Figs. 3.7B and 3.7C).
4. Remove the EpiPen® and massage the thigh for 10 seconds.

Nursing Considerations
- The child should carry the pen with him or her at all times.
- Explain to the child and family that the gray safety release on the EpiPen® should never be removed until just before use.

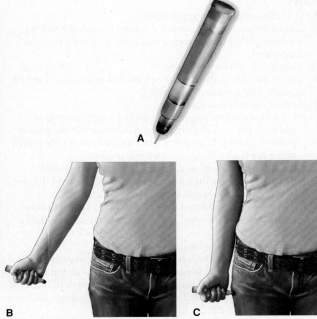

FIGURE 3.7 Using the EpiPen® or EpiPen Jr® (see steps).

- In addition, teach the child and family that the thumb, fingers, or hand should not be placed over the black tip.
- Instruct the child and family to call 911 and seek immediate medical attention after using the EpiPen®.
- Warn the child that the epinephrine may make him or her feel as if the heart is racing.

Adapted from Mylan Specialty. (2015). *How to use your EpiPen® (epinephrine injection) autoinjector.* Retrieved October 8, 2015, from https://www.epipen.com/about-epipen/how-to-use-epipen.

INSERTING A GAVAGE FEEDING TUBE

Purpose
- To provide a means for delivering nutrition to the child's functioning GI tract.

Steps

1. Verify the order for gavage feeding.
2. Gather the necessary equipment; remove formula for feeding from refrigerator if appropriate and allow it to come to room temperature.
3. Wash hands and put on gloves.
4. Inspect the child's nose and mouth for deformities that may interfere with passage of the tube.
5. Position the infant or child.
   • Position the infant supine with the head slightly elevated and with the neck slightly hyperextended so that the nose is pointed upward. If necessary, place a rolled towel or blanket under the neck to help maintain this position.
   • Assist the older child to a sitting position if appropriate.
   • Alternatively, have the parent or another person hold the child to promote comfort and reassurance.
   • Enlist the aid of additional people, such as a parent or other healthcare team member, to assist in maintaining the child's position.
6. Determine the tubing length for insertion.
   • For neonates (up to 2 weeks of age), children with short stature, or if unable to obtain an accurate height, use traditional morphologic methods to determine tubing length (Cincinnati Children's Hospital Medical Center, 2011; National Guideline Clearinghouse, 2012).
     • Measure from the tip of the nose to the earlobe to the middle of the area between the xiphoid process and umbilicus (Fig. 3.8).
     • Mark this measurement on the tube with an indelible pen or with a piece of tape.
   • According to the Agency for Healthcare Research and Quality's National Guideline Clearinghouse (2012), determining tubing length for insertion of a nasogastric tube using age-related height-based methods versus traditional morphologic, nose–ear–mid-xiphoid–umbilicus is more accurate for children greater than 2 weeks (National Guideline Clearinghouse, 2012). Refer to Table 3.2.
7. Lubricate the tube with a generous amount of sterile water or water-soluble lubricant to promote passage of the tube and minimize trauma to the child's mucosa.
8. Insert the tube into one of the nares or the mouth. Direct a nasally inserted tube straight back toward the occiput; direct an orally inserted tube toward the back of the throat.

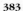

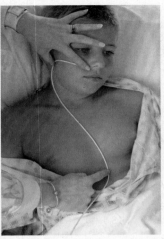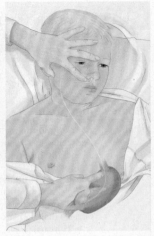

FIGURE 3.8 Traditional morphologic methods to determine gavage tubing length prior to insertion.

9. Advance the tube slowly to the designated length; encourage the child (if capable) to swallow frequently to assist with advancing the tube.
10. Watch for signs of distress, such as gasping, coughing, or cyanosis, indicating that the tube is in the airway. If these signs develop, withdraw the tube and allow the child to rest before attempting reinsertion.
11. Temporarily secure tube, remove stylet if applicable, and check for proper placement of the tube. Refer to Box 3.1.
12. Document the type of tube inserted, the length of tubing inserted, measurement of external tubing length, from nares to end of the tube, after insertion, and confirmation of placement.
13. If tubing is to remain in place, secure to child's cheek.

Nursing Considerations

• Explain the procedure to the child and parents using appropriate language geared to the child's development level. Assess for proper understanding.
• Provide an opportunity for therapeutic play for preparation for procedure and coping after the procedure. Enlist assistance from a child life specialist.

TABLE 3.2	AGE-RELATED HEIGHT-BASED (ARHB) EQUATIONS FOR PREDICTING OG/NG TUBE INSERTION LENGTHS	
Route	Age Group	Predicted Internal Distance to the Body of the Stomach Determined by:
Oral	Age ≤28 months	$16.6 + 0.183$ (height cm)
	Between ages 28 months and 100 months (8 years 4 months)	$20.1 + 0.183$ (height cm)
	Between ages 100 months (8 years 4 months) and 121 months (~10 years)	$17 + 0.218$ (height cm)
	Greater than 121 months (~10 years)	$18.5 + 0.218$ (height cm)
Nasal	Age <28 months	$17.6 + 0.197$ (height cm)
	Between ages 28 months and 100 months (8 years 4 months)	$21.1 + 0.197$ (height cm)
	Between ages 100 months (8 years 4 months) and 121 months (~10 years)	$18.7 + 0.218$ (height cm)
	Greater than 121 months (~10 years)	$21.2 + 0.218$ (height cm)

Adapted from Cincinnati Children's Hospital Medical Center (2011). *Best evidence statement (BESt). Confirmation of nasogastric/orogastric tube (NGT/OGT) placement.* Cincinnati, OH: Cincinnati Children's Hospital Medical Center. Retrieved on October 8, 2015, from http://www.cincinnatichildrens.org/assets/0/78/ 1067/2709/2777/2793/9198/ad67ab29-2a71-42a4-b78e-3d0e9710adac.pdf

- Use distraction techniques, such as relaxation and breathing, during the procedure.
- Once tube is placed, check for tube placement before every use and at least every shift. Be cautious and proactive if you have any suspicion that the tube is misplaced.
- Ensure the tube is properly secured to prevent the child from pulling it out, on purpose or inadvertently.
- Assess cheek where the tube is secured for signs of skin irritation or breakdown.

(text continues on page 386)

BOX 3.1

METHODS FOR VERIFICATION OF FEEDING TUBE PLACEMENT[a]

- Obtain radiographic confirmation of proper tube placement in children who are considered high risk for aspiration, such as children with neurologic impairment, children obtunded, sedated, unconscious, critically ill, reduced gag reflex or static encephalopathy, or when nonradiologic methods are not feasible or beside results are conflicting.
- Nonradiologic verification is used in children who are not considered high risk for aspiration, document pH of aspirate; document insertion distance and external length of tube in the chart. Mark and document the tube's exit site from the nose or mouth.
- Use bedside techniques at regular intervals to determine proper tube positioning.
- Measure pH.
  - Gastric secretions have a pH value of <5.
  - Small intestine secretions will usually have a pH value of >6, but this does not reliably predict proper tube placement.
  - A pH value of >6 can occur with respiratory or esophageal placement, with proper tube placement (gastric or intestinal) when feedings are given continuously, or if the child is receiving acid-inhibiting medications.
  - Therefore, if the pH is >5, additional assessment is warranted.
- Observe appearance of fluid aspirated from the tube (can be used in conjunction with pH testing but is not a reliable single verification method).
  - Gastric secretions are usually grassy green or clear and colorless and can have off-white or tan mucus shreds. It may also be brown-tinged if blood is present.
  - Intestinal secretions are often bile stained, light golden yellow to brownish green. They tend to be thicker and more translucent than gastric secretions.
  - Respiratory secretions can be white, yellow, straw colored, or clear.
- Instill air into the tube and then auscultate for the sound (gastric auscultation) (can be used in conjunction with other assessment methods).
- Check external markings on tube and external tube length (tube remaining from nares to the end of tube) to determine whether the tube seems to have migrated or been misplaced.

(continued on page 386)

METHODS FOR VERIFICATION OF FEEDING TUBE PLACEMENT *continued*

- Continually assess for signs indicative of feeding tube misplacement, such as unexplained gagging, vomiting, or coughing; signs and symptoms of respiratory distress; and decreased oxygen saturations.
- Review routine chest and abdominal radiographs (if obtained) to double check correct tube position.

[a]Always follow agency policy and procedures.
Adapted from Cincinnati Children's Hospital Medical Center. (2011). *Best evidence statement (BESt). Confirmation of nasogastric/orogastric tube (NGT/OGT) placement.* Cincinnati, OH: Cincinnati Children's Hospital Medical Center. Retrieved on October 8, 2015, from http://www.cincinnatichildrens.org/assets/0/78/1067/2709/2777/2793/9198/ad67ab29-2a71-42a4-b78e-3d0e9710adac.pdf

---

- Monitor intake and output closely.
- For nasogastric tubes, remove and replace in other nostril per institutional policy.
- Assess nares for skin breakdown or irritation.
- Irrigate with water per order.

NASOPHARYNGEAL OR ARTIFICIAL AIRWAY SUCTION TECHNIQUE

Description
- Suctioning manually removes secretions from the nasopharyngeal or artificial airway.
- It may be necessary in any child with airway secretions who exhibits noisy breathing and/or respiratory distress.
- Airway clearance is critical in the child with respiratory illness.

Steps
1. Make sure the suction equipment works properly before starting.
2. After washing your hands, assemble the equipment needed:
    - Appropriate-size sterile suction catheter
    - Sterile gloves
    - Supplemental oxygen
    - Sterile water-based lubricant
    - Sterile normal saline if indicated
3. Don sterile gloves, keeping dominant hand sterile and nondominant hand clean.
4. Preoxygenate the infant or child if indicated.
5. Apply lubricant to the end of the suction catheter.

6. If indicated for loosening of secretions, instill sterile saline.
7. Maintaining sterile technique, insert the suction catheter into the child's nostril or airway.
   • Insert only to the point of gagging if inserting via the nostril.
   • Insert only 0.5 cm further than the length of the artificial airway.
8. Intermittently apply suction for no longer than 10 seconds while twisting and removing the catheter.
   • Adjust the pressure range between 60 and 100 mm Hg for suctioning infants and children.
   • Use the pressure range between 40 and 60 mm Hg for suctioning premature infants.
9. Supplement with oxygen after suctioning.

PERFORMING ORTOLANI AND BARLOW MANEUVERS

Purpose
• To detect congenital developmental dysplasia of the hip.

Steps

Ortolani Maneuver
1. Place the newborn in the supine position and flex the hips and knees to 90 degrees at the hip.
2. Grasp the inner aspect of the thighs and abduct the hips (usually to ~180 degrees) while applying upward pressure (Fig. 3.9).

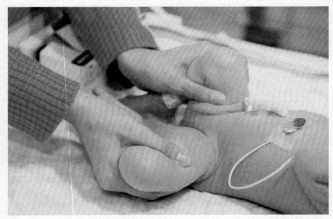

FIGURE 3.9 Ortolani maneuver.

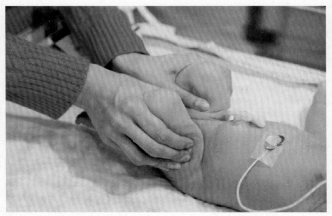

FIGURE 3.10 Barlow maneuver.

3. Listen for any sounds during the maneuver. There should be no "cluck" heard or felt when the legs are abducted. Such a sound indicates the femoral head hitting the acetabulum as the femoral head reenters the area. This suggests developmental hip dysplasia.

Barlow Maneuver

1. With the newborn still lying supine and grasping the inner aspect of the thighs (as just mentioned), adduct the thighs while applying outward and downward pressure to the thighs (Fig. 3.10).
2. Feel for the femoral head slipping out of the acetabulum; also listen and feel for a "clunk."

> **Take Note!**
> A higher-pitched "click" may occur with flexion or extension of the hip. When assessing for DDH, do not confuse this benign, adventitial sound with a true "clunk."

Nursing Considerations

- Earlier recognition of hip dysplasia with earlier harness use results in better correction of the anomaly.
- Excellent assessment skills and reporting of any abnormal findings are critical.

PERFORMING OSTOMY CARE

Description
- Ostomy care for a child can be challenging due to the child's normal growth and development as well as activity.
- Empty the ostomy pouch and measure for stool output several times per day.
- If stool is liquid, it may cause irritation and severe burn-like areas on the surrounding skin, so special attention to skin care around the ostomy site is essential.
- The ostomy pouch should be changed every 1 to 4 days.

Steps
1. Set up the equipment:
   - Warm, wet washcloths or paper towels
   - Clean pouch and clamp
   - Skin barrier powder, paste, and/or sealant
   - Pencil or pen
   - Scissors
   - Pattern to measure stoma size
2. Take off the pouch (may need to use adhesive remover or wet washcloth to ease pouch removal).
3. Observe the stoma and surrounding skin. Clean the stoma and skin as needed, allowing it to dry thoroughly.
4. Measure the stoma, mark the new pouch backing, and cut the new backing to size.
5. Apply the new pouch.

Adapted from University of California, San Francisco. (2015). *Colostomy.* Retrieved October 8, 2015 from http://pedsurg.ucsf.edu/conditions–procedures/colostomy.aspx.

Nursing Considerations
- Ensure proper fit of the ostomy appliance/pouch to avoid acidic stool contact with skin.
- Products such as powders and pastes are available to help protect the skin.
- To avoid repeated pulling of adhesive tape from skin, use a barrier wafer (e.g., Stomahesive® or Duoderm®) to attach the appliance.
- Immediately notify the physician or nurse practitioner if the stoma is not moist and pink or red, if the volume of stool output is greatly increased, or if the stoma is prolapsed or retracted.
- Consult enterostomal therapy nurse as needed.
- Perform ostomy care as needed; pouches usually need to be changed every 1 to 4 days.

ADMINISTERING MEDICATION VIA A SYRINGE PUMP

Purpose
• To provide accurate and safe administration of IV medication (Fig. 3.11)

Steps
1. Verify the medication order.
2. Gather the medication and necessary equipment and supplies.
3. Wash hands and put on gloves.
4. Attach the syringe pump tubing to the medication syringe and purge air from the tubing by gently filling the tubing with medication from the syringe.
5. Insert the syringe into the pump according to the manufacturer's directions.
6. Clean the appropriate port on the child's IV access device or tubing, flush the device or tubing if appropriate (e.g., an intermittent infusion device [saline lock or heparin lock]), and attach the syringe tubing to the IV tubing or device.
7. Set the infusion rate on the pump as ordered.

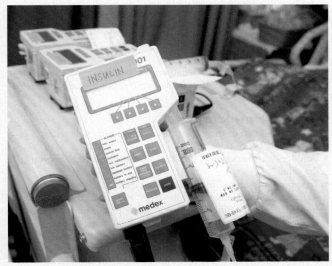

FIGURE 3.11 Syringe pump.

8. When the medication infusion is completed, flush the syringe pump tubing to deliver any medication remaining in the tubing according to institution protocol.
9. Document the procedure and the child's response to it.

Nursing Considerations

- Explain procedure to the child and family in a developmentally appropriate manner.
- If IV fluids or other medications are also infusing, assess for compatibility.
- Assess syringe tubing for date. Change tubing per institution protocol if needed.
- Ensure battery of the pump is functioning properly if unplugged.

Adapted from Bowden, V. R., & Greenberg, C. S. (2012). *Pediatric nursing procedures* (3rd ed). Philadelphia, PA: Lippincott Williams & Wilkins.

TRACHEOSTOMY CARE

Description

- Cleansing of the tracheostomy insertion site and changing of the tracheostomy tube are important for maintaining skin integrity.
- Secretions from the tracheostomy and saliva from the child's mouth tend to pool in the neck area, leading to skin breakdown.
- Perform tracheostomy care every 8 hours and as needed or according to institution protocol.

Steps

1. Gather the necessary equipment:
   - Cleaning solution
   - Gloves
   - Precut gauze pad
   - Cotton-tipped applicators
   - Clean tracheostomy ties
   - Scissors
   - Extra tracheostomy tube in case of accidental dislodgement
2. Position the infant/child supine with a blanket or towel roll to extend the neck.
3. Open all packaging and cut tracheostomy ties to appropriate length if necessary.
4. Cleanse around the tracheostomy site with prescribed solution (half-strength hydrogen peroxide or acetic acid, or normal saline; teach parents to use soap and water at home) and cotton-tipped applicators, working from just around the tracheostomy tube outward.

5. Rinse with sterile water and cotton-tipped applicator in similar fashion.
6. Place the precut sterile gauze under the tracheostomy tube.
7. With the assistant holding the tube in place, cut the ties and remove from the tube.
8. Attach the clean ties to the tube and tie or secure in place with Velcro.

Nursing Considerations

- Always keep additional tracheostomy ties and an additional tracheostomy tube at the child's bedside in case of an emergency.
- Attempt to keep the tracheostomy site area and neck free from secretions in between tracheostomy care sessions to decrease skin integrity impairment.

APPLYING THE URINE BAG

Purpose

- A urine bag may be used for collection of urine specimens in infants and toddlers who are not yet toilet trained.
- A sterile urine bag is required for a urine culture and a clean bag for routine urinalysis. A 24-hour urine collection bag is also available.

Steps

1. Cleanse the perineal area well and pat dry (Fig. 3.12A). If a culture is to be obtained, cleanse the genital area with povidone–iodine (Betadine) or per institutional protocol.
2. Apply benzoin around the scrotum or the vulvar area to aid with urine bag adhesion.
3. Allow the benzoin to dry.
4. Apply the urine bag.
   - For boys: Ensure that the penis is fully inside the bag; a portion of the scrotum may or may not be inside the bag, depending upon scrotal size.
   - For girls: Apply the narrow portion of the bag on the perineal space between the anal and vulvar areas first for best adhesion and then spread the remaining adhesive section (Fig. 3.12B).
5. Tuck the bag downward inside the diaper to discourage leaking.
6. Check the bag frequently for urine (Fig. 3.12C).

Nursing Considerations

- When possible, the urine bag collection method should be used as a method of less traumatic urine collection (as compared with catheterization).
- Appropriate cleansing is critical when a urine culture is needed.

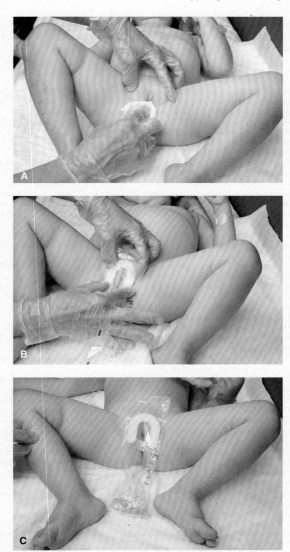

FIGURE 3.12 Applying the urine bag. **A:** Cleansing the perineal area. **B:** Spreading adhesive section over perineal space. **C:** Checking the bag for urine.

• Frequent checking of the bag is absolutely necessary to increase chances of successful collection of the specimen, rather than leakage of urine, which results in dislodging of the bag.

REFERENCES

Abdallah, H. (2015). *About the children's heart institute*. Retrieved October 8, 2015, from http://www.childrenheartinstitute.org/testing/testhome.htm.

American Academy of Pediatrics, Committee on Pediatric Emergency Medicine, & Committee on Bioethics. (2011). Consent for emergency medical services for children and adolescents. *Pediatrics, 128*(2), 427–433.

American Diabetes Association. (2014). Standards of medical care in diabetes—2014. *Diabetes Care, 37*(suppl 1), S14–S80.

Bowden, V. R., & Greenberg, C. S. (2012). *Pediatric nursing procedures* (3rd ed.). Philadelphia, PA: Lippincott Williams & Wilkins.

Centers for Disease Control and Prevention. (2015). *Newborn screening: importance of newborn screening*. Retrieved on October 8, 2015, from http://www.cdc.gov/ncbddd/newbornscreening/

Cincinnati Children's. (2015). *Enema administration*. Retrieved October 8, 2015, from http://www.cincinnatichildrens.org/health/e/enema/.

Cincinnati Children's Hospital Medical Center. (2011). *Best evidence statement (BESt). Confirmation of nasogastric/orogastric tube (NGT/OGT) placement*. Cincinnati, OH: Cincinnati Children's Hospital Medical Center. Retrieved on October 8, 2015, from http://www.cincinnatichildrens.org/assets/0/78/1067/2709/2777/2793/9198/ad67ab29-2a71-42a4-b78e-3d0e9710adac.pdf

Deutsch, E. S. (2010). Tracheostomy: Pediatric considerations. *Respiratory Care, 55*(8), 1082–1090.

Dowshen, S. (2014). *Stool tests*. Retrieved October 8, 2015, from http://www.kidshealth.org/parent/general/sick/labtest8.html

Fischbach, F. T., & Dunning III, M. B. (2015). *A manual of laboratory and diagnostic tests* (9th ed.). Philadelphia, PA: Wolters Kluwer Health/Lippincott Williams & Wilkins.

Florida Children's Hospital, Child Life Department. (n.d.). *Suggested vocabulary to use with children*. Orlando, FL: Author.

Fouzas, S., Priftis, K. N., & Anthracopoulos, M. B. (2011). Pulse oximetry in pediatric practice. *Pediatrics, 128*, 740–752.

March of Dimes. (2015). *Newborn screening*. Retrieved October 8, 2015, from http://www.marchofdimes.org/baby/newborn-screening-tests-for-your-baby.aspx

Morrow, B. M., & Argent, A. C. (2008). A comprehensive review of pediatric endotracheal suctioning: Effects, indications, and clinical practice. *Pediatric Critical Care Medicine, 9*(5), 465–477.

Mount Nittany Medical Center. (2013). *When your son needs surgery for hypospadias*. Retrieved October 8, 2015, from http://www.mountnittany.org/articles/healthsheets/11970

Mylan Specialty. (2015). *How to use your EpiPen® (epinephrine injection) autoinjector*. Retrieved October 8, 2015, from https://www.epipen.com/about-epipen/how-to-use-epipen.

National Asthma Education and Prevention Program. (2007). *Expert panel report 3: Guidelines for the diagnosis and management of asthma* (NIH Publication No. 07–4051). Bethesda, MD: National Institutes of Health, National Heart, Lung and Blood Institute.

National Guideline Clearinghouse. (2012). *Best evidence statement (BESt). Confirmation of nasogastric tube placement in pediatric patients*. Retrieved October 8, 2015, from http://www.guideline.gov/content.aspx?id=35117

Pickering, L. K. (Ed.). (2012). *Red book: 2012 report of the committee on infectious diseases* (29th ed.). Elk Grove Village, IL: American Academy of Pediatrics.

Schechter, M. S. (2007). Airway clearance applications in infants and children. *Respiratory Care, 52*(10), 1382–1391.

Sheth, K. (2015). *Nerve conduction velocity.* Retrieved October 8, 2015 from http://www.nlm.nih.gov/medlineplus/ency/article/003927.htm

University of California, San Francisco. (2015). *Colostomy.* Retrieved October 8, 2015 from http://pedsurg.ucsf.edu/conditions–procedures/colostomy.aspx

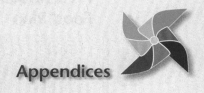

Appendices

Appendix A Healthy Eating for Preschoolers Daily Food Plan

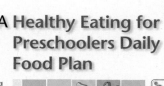

Healthy Eating for preschoolers — Daily Food Plan

Use this Plan as a general guide.

- These food plans are based on average needs. Do not be concerned if your child does not eat the exact amounts suggested. Your child may need more or less than average. For example, food needs increase during growth spurts.
- Children's appetites vary from day to day. Some days they may eat less than these amounts; other days they may want more. Offer these amounts and let your child decide how much to eat.

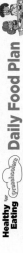

Food group	2 year olds	3 year olds	4 and 5 year olds	What counts as:
Fruits	1 cup	1 - 1½ cups	1 - 1½ cups	**½ cup of fruit?** ½ cup mashed, sliced, or chopped fruit ½ cup 100% fruit juice ½ medium banana 4-5 large strawberries
Vegetables	1 cup	1½ cups	1½ - 2 cups	**½ cup of veggies?** ½ cup mashed, sliced, or chopped vegetables 1 cup raw leafy greens ½ cup vegetable juice 1 small ear of corn
Grains Make half your grains whole	3 ounces	4 - 5 ounces	4 - 5 ounces	**1 ounce of grains?** 1 slice bread 1 cup ready-to-eat cereal flakes ½ cup cooked rice or pasta 1 tortilla (6" across)
Protein Foods	2 ounces	3 - 4 ounces	3 - 5 ounces	**1 ounce of protein foods?** 1 ounce cooked meat, poultry, or seafood 1 egg 1 Tablespoon peanut butter ¼ cup cooked beans or peas (kidney, pinto, lentils)
Dairy Choose low-fat or fat-free	2 cups	2 cups	2½ cups	**½ cup of dairy?** ½ cup milk 4 ounces yogurt ¾ ounce cheese 1 string cheese

Some foods are easy for your child to choke on while eating. Stay back, watch, and offer foods, such as popcorn, nuts, seeds, and hard candy. Cut up foods such as hot dogs, grapes, and carrots into pieces smaller than the size of your child's throat—about the size of a nickel.

There are many ways to divide the Daily Food Plan into meals and snacks. View the "Meal and Snack Patterns and Ideas" to see how these amounts might look on your preschooler's plate at www.choosemyplate.gov/preschoolers.html

Healthy Eating for preschoolers

Get your child on the path to healthy eating.

Focus on the meal and each other. Your child learns by watching you. Children are likely to copy your table manners, your likes and dislikes, and your willingness to try new foods.

Offer a variety of healthy foods. Let your child choose how much to eat. Children are more likely to enjoy a food when eating it is their own choice.

Be patient with your child. Sometimes new foods take time. Give children a taste at first and be patient with them. Offer new foods many times.

Let your children serve themselves. Teach your children to take small amounts at first. Let them know they can get more if they are still hungry.

Cook together.
Eat together.
Talk together.
Make meal time family time.

ChooseMyPlate.gov

FNS-457
October 2012
USDA is an equal opportunity provider and employer.

Source: U.S. Department of Agriculture Food and Nutrition Service. (2012). *Healthy eating for preschoolers*. Retrieved October 6, 2015 from http://www.choosemyplate.gov/sites/default/files/audiences/HealthyEatingForPreschoolers-MiniPoster.pdf

Appendix B MyPlate

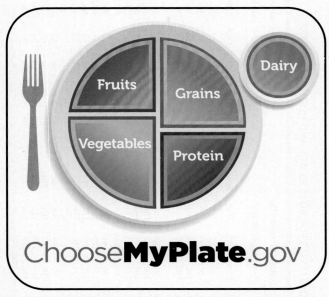

Choose**MyPlate**.gov

From United States Department of Agriculture, ChooseMyPlate.gov; retrieved from http://www.choosemyplate.gov/print-materials-ordering/graphic-resources.html

Appendix C Blood Pressure Charts

TABLE B.1 BLOOD PRESSURE LEVELS FOR BOYS BY AGE AND HEIGHT PERCENTILE

Age (Year)	BP Percentile →	Systolic BP (mm Hg) ← Percentile of Height →							Diastolic BP (mm Hg) ← Percentile of Height →						
		5th	10th	25th	50th	75th	90th	95th	5th	10th	25th	50th	75th	90th	95th
1	50th	80	81	83	85	87	88	89	34	35	36	37	38	39	39
	90th	94	95	97	99	100	102	103	49	50	51	52	53	53	54
	95th	98	99	101	103	104	106	106	54	54	55	56	57	58	58
	99th	105	106	108	110	112	113	114	61	62	63	64	65	66	66
2	50th	84	85	87	88	90	92	92	39	40	41	42	43	44	44
	90th	97	99	100	102	104	105	106	54	55	56	57	58	58	59
	95th	101	102	104	106	108	109	110	59	59	60	61	62	63	63
	99th	109	110	111	113	115	117	117	66	67	68	69	70	71	71
3	50th	86	87	89	91	93	94	95	44	44	45	46	47	48	48
	90th	100	101	103	105	107	108	109	59	59	60	61	62	63	63
	95th	104	105	107	109	110	112	113	63	63	64	65	66	67	67
	99th	111	112	114	116	118	119	120	71	71	72	73	74	75	75
4	50th	88	89	91	93	95	96	97	47	48	49	50	51	51	52
	90th	102	103	105	107	109	110	111	62	63	64	65	66	66	67
	95th	106	107	109	111	112	114	115	66	67	68	69	70	71	71
	99th	113	114	116	118	120	121	122	74	75	76	77	78	78	79

Age															
5	50th	90	91	93	95	96	98	98	50	51	52	53	54	55	55
	90th	104	105	106	108	110	111	112	65	66	67	68	69	69	70
	95th	108	109	110	112	114	115	116	69	70	71	72	73	74	74
	99th	115	116	118	120	121	123	123	77	78	79	80	81	81	82
6	50th	91	92	94	96	98	99	100	53	53	54	55	56	57	57
	90th	105	106	108	110	111	113	113	68	68	69	70	71	72	72
	95th	109	110	112	114	115	117	117	72	72	73	74	75	76	76
	99th	116	117	119	121	123	124	125	80	80	81	82	83	84	84
7	50th	92	94	95	97	99	100	101	55	55	56	57	58	59	59
	90th	106	107	109	111	113	114	115	70	70	71	72	73	74	74
	95th	110	111	113	115	117	118	119	74	74	75	76	77	78	78
	99th	117	118	120	122	124	125	126	82	82	83	84	85	86	86
8	50th	94	95	97	99	100	102	102	56	57	58	59	60	60	61
	90th	107	109	110	111	114	115	116	71	72	72	73	74	75	76
	95th	111	112	114	116	118	119	120	75	76	77	78	79	79	80
	99th	119	120	122	123	125	127	127	83	84	85	86	87	87	88
9	50th	95	96	98	100	102	103	104	57	58	59	60	61	61	62
	90th	109	110	112	114	115	117	118	72	73	74	75	76	76	77
	95th	113	114	116	118	119	121	121	76	77	78	79	80	81	81
	99th	120	121	123	125	127	128	129	84	85	86	87	88	88	89
10	50th	97	98	100	102	103	105	106	58	59	60	61	61	62	63
	90th	111	112	114	115	117	119	119	73	73	74	75	76	77	78
	95th	115	116	117	119	121	122	123	77	78	79	80	81	81	82
	99th	122	123	125	127	128	130	130	85	86	87	88	88	89	90

(Continued)

TABLE B.1 BLOOD PRESSURE LEVELS FOR BOYS BY AGE AND HEIGHT PERCENTILE (continued)

Age (Year)	BP Percentile →	Systolic BP (mm Hg) ← Percentile of Height →							Diastolic BP (mm Hg) ← Percentile of Height →						
		5th	10th	25th	50th	75th	90th	95th	5th	10th	25th	50th	75th	90th	95th
11	50th	99	100	102	104	105	107	107	59	59	60	61	62	63	63
	90th	113	114	115	117	119	120	121	74	74	75	76	77	78	78
	95th	117	118	119	121	123	124	125	78	78	79	80	81	82	82
	99th	124	125	127	129	130	132	132	86	86	87	88	89	90	90
12	50th	101	102	104	106	108	109	110	59	59	60	62	63	63	64
	90th	115	116	118	120	121	123	123	74	75	75	76	77	78	79
	95th	119	120	122	123	125	127	127	78	79	79	81	82	82	83
	99th	126	127	129	131	133	134	135	86	86	87	89	90	90	91
13	50th	104	105	106	108	110	111	112	60	60	61	62	63	64	64
	90th	117	118	120	122	124	125	126	75	75	76	77	78	79	79
	95th	121	122	124	126	128	129	130	79	79	80	81	82	83	83
	99th	128	130	131	133	135	136	137	87	87	88	89	90	91	91
14	50th	106	107	109	111	113	114	115	60	61	62	63	64	65	65
	90th	120	121	123	125	126	128	128	75	76	77	78	79	79	80
	95th	124	125	127	128	130	132	132	80	80	81	82	83	84	84
	99th	131	132	134	136	138	139	140	87	88	89	90	91	92	92

Age	BP Percentile														
15	50th	109	110	112	113	115	117	117	61	62	63	64	65	66	66
	90th	122	124	125	127	129	130	131	76	77	78	79	80	81	81
	95th	126	127	129	131	133	134	135	81	81	82	83	84	85	85
	99th	134	135	136	138	140	142	142	88	89	90	91	92	93	93
16	50th	111	112	114	116	118	119	120	63	63	64	65	66	67	67
	90th	125	126	128	130	131	133	134	78	78	79	80	81	82	82
	95th	129	130	132	134	135	137	137	82	83	83	84	85	86	87
	99th	136	137	139	141	143	144	145	90	90	91	92	93	94	94
17	50th	114	115	116	118	120	121	122	65	66	66	67	68	69	70
	90th	127	128	130	132	134	135	136	80	80	81	82	83	84	84
	95th	131	132	134	136	138	139	140	84	85	86	87	87	88	89
	99th	139	140	141	143	145	146	147	92	93	93	94	95	96	97

BP: blood pressure. 90th to 95th percentile: prehypertension; 95th to 99th percentile: stage 1 hypertension; >99th percentile: stage 2 hypertension.

Adapted from U.S. Department of Health and Human Services, National Institutes of Health, National Heart, Lung, and Blood Institute. (2005). *The fourth report on the diagnosis, evaluation, and treatment of high blood pressure in children and adolescents* (NIH Publication No. 05–5267). Washington, DC: U.S. Department of Health and Human Services.

TABLE B.2 BLOOD PRESSURE LEVELS FOR GIRLS BY AGE AND HEIGHT PERCENTILE

Age (Year)	BP Percentile →	Systolic BP (mm Hg) ← Percentile of Height →							Diastolic BP (mm Hg) ← Percentile of Height →						
		5th	10th	25th	50th	75th	90th	95th	5th	10th	25th	50th	75th	90th	95th
1	50th	83	84	85	86	88	89	90	38	39	39	40	41	41	42
	90th	97	97	98	100	101	102	103	52	53	53	54	55	55	56
	95th	100	101	102	104	105	106	107	56	57	57	58	59	59	60
	99th	108	108	109	111	112	113	114	64	64	65	65	66	67	67
2	50th	85	85	87	88	89	91	91	43	44	44	45	46	46	47
	90th	98	99	100	101	103	104	105	57	58	58	59	60	61	61
	95th	102	103	104	105	107	108	109	61	62	62	63	64	65	65
	99th	109	110	111	112	114	115	116	69	69	70	70	71	72	72
3	50th	86	87	88	89	91	92	93	47	48	48	49	50	50	51
	90th	100	100	102	103	104	106	106	61	62	62	63	64	64	65
	95th	104	104	105	107	108	109	110	65	66	66	67	68	68	69
	99th	111	111	113	114	115	116	117	73	73	74	74	75	76	76
4	50th	88	88	90	91	92	94	94	50	50	51	52	52	53	54
	90th	101	102	103	104	106	107	108	64	64	65	66	67	67	68
	95th	105	106	107	108	110	111	112	68	68	69	70	71	71	72
	99th	112	113	114	115	117	118	119	76	76	76	77	78	79	79

		89	90	91	93	94	95	96	52	53	53	54	55	55	56
5	50th	89	90	91	93	94	95	96	52	53	53	54	55	55	56
	90th	103	103	105	106	107	109	109	66	67	67	68	69	69	70
	95th	107	107	108	110	111	112	113	70	71	71	72	73	73	74
	99th	114	114	116	117	118	120	120	78	78	79	79	80	81	81
6	50th	91	92	93	94	96	97	98	54	54	55	56	56	57	58
	90th	104	105	106	108	109	110	111	68	68	69	70	70	71	72
	95th	108	108	110	111	113	114	115	72	72	73	74	74	75	76
	99th	115	116	117	119	120	121	122	80	80	80	81	82	83	83
7	50th	93	93	95	96	97	99	99	55	56	56	57	58	58	59
	90th	106	107	108	109	111	112	113	69	70	70	71	72	72	73
	95th	110	111	112	113	115	116	116	73	74	74	75	76	76	77
	99th	117	118	119	120	122	123	124	81	81	82	82	83	84	84
8	50th	95	95	96	98	99	100	101	57	57	57	58	59	60	60
	90th	108	109	110	111	113	114	114	71	71	71	72	73	74	74
	95th	112	112	114	115	116	118	118	75	75	75	76	77	78	78
	99th	119	120	122	122	123	125	125	82	82	83	83	84	86	86
9	50th	96	97	98	100	101	102	103	58	58	58	59	60	60	61
	90th	110	110	112	113	114	116	116	72	72	72	73	74	74	75
	95th	114	114	115	117	118	119	120	76	76	76	77	78	78	79
	99th	121	121	123	124	125	127	127	83	83	84	84	85	86	87
10	50th	98	99	100	102	103	104	105	59	59	59	60	61	62	62
	90th	112	112	114	115	116	118	118	73	73	73	74	75	76	76
	95th	116	116	117	119	120	121	122	77	77	77	78	79	80	80
	99th	123	123	125	126	127	129	129	84	84	85	86	86	87	88

(Continued)

TABLE B.2   BLOOD PRESSURE LEVELS FOR GIRLS BY AGE AND HEIGHT PERCENTILE (continued)

Age (Year)	BP Percentile →	Systolic BP (mm Hg) ← Percentile of Height →							Diastolic BP (mm Hg) ← Percentile of Height →						
		5th	10th	25th	50th	75th	90th	95th	5th	10th	25th	50th	75th	90th	95th
11	50th	100	101	102	103	105	106	107	60	60	60	61	62	63	63
	90th	114	114	116	118	118	119	120	74	74	74	75	76	77	77
	95th	118	118	119	121	122	123	124	78	78	78	79	80	81	81
	99th	125	125	126	128	129	130	131	85	85	86	87	87	88	89
12	50th	102	103	104	105	107	108	109	61	61	61	62	63	64	64
	90th	116	116	117	119	120	121	122	75	75	75	76	77	78	78
	95th	119	120	121	123	124	125	126	79	79	79	80	81	82	82
	99th	127	127	128	130	131	132	133	86	86	87	88	88	89	90
13	50th	104	105	106	107	109	110	110	62	62	62	63	64	65	65
	90th	117	118	119	121	122	123	124	76	76	76	77	78	79	79
	95th	121	122	123	124	126	127	128	80	80	80	81	82	83	83
	99th	128	129	130	132	133	134	135	87	87	88	89	89	90	91
14	50th	106	106	107	109	110	111	112	63	63	63	64	65	66	66
	90th	119	120	121	122	124	125	125	77	77	77	78	79	80	80
	95th	123	123	125	126	127	129	129	81	81	81	82	83	84	84
	99th	130	131	132	133	135	136	136	88	88	89	90	90	91	92

Age	BP percentile														
15	50th	107	108	109	110	111	113	113	64	64	64	65	66	67	67
	90th	120	121	122	123	125	126	127	78	78	78	79	80	81	81
	95th	124	125	126	127	129	130	131	82	82	82	83	84	85	85
	99th	131	132	133	134	136	137	138	89	89	89	90	91	92	93
16	50th	108	108	110	111	112	114	114	64	64	65	65	66	67	68
	90th	121	122	123	124	126	127	128	78	78	78	79	80	81	82
	95th	125	126	127	128	130	131	132	82	82	82	83	84	85	86
	99th	132	133	134	135	137	138	139	90	90	90	90	91	92	93
17	50th	108	109	110	111	113	114	115	64	65	65	66	66	67	68
	90th	122	122	123	125	126	127	128	78	79	79	80	80	81	82
	95th	125	125	127	129	130	131	132	82	83	83	84	85	85	86
	99th	133	133	134	136	137	138	139	90	90	90	91	91	93	93

BP, blood pressure. 90th to 95th percentile: prehypertension; 95th to 99th percentile: stage 1 hypertension; >99th percentile: stage 2 hypertension.

Adapted from U.S. Department of Health and Human Services, National Institutes of Health, National Heart, Lung, and Blood Institute. (2005). *The fourth report on the diagnosis, evaluation, and treatment of high blood pressure in children and adolescents* (NIH Publication No. 05–5267). Washington, DC: U.S. Department of Health and Human Services.

Appendix D Growth Charts

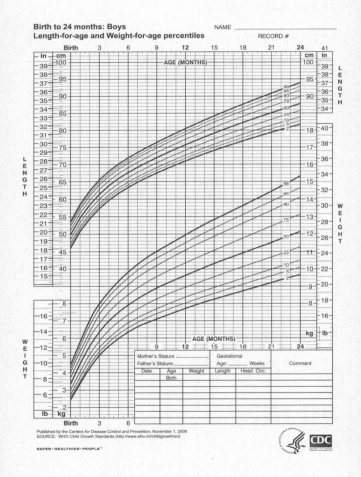

Birth to 24 months: Boys
Length-for-age and Weight-for-age percentiles

NAME _____

RECORD # _____

Published by the Centers for Disease Control and Prevention, November 1, 2009
SOURCE: WHO Child Growth Standards (http://www.who.int/childgrowth/en)

SAFER · HEALTHIER · PEOPLE™

CDC

Birth to 24 months: Girls
Length-for-age and Weight-for-age percentiles

NAME _____

RECORD # _____

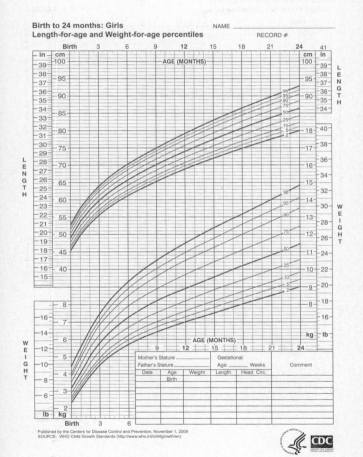

Published by the Centers for Disease Control and Prevention, November 1, 2009
SOURCE: WHO Child Growth Standards (http://www.who.int/childgrowth/en)

Birth to 24 months: Boys
Head circumference-for-age and
Weight-for-length percentiles

NAME _____

RECORD # _____

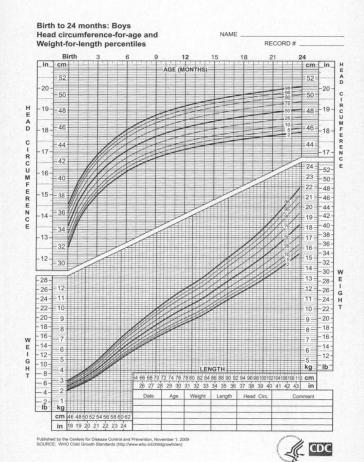

Published by the Centers for Disease Control and Prevention, November 1, 2009
SOURCE: WHO Child Growth Standards (http://www.who.int/childgrowth/en)

Birth to 24 months: Girls
Head circumference-for-age and
Weight-for-length percentiles

NAME _____

RECORD # _____

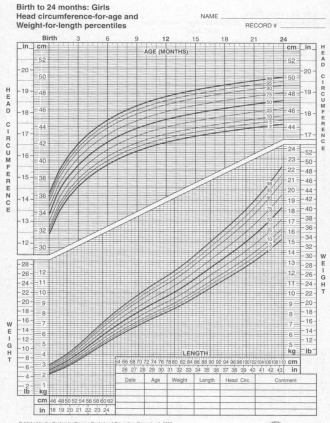

Date	Age	Weight	Length	Head Circ.	Comment

Published by the Centers for Disease Control and Prevention, November 1, 2009
SOURCE: WHO Child Growth Standards (http://www.who.int/childgrowth/en)

2 to 20 years: Boys
Stature-for-age and Weight-for-age percentiles

NAME

RECORD #

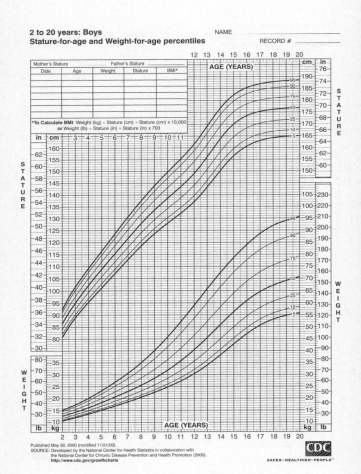

Published May 30, 2000 (modified 11/21/00).
SOURCE: Developed by the National Center for Health Statistics in collaboration with
the National Center for Chronic Disease Prevention and Health Promotion (2000).
http://www.cdc.gov/growthcharts

2 to 20 years: Girls
Stature-for-age and Weight-for-age percentiles

NAME _____

RECORD # _____

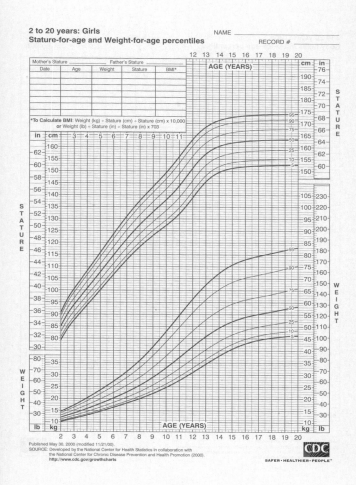

Published May 30, 2000 (modified 11/21/00).
SOURCE: Developed by the National Center for Health Statistics in collaboration with
the National Center for Chronic Disease Prevention and Health Promotion (2000).
http://www.cdc.gov/growthcharts

SAFER · HEALTHIER · PEOPLE™

2 to 20 years: Boys
Body mass index-for-age percentiles

NAME _____

RECORD # _____

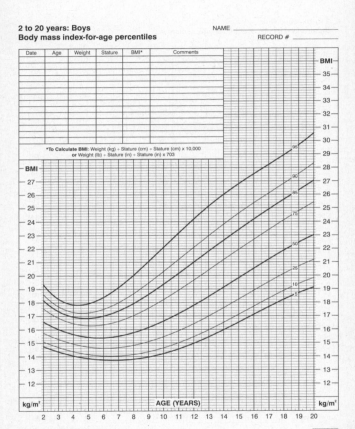

*To Calculate BMI: Weight (kg) ÷ Stature (cm) ÷ Stature (cm) x 10,000
or Weight (lb) ÷ Stature (in) ÷ Stature (in) x 703

Published May 30, 2000 (modified 10/16/00).

SOURCE: Developed by the National Center for Health Statistics in collaboration with
the National Center for Chronic Disease Prevention and Health Promotion (2000).
http://www.cdc.gov/growthcharts

2 to 20 years: Girls
Body mass index-for-age percentiles

NAME _____

RECORD # _____

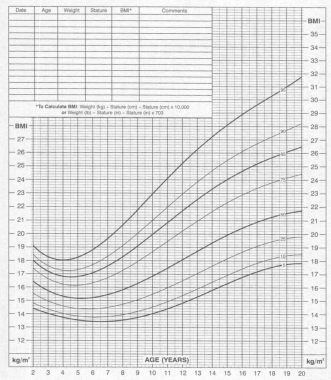

Date	Age	Weight	Stature	BMI*	Comments

*To Calculate BMI: Weight (kg) ÷ Stature (cm) ÷ Stature (cm) x 10,000
or Weight (lb) ÷ Stature (in) ÷ Stature (in) x 703

Published May 30, 2000 (modified 10/16/00).
SOURCE: Developed by the National Center for Health Statistics in collaboration with
the National Center for Chronic Disease Prevention and Health Promotion (2000).
http://www.cdc.gov/growthcharts

CDC
SAFER · HEALTHIER · PEOPLE™

Appendix E Temperature Conversions

To convert Fahrenheit to Celsius, subtract 32 from the temperature in Fahrenheit and then divide by 1.8; to convert Celsius to Fahrenheit, multiply the temperature in Celsius by 1.8 and then add 32.

$$(F - 32) - 1.8 = \text{degrees Celsius}$$
$$(C \times 1.8) - 32 = \text{degrees Fahrenheit}$$

Degrees Fahrenheit (°F)	Degrees Celsius (°C)	Degrees Fahrenheit (°F)	Degrees Celsius (°C)
89.6	32	100.8	38.2
91.4	33	101	38.3
93.2	34	101.2	38.4
94.3	38.6	101.4	38.6
95	35	101.8	38.8
95.4	35.2	102	38.9
96.2	35.7	102.2	39
96.8	36	102.6	39.2
97.2	36.2	102.8	39.3
97.6	36.4	103	39.4
98	36.7	103.2	39.6
98.6	37	103.4	39.7
99	37.2	103.6	39.8
99.3	37.4	104	40
99.7	37.6	104.4	40.2
100	37.8	104.6	40.3
100.4	38	104.8	40.4
		105	40.6

Appendix F Weight Conversions

Neonate and Infant Weight Conversion
Use this table to convert from pounds and ounces to grams when weighing neonates of infants.

Pounds	Ounces															
	0	1	2	3	4	5	6	7	8	9	10	11	12	13	14	15
0	—	28	57	85	113	142	170	198	227	255	283	312	340	369	397	425
1	454	484	510	539	567	595	624	652	680	709	737	765	794	822	850	879
2	907	936	964	992	1021	1049	1077	1106	1134	1162	1191	1219	1247	1276	1304	1332
3	1361	1389	1417	1446	1474	1503	1531	1559	1588	1616	1644	1673	1701	1729	1758	1786
4	1814	1843	1871	1899	1928	1956	1984	2013	2041	2070	2098	2126	2155	2183	2211	2240
5	2268	2296	2325	2353	2381	2410	2438	2466	2495	2523	2551	2580	2608	2637	2665	2693
6	2722	2750	2778	2807	2835	2863	2892	2920	2948	2977	3005	3033	3062	3090	3118	3147
7	3175	3203	3230	3260	3289	3317	3345	337	3402	3430	3459	3487	3515	3544	3572	3600
8	3629	3657	3685	37414	3742	3770	3799	3827	3856	3884	3912	3941	3969	3997	4026	4054
9	4082	4111	4139	4167	4196	4224	4252	4281	4309	4337	4366	4394	4423	4451	4479	4508
10	4536	4564	4593	4621	4649	4678	4706	4734	4763	4791	4819	4848	4876	4904	4933	4961
11	4990	5018	5046	5075	5103	5131	5160	5188	5216	5245	5273	5301	5330	5358	5386	5415
12	5443	5471	5500	5528	5557	5585	5613	5642	5672	5698	5727	5755	5783	5812	5840	5868
13	5897	5925	5953	5982	6010	6038	6067	6095	6123	6152	6180	6209	6237	6265	6294	6322
14	6350	6379	6407	6435	6464	6492	6520	6549	6577	6605	6634	6662	6690	6719	6747	6776
15	6804	6832	6860	6889	6917	6945	6973	7002	7030	7059	7087	7115	7144	7172	7201	7228

Weight Conversion

To convert a patient's weight in pounds to kilograms, divide the number of pounds by 2.2 kg. to convert a patient's weight in kilograms to pounds, multiply the number of kilograms by 2.2 lb.

Pounds	Kilograms	Pounds	Kilograms
10	**4.5**	160	72.6
20	**9**	170	77.1
30	**13.6**	180	81.6
40	**18.1**	190	86.2
50	**22.7**	200	9038
60	**27.2**	210	95.5
70	**31.8**	220	100
80	**36.3**	230	104.5
90	**40.9**	240	109.1
100	**45.4**	250	113.6
110	**49.9**	260	118.2
120	**54.4**	270	122.7
130	**59**	280	127.3
140	**63.5**	290	131.8
150	**68**	300	136.4

Index

Note: Page numbers followed by 'b' indicates box, 'c' indicates chart, 'f' indicates figure, and 't' indicates table.